MORECAMBE BAY HOSPITALS NHS TRUST

Rheumatology Nursing

D0277278

hs

THL

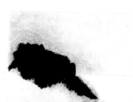

Rheumatology Nursing

A Creative Approach 2nd edition

Edited by
JACKIE HILL

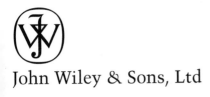

John Wiley & Sons, Ltd

Other Wiley Editorial Offices

John Wiley & Sons Inc., 111 River Street, Hoboken, NJ 07030, USA

Jossey-Bass, 989 Market Street, San Francisco, CA 94103-1741, USA

Wiley-VCH Verlag GmbH, Boschstr. 12, D-69469 Weinheim, Germany

John Wiley & Sons Australia Ltd, 42 McDougall Street, Milton, Queensland 4064, Australia

John Wiley & Sons (Asia) Pte Ltd, 2 Clementi Loop #02-01, Jin Xing Distripark, Singapore 129809

John Wiley & Sons Canada Ltd, 22 Worcester Road, Etobicoke, Ontario, Canada M9W 1L1

Wiley also publishes its books in a variety of electronic formats. Some content that appears in print may not be available in electronic books.

Library of Congress Cataloging-in-Publication Data
Rheumatology nursing : a creative approach / edited by Jackie Hill. – 2nd ed.
    p.   ;   cm.
    Includes bibliographical references and index.
    ISBN-13: 978-0-470-01961-0
    ISBN-10: 0-470-01961-1
    1. Musculoskeletal system–Diseases–Nursing.   2. Arthritis–Nursing.
3. Rheumatism–Nursing.   I. Hill, Jacqueline, 1946–
    [DNLM: 1. Rheumatic Diseases–nursing.   2. Orthopedic Nursing–methods.
    WY 157.6 R472 2006]
    RC925.5.R48 2006
    616.7'23 dc22

                                                                                2005029943

British Library Cataloguing in Publication Data
A catalogue record for this book is available from the British Library
ISBN-13   978-0-470-01961-0
ISBN-10   0-470-01961-1

Typeset by SNP Best-set Typesetter Ltd., Hong Kong
Printed and bound in Great Britain by TJ International Ltd, Padstow, Cornwall

This book is printed on acid-free paper responsibly manufactured from sustainable forestry in which at least two trees are planted for each one used for paper production.

Contents

SECTION 3   THERAPEUTIC INTERVENTIONS

The multifaceted nature of rheumatic diseases requires a combination of therapies. In addition to conventional treatments such as drug therapy and surgery, this section includes complementary therapeutic interventions such as aromatherapy and acupuncture. Continuing the theme of empowering and working in partnership with the patient, this chapter is underpinned by a chapter on patient education.

SECTION 4   PRIMARY AND PAEDIATRIC CARE

A person with a rheumatic disease is often cared for in both the primary and secondary sector. This 'shared care' makes an important contribution to the patient's well-being but requires adequate support mechanisms to function efficiently. The factors necessary to implement effective shared-care schemes are discussed in detail. The final chapter concerns children and young people. Although children with rheumatic diseases share many of the problems faced by adults, they and their families also confront many discrete additional problems. The chapter on paediatric care provides a description of the classification of Juvenile Idiopathic Arthritis and its treatments, and describes the educational and psychological needs of this vulnerable group.

About the Editor

Jackie Hill is an arc Senior Lecturer in Rheumatology Nursing and Co-Director of the Academic and Clinical Unit for Musculoskeletal Nursing (ACUMeN). She has worked in the field of rheumatology for over 25 years as both a clinician and an academic and has gained an international reputation as a leader in the development of the specialty. She has undertaken some of the seminal research into outcomes from rheumatology nursing care and published widely on the subject. She is an Associate Editor of the journal Musculoskeletal Care and holds the office of President of British Health Professionals Rheumatology (BHPR).

Contributors

Mrs Valerie Arthur M Phil, RGN
Clinical Nurse Specialist in Rheumatology (retired)
University Hospital
Birmingham, UK

Miss Domini Bryer RGN, Dip N, BSc (Hons), MA
Biologics Nurse Specialist in Rheumatology
Regional Rheumatology Centre
Day Case Unit/Ward 8
Chapel Allerton Hospital
Leeds, West Yorkshire, UK

Mrs Jill Byrne RGN, SCM, MSc
Director of Nursing and Midwifery
Stockport NHS Foundation Trust
Stepping Hill Hospital
Stockport, Cheshire, UK

Mrs Anne Cawthorn, MSc, BSc, RGN, Dip N, Dip Aromatherapy
Lecturer in Nursing/Psychotherapy Practitioner
School of Nursing
University of Manchester
Christie Hospital
Manchester, UK

Mrs Maureen Cox, RGN, MSc, Dip N, SCM, ONC
Clinical Nurse Specialist in Rheumatology
Nuffield Orthopaedic Centre
Headington
Oxford, UK

Mrs Mandy Edwards SRN, BSc (Hons), FETC
Specialist Practitioner, Practise Nurse
Bilbrook Medical Centre
Bilbrook
Staffordshire, UK

Mrs Pauline Fitzgerald RGN, BSc (Hons), Nursing Studies
Senior Sister
Ward 2, Rheumatology
Chapel Allerton Hospital
Leeds, West Yorkshire, UK

Jackie Hill PhD, MPhil, RN, FRCN
arc Senior Lecturer in Rheumatology Nursing
and Co-Director of the Academic and Clinical Unit for Musculoskeletal
Nursing (ACUMeN)
Academic Unit of Musculoskeletal Diseases
University of Leeds
Chapel Allerton Hospital
Leeds, West Yorkshire, UK

Mrs Gill Jackson, RGN, RSCN
Children's Rheumatology Nurse Specialist
A Floor, Clarendon Wing
Leeds General Infirmary
Leeds, West Yorkshire, UK

Mr Peter Mackereth MA Cert Ed, RNT, RGN, Dip. Nursing
Clinical Lead & Lecturer Complementary Therapies
Christie Hospital NHS Trust & Salford University
Manchester, UK

Mrs Susan Oliver RGN, MSc
Independent Nurse Specialist Rheumatology
Litchdon Medical Centre, North Devon
and 10 Harley Street, London, UK

Mrs Naomi Reay RGN, RSCN, DN, SRCh, BSc (Hons), MA
Clinical Nurse Specialist Raynauds and Scleroderma
Department of Rheumatology and Rehabilitation
University of Leeds
Leeds, West Yorkshire, UK

Dr Sarah Ryan, RGN, PhD, MSc, BSc, FRCN
Nurse Consultant Rheumatology
Haywood Hospital
Stoke on Trent, Staffordshire, UK

Mrs Sally Smith, RN (DiP HE) BSc (Hons)
Raynauds & Scleroderma Nurse Specialist
Rheumatology Department
Chapel Allerton Hospital
Leeds, West Yorkshire, UK

Mrs Christine White RGN
Rheumatology Nurse Specialist (retired)
Mid Yorkshire Hospital Trust
Wakefield
West Yorkshire, UK

Jo White, RGN, MA
Clinical Nurse Specialist in Rheumatology
Rheumatology Department
Leeds General Infirmary
Leeds, West Yorkshire, UK

Acknowledgements

I would like to thank all the nurses and patients who have shared their knowledge and experience with me over the years, but a few individuals need special thanks.

Firstly, I would like to thank my fellow 'scribes' many of whom are renowned experts in their chosen topics and all have been keen to share their knowledge.

Anne Bassett deserves my thanks and a medal for her guidance and unbelievable forbearance.

Helen Greenwood has spent many hours checking references and co-ordinating changes, all well beyond the call of duty!

Finally, I have to give my love and thanks to my husband Geoff whose unbelievable tolerance is something to behold and whose 'household management skills' have improved no end whilst I was editing this second edition.

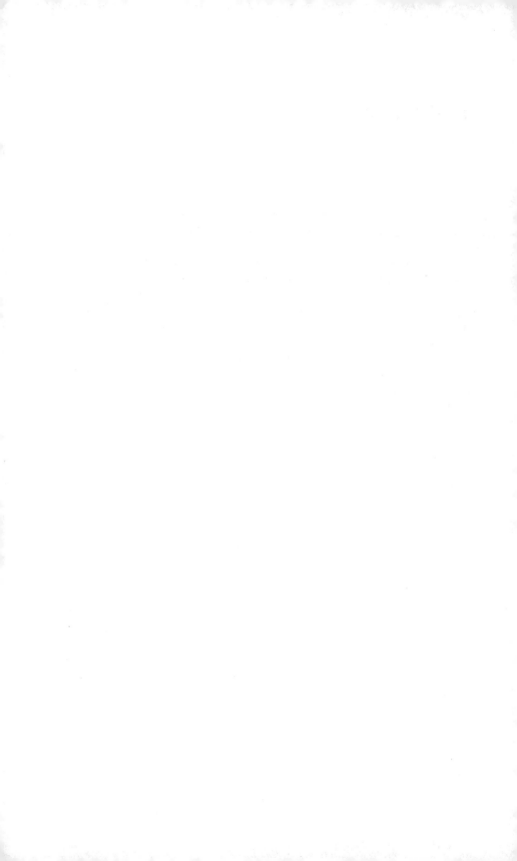

Preface

Musculoskeletal diseases are the most common causes of disability in developed countries throughout the world, and in the United Kingdom, a significant rheumatic disease affects one in seven of the population. They also affect people from all walks of life and of all age groups including babies and the very elderly. Rheumatic diseases are so common that it is inevitable that every nurse will at some time provide care for a rheumatic patient. It is therefore essential that they have some knowledge of rheumatology nursing. Historically this knowledge has been difficult to acquire as there is a paucity of textbooks specifically about rheumatology nursing, and therefore the aim of this book is to fill this gap.

The essence of rheumatology nursing is the 'Three E's'; educating, empowering and enabling our patients. This requires the nurse to work in partnership with the patient and their carers and to adopt a holistic approach to care. This approach is acknowledged in each chapter by the seventeen experienced senior nurses who have written this edition.

The book is intended primarily for nurses working at post basic level, but it will also be a useful resource for pre-registered nurses. It is also intended to accommodate continuing nurse education and this is emphasised by the inclusion of aims and intended learning outcomes at the beginning of each chapter, and action points for practice at the end.

The book aims to enhance all aspects of nursing practice and will be particularly helpful to nurses working in the fields of rheumatology, orthopaedic surgery and in general practice. It will also prove useful to nurses caring for patients on geriatric or general medical and surgical wards as rheumatic disease is often a secondary diagnosis. This new edition includes a chapter on the care of children and juveniles with Juvenile Idiopathic Arthritis. This specialist subject was omitted from the first edition but it has been included for completeness.

The book is in four sections. The first sets the scene and comprises four chapters. Chapter one discusses the underlying principles of rheumatology nursing and focuses on the benefits of adopting a therapeutic rather than a purely supportive approach to care delivery. The next two chapters are devoted to the diseases, their diagnoses and their effect on the immune system. Chapter four outlines the various biochemical, haematological, clinical and other assessments used to diagnose and assess the patient's outcome.

The second section of the book comprises six chapters all of which address the patient's problems. The chapters include effective interventions that help relieve symptoms such as pain and stiffness, fatigue and sleep disturbance and the psychological and social effects. The effects of rheumatic diseases on the skin are explored and also included is a discussion of the relationship between skin integrity and nutrition and a summary of the effectiveness of dietary supplementation on the rheumatic diseases. Pain, disability and changes in body image can have a profound effect on both sexual function and pregnancy and this is explored in detail. One chapter is devoted to the role of the multidisciplinary team and the care they provide.

The third section of the book focuses on therapeutic interventions. The chapter on medications includes up-to-date information on new developments such as biologic therapies. Other chapters included are complementary therapies and caring for the patient undergoing surgical interventions. Teaching patients about their disease and its treatments is the foundation upon which successful management programmes are built and no book on caring for the rheumatology patient would be complete without a chapter on patient education. Various approaches to patient teaching are discussed and methods of assessing and writing educational material are described.

The fourth section focuses on primary care and paediatric care.

Rheumatology as a speciality has often been described as one of the Cinderella Services; it is not seen as a glamorous, emotive or technical branch of nursing. However, to those of us who work in it and love it, nursing the patient with a rheumatic disease is a truly stretching and satisfying experience. Although essential, our nurturing nursing skills alone will not provide the quality of service that our patients deserve. The aim of providing a high quality rheumatology nursing service will be achieved only through great depth and breadth of knowledge; this book represents one step on the road to realising that aim.

I Setting the Scene

1 The Principles, Practice and Evolution of Rheumatology Nursing

S. RYAN
Haywood Hospital, Staffordshire, UK

J. HILL
University of Leeds, West Yorkshire, UK

The aim of this chapter is to provide an understanding of the important contribution that therapeutic nursing can make to a patient living with a chronic rheumatological condition. After reading this chapter the reader should be able to:

- describe the key elements of nursing and explain why they are important to a patient with a rheumatological condition;
- discuss the skills and qualities required for the nurse to enter into a therapeutic relationship;
- describe the difference between supportive and therapeutic nursing and provide examples to illustrate this;
- discuss the actual and potential barriers to therapeutic practice;
- outline the components of the nurse consultant role.

DEFINITIONS OF NURSING

The most widely known definition of nursing is that of Henderson (1966) who states that 'the unique function of the nurse is to assist the individual sick or well in the performance of those activities contributing to health or its recovery (or to a peaceful death) that he would perform unaided if he had the necessary strength, will or knowledge, and to do this in such a way as to help him gain independence as rapidly as possible'. Although this definition is not new, it contains the elements relevant to today's health care with its emphasis on empowerment, rehabilitation, education and self-management.

Rheumatology Nursing: A Creative Approach, 2nd edn. Edited by Jackie Hill.
Copyright 2006 by John Wiley & Sons, Ltd.

Health and illness are not static but dynamic entities, fluctuating in response to many internal and external influences. The role that the nurse assumes will be governed by the patient's perceived need at any particular time. Shaul (1995) in a qualitative study, identified four defined stages that patients encountered as they adjusted to living with rheumatoid arthritis (RA). These included:

- becoming aware (Symptoms became persistent and impacted work, the family and mood.);
- seeking medical help;
- learning to live with it (Through experience, the individual develops different coping strategies that equate with their context.);
- mastery (The individual adapts and lives with the symptoms.).

CARING

Caring is one of the most important values of the nursing profession. Although often referred to as a basic requirement, there is nothing basic about high quality nursing care. The term 'basic care' has been used and interpreted incorrectly to the detriment of the profession. Nursing requires a combination of:

- knowledge
- understanding
- expertise.

Identifying and meeting the needs of patients who are unable to care fully for themselves involves having regard for people as individuals and being concerned about what happens to them (Malin and Teasdale, 1991). The process of caring comprises elements of both action and emotion. However, in practice the action element frequently dominates, as the nurse concentrates on the patient's physical needs (May, 1991; Henderson, 1994). This can result in a neglect of the emotional needs that have been shown to be the predominating factor influencing the experience of good or bad care as perceived by patients (Smith, 1992).

An overemphasis on the physical manifestation of rheumatoid arthritis (RA) such as synovitis of the small joints, without consideration of the effects the condition has on the individual's lifestyle, will not provide comprehensive care and may well be harmful. RA can impact on the patient's social activity with over 50% of patients experiencing social isolation (Yelin and Callahan, 1995). If no one has explored the emotional impact of chronic illness with the patient, they may find themselves bewildered, and unsure of where to turn for help and advice. It is common for patients with a chronic condition to experience a plethora of emotions including:

- shock
- anger
- grief
- depression.

It is essential that the nurse has the necessary support and education to provide the emotional elements of care; otherwise care will not be holistic, meaningful or relevant to the patient.

THE ELEMENTS OF NURSING

The key elements or functions of nursing can be seen in Table 1.1. The main link between the elements is the nature of the relationship between the nurse and the patient.

Once problems have been identified, a plan of care will be formulated which incorporates the patient's identified needs. Chronic conditions have a global impact on the patient's life; living with a rheumatological illness will affect not only the individual but also their family and significant others (Ryan, 1996a). The social implications of rheumatological illness are discussed in Chapter 7.

As well as a sound knowledge base, the nurse will require the ability to understand exactly what physical disability means to each individual (Powell, 1991). For instance, a mother with active inflammation in her hands may be prevented from lifting her child, causing feelings of guilt and anxiety. She must be allowed to express her feelings and be given support and advice about practical measures such as lying on the bed to cuddle her child. For others, inflammatory changes in the hands may affect their ability to work, causing depression and poor self-esteem. Counselling will be required to support the individual through this life crisis, but until the nurse is able to appreciate and understand the impact of illness from the patient's perspective, they will not be able to offer care from a humanistic viewpoint.

Table 1.1 Nursing functions (Wilson-Barnett 1984)

- Understanding illness and treatment from the patient's viewpoint
- Providing continuous psychological care during illness and critical events
- Helping people cope with illness or potential health problems
- Providing comfort
- Coordinating treatment and other events affecting the patient

Essentially, nursing is a social activity. The nurse will need to possess good communication skills and a level of understanding and knowledge about the complex nature of rheumatological illness to be able to offer a complete care package.

THE PHILOSOPHY OF NURSING

A philosophy of practice is essential. It should provide a clear outline of what nurses perceive to be important and central to their practice. This ensures a continuity of approach and can unify the team and ensure that care is practised from a shared understanding with an identified purpose. If nurses working within a clinical area do not share a common purpose, disunity and fragmentation of care can occur. To be meaningful, the philosophy should be derived from those working in both primary and secondary care. Each clinical area will need to determine and develop the beliefs that shape present practice. A philosophy imposed by the wider organisation without the necessary consultation will probably fail in its objective. A rheumatology philosophy of care can be divided into four interlinked and complementary areas (Figure 1.1). Underpinning each area is the patient as the central focus of care delivery.

BELIEFS RELATING TO HEALTH

Health is the state in which the individual has adapted to physical, psychological and/or social imbalances and is able to cope with their arthritis in a positive and constructive manner. In the context of rheumatological conditions, health does not mean the removal of all symptoms, as this would be an unre-

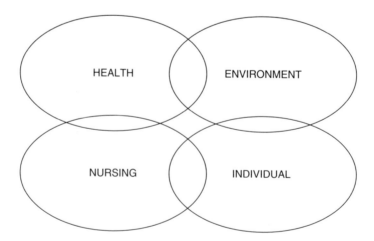

Figure 1.1 The rheumatology philosophy of care.

alistic outcome and an unfair burden to place on patients. Health and illness are not static entities, many rheumatological conditions are characterised by flares and remissions and the patient will require advice, support, guidance, motivation and education to deal with problems presented by each new phase of their illness.

BELIEFS RELATING TO THE ENVIRONMENT

The hospital

The hospital environment is alien to most people and can cause anxiety and loss of confidence. To counter this, a person needs to believe that they can influence care management (Tones, 1991) even if the belief is illusory, and participate actively at all levels. Neglect of the patient's individual concerns and perceptions can lead to isolation and the adoption of poor coping mechanisms. Nursing must create a positive atmosphere that will address both internal and external issues. If the orientation of the ward is committed to task delivery with little emphasis on interpersonal communication, the patient will be unable to explore their emotions to the detriment of their health and acceptance of their condition. Work by Edwards *et al.* (2001) has demonstrated that when patients are nursed on specialist rheumatology wards they report increased confidence in the nurses' ability and knowledge, whilst patients nursed on non-specialist wards reported a lack of understanding regarding their arthritis.

The community

As resources are increasingly diverted to the community, a person with arthritis may have reduced access to the specialist multidisciplinary hospital team. It is therefore necessary that nursing expertise moves into the community. A community rheumatology nurse can act as the interface between primary and secondary care. The rheumatology nurse can liaise with practice nurses and other community workers to promote a greater understanding of the needs of the patients and to ensure continuity of care. Practice nurses are conducting assessment clinics (Dargie and Proctor, 1994) and monitoring second line disease-modifying drugs. It is important that primary care is supported by the secondary care service, and that community nursing staff have easy access to their hospital colleagues. In this way, the patient can be given ready access to whichever service best matches their need. Aspects of seamless care are discussed in Chapter 16.

BELIEFS RELATING TO THE INDIVIDUAL PATIENT

The beliefs that the rheumatology nurse holds toward the patient have important impact on the care provided. Viewing patients according to the following beliefs is essential to underpinning quality care provision.

The individual is a person with an ongoing health related problem. The individual should not be depowered, but encouraged to share their own valuable knowledge store, which is essential to their care.

The individual will bring their own lay beliefs and life experience to all situations. These are usually consistent over time and pertinent to the individual concerned (Donovan, 1991). They need to be shared with the nurse, as they will influence the success and acceptance of care management. For instance, if a patient believes that exercise damages the joints, this needs discussing so that the patient can incorporate new information into their existing knowledge. In this instance, advice will be required about the type and amount of exercise needed and the anticipated outcome, enabling the patient to make an informed choice and contribute to the decision-making process.

Patient autonomy should be the overriding principle that guides nursing practice. Paternalism is based on the principle of beneficence (*i.e.* the professional knows best) and is frequently used to justify actions such as forcing treatment on the individual for the individual's supposed good. Use of the principle of autonomy to guide nursing decision-making will remove the passivity and dependency implicit in paternalism. A heavy reliance on professional beneficence can unintentionally remove the rights or abilities of patients to participate in their own care.

The individual has the right to be an active rather than passive recipient of care if they wish. However, to assume that all patients wish to be empowered is not adopting an individualized approach. Research by Waterworth and Luker (1990) showed that some patients were 'reluctant collaborators in care'. They wished to leave decision-making to the nurse, regarding their own involvement as neglect of care. By carrying out an individual assessment, the nurse will recognise the patient's perceived needs and plan care accordingly. Some patients may prefer a partial involvement rather than a full contributing and participating role. This should be respected and reflected in care management. It will take time for patients to learn about their condition, and reliance on the nurse at a time of crisis, may be necessary for adaptation. As the therapeutic relationship develops, the patient may feel more able to contribute to care decisions. Nevertheless, the emergence of a new stressor such as a reduction in mobility may return the patients to a heightened state of dependency.

The patient is not an isolated being but lives as part of a social network. Any decisions concerning their care should incorporate the needs, values and expectations of these significant others. The individual has many social and occupational roles and the effects of illness must be addressed in a holistic manner.

The individual's values, perceptions and expectations will be central to care planning and the success of care interventions.

BELIEFS RELATING TO NURSING

Carr (2001) defined the following beliefs:

- Nursing enables the patient to manage their condition, lead as full a life as possible and make informed choices.
- Nursing makes a difference to the patient.
- Nursing supports, enables, cares for and educates the patient.
- Nursing provides a high quality service.

EMPOWERMENT

The concept of empowerment is central to the provision of patient-focused care. Tones (1991) defines empowerment as the 'process whereby an individual or community of individuals acquires power' (*i.e.*, the capacity to control other people and resources). An empowerment approach to health recognises the rights of individuals and communities to identify their own health needs, to make their own health choices and to take action to achieve them (Wallerstein and Bernstein, 1988). This is a rather utopian viewpoint, as the ability to make health choices necessitates active participation in the nurse/patient relationship and equality of access to the possible intervention, which may not always be possible. For example, a young mother with rheumatoid arthritis may not be able to attend a pain management programme because of her inability to use public transport. However, there is some merit in Wallerstein's contribution, as it challenges the traditional view of the passive patient, placing the patient (in this definition) in a more active role. Empowerment necessitates a relinquishing of the power held by the health care professional or a sharing of power on a more equal basis.

Empowerment is a complicated subject, so much so that some authors (Gibson, 1991) have found it easier to define it by the consequences of its absence, namely:

- powerlessness
- helplessness
- hopelessness
- alienation.

The combination of an internal locus of control and a belief in powerful others can be of benefit (Wallston, 1995). For instance, the patient may respect the information offered by the nurse, but will judge its relevance against what is meaningful to them. If the nurse recommends an increase in exercise, they will experiment and balance the perceived benefits against time that could be spent on other activities. A person who believes only in powerful others, will preclude individual judgement and prevent an individual assessment of whether the situation is within their personal control.

Empowerment comprises three elements:

- responsibility
- accountability
- risk taking.

Responsibility can be allocated to a person, but unless the person accepts the responsibility they are powerless to act. It may also be the case that an individual is willing to take responsibility, but social and political constraints prevent this. Tones (1991) states that acceptance of responsibility will be determined by the extent to which an individual possesses competence, skills and/or the belief that they are capable of controlling central aspects of their lives and overcoming environmental barriers.

THERAPEUTIC NURSING

Therapeutic nursing has been defined as 'that practice where the nurse has made a positive difference to a patient or client's health state, and where he or she is aware of how and why this positive health difference has occurred' (Powell, 1991). Four main areas (Table 1.2) in which nursing can be seen to be therapeutic have been highlighted by MacMahon and Pearson (1991).

Rheumatoid arthritis is an incurable condition but the goal of well-being remains realistic. Supportive nursing has a role to play as the aim of many of the interventions (both medical and nursing) is to limit the potential for further deformity and disability. One example is disease-modifying drug therapy such as methotrexate or gold injections. However, to adopt an exclusively supportive approach would be detrimental to the patient, as it does not allow the patient to participate in the control of their management. Control is retained by the nurse, stifling any attempt by the patient to take an active part in their care.

Some nurses do not wish to develop a therapeutic relationship with patients (Salvage, 1990) and others do not value working with patients whose conditions are not amenable to cure (Nolan and Nolan, 1995).

Table 1.2 Areas of therapeutic nursing

- Nurse/patient relationship
- Conventional nursing interventions, *e.g.*, pressure-area care
- Unconventional nursing interventions, *e.g.*, practices taken from therapies
- Patient teaching

In order to improve the patient's well-being the nurse must play the roles of:

- educator
- guide
- motivator
- supporter.

The satisfaction obtained when the patient and the nurse grow together, will help to remove some of the negative perceptions that nurses sometimes acquire when caring for patients with long-term needs.

THE NURSE/PATIENT RELATIONSHIP

Salvage (1990) has questioned whether patients desire a close relationship if their immediate concern is relief from pain and discomfort. This may be relevant to patients experiencing acute illness, but in chronic conditions it takes time and close cooperation to cope with pain that cannot be alleviated. This is where individual patient assessment is so important. It should be remembered that some patients may not perceive benefits from developing a relationship, and so long as the patient is aware of how to renew or establish contact should a problem occur, this view must be respected.

PATIENT PERCEPTIONS

Some patients with rheumatoid arthritis have a negative concept of the future that persists even after their condition is in remission (Hewlett, 1994). The nurse should identify and address any problems perceived by the patient in the initial assessment. If the patient is convinced that the future means a wheelchair existence, it is not helpful to be told that only 5% of people with rheumatoid arthritis require a wheelchair. Patients require acknowledgement of their problems and explanations provided within their own context (Donovan and Blake, 2000).

The concept of shared care, where the patients take responsibility for their condition with support and guidance of a named nurse, offers the best way forward. Patients who believe they can influence their condition will report fewer physical problems and enhanced well-being (Newman, 1993).

Adopting a holistic humanistic approach to care requires a change from the supportive role of doing for the patient, to a therapeutic approach which necessitates enabling the patient to feel in control (Chapter 5). For instance, if the patient's main problem is that of pain, the nurse can have a therapeutic input by establishing in conjunction with the patient, the pattern, type and severity of the discomfort, whether or not it is related to activity, and the apprehensions and anxieties associated with it. This is a two way process, first achieving clarification of the problems from the patient's perspective and then working in partnership to minimise the stressor. By the use of empathy, respect and trust nurses enable patients to believe in their decisions.

It is also essential to encourage those who have value in the patient's life to participate in care management. For example, rest is an important part of the treatment for a patient with a systemic condition such as rheumatoid arthritis in which both physical and emotional fatigue can occur. If the family is unaware of this, pressure may be placed on the patient to abandon resting. This can be avoided if the family learns the role of rest in the management of the condition. If there is an absence of shared understanding within the family, the patient may try to disguise their limitations resulting in increased symptoms and a reduced quality of life.

BARRIERS TO THERAPEUTIC PRACTICE

THE VIEW OF NURSING

Some nursing activities, such as assisting a patient to bathe, are often considered to be basic or menial where in fact they are essential to a patient's well-being. Technical skills are associated with greater status and are therefore deemed to be more important than basic care skills. Therapeutic nursing will include technical skills, but at its core is the realisation of the value of expressive skills (Wright, 1991) which include the ability to:

- be with the patient
- provide comfort
- provide education
- provide the emotional element of care.

Within the framework of therapeutic practice, no act of care having relevance to the patient can be described as menial. Indeed high technology skills without the addition of high touch skills have little meaning for the patient concerned (Wright, 1991). The importance of these expressive skills must be emphasised and should therefore be taught at both basic and post-basic level. A nurse engaged in therapeutic practice will relate to the patient as an individual, adopting a combination of skills that are perceived to be beneficial and to solve the patient's problems. Nursing should not be embarrassed by this caring element, but should strongly endorse it as the component which the patient directly relates to the success of their nursing care (Smith, 1992). The challenge to nurses is to combine both technical and comprehensive skills into a healing whole which serves the patient (Wright, 1991).

EMOTIONAL INVOLVEMENT

It has been suggested that nurses do not want to develop the relationship required to nurse patients with a chronic, or indeed an acute, illness. A study of communication between nurses and patients on a surgical ward found that nurses in close relationships concentrated on medical treatment rather than emotional need (Macleod Clarke, 1983). To some nurses, working with patients who have ongoing needs offers little job satisfaction because they are unable to sustain a sense of therapeutic optimism (Evers, 1991; Reed and Bond, 1991; Reed and Watson, 1994). It is possible that rather than working in partnership with the patient to establish shared objectives, nurses set themselves unrealistic care objectives from their own frame of reference. Establishing and being committed to a relationship is demanding as it is necessary to give of one's self to develop the trust needed for partnerships to grow. To encourage this depth of involvement or emotional labour (Smith, 1992), a nurse needs to work within a supportive framework with an assigned supervisor to assist with personal and professional development. Wright (1986) has stated that all nurses need the opportunity to:

• share feelings
• express views
• raise questions relating to practice in a structured fashion.

WORK ENVIRONMENT

The culture in which nurses work does not encourage them to spend time talking to patients, but time is essential if a relationship is to develop. There is still emphasis on achieving tasks rather than engaging in therapeutic interventions, and emphasis on a growth of support workers at the expense of qualified nurses. If these trends continue, it is questionable whether it will remain possible for a relationship to develop on anything but a superficial level.

In some hospitals, the outpatient department may be the only environment where the patient with a chronic disease is cared for, and so all newly diagnosed patients should be referred to a rheumatology nurse to begin the process of therapeutic care. A realistic personal profile of care should be established which could be used by other key workers, such as the physiotherapist or practice nurse, so maintaining the continuity of care between the secondary and primary health care sections. Care profiling and planning needs to be dynamic, otherwise it will raise expectations and then cause dissatisfaction if identified needs are not met.

Therapeutic nursing requires a nonhierarchical method of care delivery that enables nurses to be involved in the decision-making process and places them in a position where they can develop a partnership with the patient. The philosophy of the work environment is of vital importance because if the nursing team is not committed to developing a relationship, a relationship will not occur. The belief that therapeutic practice is of mutual benefit will only become reality if it is actively fostered and reinforced by the organisation that delivers care. A routinised and ritualistic approach will not serve the needs of the patients.

THE DEVELOPING ROLE OF THE RHEUMATOLOGY NURSE

Rheumatology nursing has been evolving over many years, but due to the absence of a formal group or network through which nurses working with rheumatology patients could share and increase their knowledge and skills, its progress remained unappreciated until the early 1980s. This situation was resolved when, after many months of negotiation, the Royal College of Nursing (RCN) agreed to the establishment of the Rheumatology Forum (RF). The inaugural meeting of the RCN RF was held in Manchester in 1981. It was a significant event because it finally conferred acknowledgement that rheumatology nursing was a speciality in its own right, and this paved the way to future development.

The driving force behind the founding of the RCN RF was a rheumatology nurse called Vickie Stephenson. However, her vision did not stop there. She knew that nurses contributed unique care to rheumatology patients, but also acknowledged that they work as part of a multidisciplinary team, not in isolation. Although rheumatologists had their own association, the British Society of Rheumatology (BSR), nonmedical health professionals did not. Ms. Stephenson envisaged a new organisation, British Health Professionals in Rheumatology (BHPR), and played a significant role in its establishment in 1985.

Both the RCN RF and BHPR have gone from strength to strength, and it is largely due to them that roles are evolving rapidly and the work of nonmedical health professionals is acknowledged as being central to successful outcomes for rheumatology patients.

The intervening years since the inception of these two organisations have seen many innovations in care. The most significant events in nursing have been the establishment and growth of:

- nurse-led clinics
- consultant nurse role
- academic rheumatology posts for nonmedical health professionals.

THE EVOLUTION OF RHEUMATOLOGY NURSING ROLES

Although nurse-led clinics existed in a number of areas of chronic disease in the United Kingdom, it was not until the 1980's that they began to emerge in rheumatology. The first clinics began when nurses working on clinical drugs trials in Leeds began taking on responsibility for more patient-centred care (Bird *et al.*, 1980). They monitored disease progress and provided education and support to the patients and their families. Once the clinical trial was completed, normal practice was for the nurse to return the patient to the medical clinics. However, many of these patients began to request referrals for nursing consultations because they appreciated the supportive, educational approach provided by these nurses. By 1981, the first publications about nurse-led rheumatology clinics in the United Kingdom began to appear (Bird *et al.*, 1981; Bird, 1983; Hill, 1985), followed by the first descriptive research on patients' evaluations of the care they received from the nurse (Hill, 1986). During the following two decades nurse-led care in all specialities, including rheumatology, has grown exponentially. There are a number of reasons for this and they include:

- an ever-increasing outpatient workload;
- reduction in the working hours of junior hospital doctors;
- pressure from government;
- willingness of nurses to innovate and advance their practice.

Over the years a number of descriptive papers have been published which outline the care that rheumatology nurses provide (Ryan and Oliver, 2002; Oliver and Mooney, 2002; Sutcliffe, 1999; Ryan, 1996b; Arthur, 1994). Research has also begun to emerge demonstrating the efficacy of care from nurse-led clinics (Hill *et al.*, 2003a; Hill *et al.*, 1994) and some of these results have been replicated in mainland Europe (Tijhuis *et al.*, 2002; Temmink *et al.*, 2001). As roles evolve, research is slowly progressing, although much work remains to be done. For instance the efficacy of the consultant nurse in rheumatology has yet to be evaluated, as has the role of the biologics nurse specialist.

NURSE-LED CLINICS

Nurse-led clinics are usually the domain of clinical nurse specialists and these nurses normally practise from rheumatology outpatient clinics alongside their medical colleagues. The setting up of such clinics and the care they provide is explained in detail by Hill and Pollard (2004).

The nursing role is essentially expressive in nature (Hill, 1992), consisting of a combination of skills including:

- caring
- helping
- supporting
- teaching

- comforting
- guiding.

Nurse-led clinics provide nurses with the opportunity to use the knowledge and communication skills that they possess, and to take a holistic approach to care utilising the standards advocated by the RCN RF (2001). These standards incorporate the physical, psychological, social, spiritual and sexual needs of the patient. A survey of practice in nurse-led rheumatoid arthritis clinics (Ryan and Hill, 2004) demonstrated that nurses are engaged in:

- monitoring of disease status
- emotional support
- patient education
- management of stable disease
- management of patients on biologic therapies.

Approximately 20% of nurse specialists engage in extended clinical roles such as recommending treatment changes to the rheumatologist and general practitioner, and the administration of joint injections. Many also undertake research and teaching (Carr, 2001).

It is essential that the role of the nurse working within this sphere remains firmly rooted in patient need and that all role expansion focuses on the patients' care. Unless this happens, there is a danger that the nurse could be viewed as a medical assistant instead of being at the forefront of developing their own profession in the interests of their patient group. Nursing requires strong leadership. It would be a tragedy if nursing were to be subsumed and lose its identity in a medically orientated alliance. The nursing profession needs to be clear as to what constitutes nursing and the necessity for both a physical and emotional element in nursing practice.

The value of a clinic run on true nursing principles was demonstrated by Hill *et al.* (1994). This study was an evaluation of the effectiveness, safety and acceptability of a nurse practitioner in a rheumatology outpatient clinic. It consisted of a single blind parallel group study, in which 70 patients with rheumatoid arthritis were randomly allocated to the care of either the nurse practitioner or consultant rheumatologist. One of the most noticeable aspects of the research was the marked difference in the referral patterns of the two practitioners, with the rheumatology nurse practitioner making greater use of the other members of the multidisciplinary team, such as the occupational therapist and physiotherapist. This study also reinforced the view that one of the primary roles of the nurse working with patients with rheumatological conditions is that of educator. Education is required to increase the patient's cognitive understanding and to impart knowledge of self-management techniques such as exercise regimes. The knowledge shared with patients was well-received and there was a greater improvement in knowledge and satisfaction with care than in the rheumatologist's group. Education is time consuming and this was reflected in the fact that over the study period the nurse practitioner saw fewer patients than the consultant. However, the patients in the nursing cohort showed greater reductions in pain and depression compared to those patients in the consultant's group. The nurse was shown to be a safe practitioner who was able to initiate and interpret clinical and laboratory data. These results were encouraging and demonstrated the effective and safe contribution the nurse can make to the care of rheumatology patients with a diversity of needs. Subsequently, this work has been replicated in the United Kingdom with similarly excellent results (Hill *et al.*, 2003a).

NURSE CONSULTANT

1998 saw the introduction of nurse consultant posts across England (DoH, 1999a) providing the opportunity to define and expand the career pathway, whilst allowing experienced nurses to remain in clinical care. Prior to the introduction of this new role the pinnacle of clinical progression was reached at nurse specialist level and nurses seeking further career advancement had to consider entering education or management. Unlike clinical nurse specialist roles, nurse consultant posts have defined criteria regarding role function. These include:

* expert practice
* professional leadership and consultancy
* education, training and development
* research.

These criteria provide a clear framework by which to structure role development. The only component that has a stated time allocation is that of expert practice, where it is specified that 50% of time must involve clinical care. This clear emphasis on clinical care is important as it conveys to the wider community that providing effective care for patients is at the heart of nursing practice. The distribution of time spent on the other role functions is determined by the needs of the local population, the knowledge and skills of the individual nurses and the environment in which the post is placed.

One of the entry criteria for these posts is a master's level qualification; the first time a nursing role has been equated with an academic level. The Nursing and Midwifery Council is currently working towards ensuring that all nurses practising at specialist level have a recognised academic qualification.

Although many clinical nurses will welcome the opportunity to retain their clinical skills and develop their education and research roles, the creation of consultant nurse posts has not been without problems. They were introduced with no specific funding, which has led to many positions being filled by the existing nurse specialist without the nurse specialist being replaced. The creation of these new posts should not be at the expense of other essential senior clinical roles.

Early evaluation of the first 451 posts (Guest, 2001) highlighted the lack of organisational support and role ambiguity that many nurse consultants were experiencing. These roles clearly require strategic influence and support from appropriate mentors. It was also found that the role component with the lowest level of involvement was that of research, which is not surprising as many senior clinical nurses have little preparation in research skills.

ACADEMIC RHEUMATOLOGY POSTS FOR NONMEDICAL HEALTH PROFESSIONALS

Although some research has been carried out within the speciality of rheumatology nursing, a great deal more is required. The reasons for this omission are numerous and include:

- The complexity and multifaceted nature of nursing make it difficult to define and research (Ryan, 1998).
- Nurses working in clinical practice have little time for research.
- Few nurses are trained to undertake major research projects.
- Although there are a number of academic nursing departments in the United Kingdom, unless the department includes an academic with a special interest in rheumatology, there is little expert support for those who wish to undertake research in this area of nursing.

THE ARTHRITIS RESEARCH CAMPAIGN (ARC) INITIATIVE

These problems were recognised by the charity the Arthritis Research Campaign (arc), which funds a number of educational and research projects. In 1999, arc made the decision to establish a small number of academic posts at the level of senior lecturer/lecturer for nonmedical health professionals. The posts were targeted at rheumatology health professionals with a commitment to research, but arc was not prescriptive and it was left open to the applicants to put forward their own ideas. Successful applicants were to be funded for five years and it was expected that the host institution would secure the posts after this time. arc stipulated that applicants:

- must be working in a department of rheumatology actively involved in academic clinical research;
- would collaborate with a second academic department that was involved in nonmedical research such as nursing or physiotherapy.

Two calls for applications were made over two years. From these five grants were awarded; three went to nurses, one to a physiotherapist and one to a podiatrist. One of the successful bids came from Leeds. This application outlined a programme of research and educational activities, but more importantly it provided a clear vision of how academic rheumatology nursing could develop in the future. The long-term strategy was to develop an academic nursing department, which would ultimately justify the inauguration of a Professor of Musculoskeletal Nursing; a world first. It was envisaged that the new nursing department would build on the existing national and international reputation of the nurses working for the Academic Unit of Musculoskeletal and Rehabilitation Medicine in Leeds, to develop both nursing practice and research. The inauguration of an academic nursing unit would provide the stability required to develop a long-term research strategy. It would also allow longer-term projects to be planned and undertaken and provide the environment in which to nurture future nurse researchers and practitioners. This was the birth of the Academic and Clinical Unit for Musculoskeletal Nursing (ACUMeN).

ACUMeN

ACUMeN is a tripartite collaboration between two departments of Leeds University; the Academic Unit of Musculoskeletal and Rehabilitation Medicine and the Department of Healthcare, and Leeds Teaching Hospitals Trust (Hill *et al.*, 2003b). The combined approach undertaken in developing ACUMeN was and remains timely. The need for collaborations and partnerships between practice settings and universities in all healthcare disciplines has been a consistent theme of a number of recent government documents such as 'Making a Difference' (DoH, 1999b), the 'NHS Plan' (DoH, 2000) and 'Shifting the Balance of Power in the NHS' (DoH, 2001). In nursing, these collaborations are predicated on the view that ideas are most easily and frequently generated at the intersection of practice, education and research. On a broader front, collaboration is central to clinical effectiveness and consequently addresses the Clinical Governance agenda (DoH, 1999c) in that it enhances:

- leadership development
- patient care
- promotion, maintenance and evaluation of best practice
- professional development
- the culture of the organization.

The structure of ACUMeN

The organisational structure of ACUMeN is shown in Figure 1.2. The three directors are responsible for the day-to-day operation of the unit. Although the overall responsibility is shared, each director has a principal responsibility for one of the three domains that are encompassed by ACUMeN:

- research
- education
- practice.

The directors are accountable to and sit on a steering committee comprised of a representative from each of the collaborating departments. This group determines the overall direction of ACUMeN policy.

The project group meets four times a year to discuss new projects, progress and problems that arise. It comprises co-directors, nurses, rheumatologists, representatives from therapy services, educationalists and patients. Input from these individuals is seen as paramount to the successful implementation of ACUMeNs programme.

The objectives of ACUMeN

ACUMeN aims to:

- produce a long-term programme to demonstrate the contribution of nursing to health care and patient well-being;
- derive a programme of clinical research which will address local as well as national and international needs;
- provide a focus for clinical teaching;
- integrate research, practice and education and so develop a model for an integrated clinical and academic nursing career structure;
- foster multidisciplinary collaboration and working practices;
- develop a model for the integration of research, education and practice in nursing between the University of Leeds and the Leeds Teaching Hospitals Trust;
- develop a model for the involvement of users in the development of research, education and practice programmes.

ACUMeN was launched in March 2003 and within two years academic secretaries, two PhD nursing students and two research assistants had come into post. A 20 credit, level 3 rheumatology course had been successfully developed and run, and ACUMeN had become a designated teaching centre for a new arc masters course. A Practice Development Unit was also being established on the rheumatology ward at Chapel Allerton Hospital, and the nurses within the rheumatology unit had become much more research-aware than previously. It remains to be seen whether the aim of the inauguration of a Professor of Musculoskeletal Nursing materialises, but the foundation stones for such a post are clearly being laid.

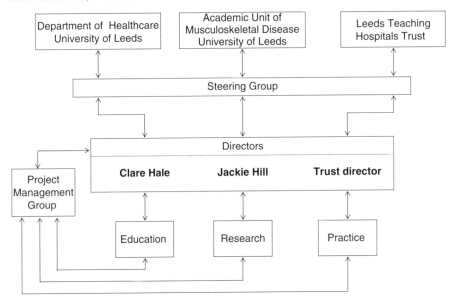

Figure 1.2 The organisational structure of ACUMeN.

ACTION POINTS FOR PRACTICE

- Review the philosophy of care in your clinical area. Does it encourage therapeutic practice?
- Conduct a patient-focus group in your clinical area to identify the beliefs of patients regarding their nursing service.
- Identify the skills needed for nurses to engage in therapeutic practice.
- Conduct a literature review of nurse-led clinics and identify areas for future research.

REFERENCES

Arthur V (1994) Nursing care of patients with rheumatoid arthritis. *British Journal of Nursing* 3:325–331.

Bird HA, Wright V, Galloway D (1980) Clinical metrology- a future career grade? *Lancet* 2:138–140.

Bird HA, Leatham P, Le Gallez P (1981) Clinical metrology. *Nursing Times* 77:1926–1927.

Bird HA (1983) Divided rheumatology care: the advent of the nurse practitioner? *Annals of the Rheumatic Diseases* 42:354–355.

Carr A (2001) Defining the extended clinical role for allied health professionals in rheumatology. Chesterfield, *ARC Conference Proceedings* No12.

Dargie L, Proctor J (1994) Setting up an arthritis clinic. *Community Outlook* 4(7):14–17.

Department of Health (1999a) Nurse, midwives and health visitor consultants: establishing posts and making appointments. *Health Service Circular* 1999/217. London, Department of Health.

Department of Health (1999b) *Strengthening the nursing, midwifery and health visiting contribution to health and healthcare.* London, Department of Health.

Department of Health (1999c) *Quality in the new NHS.* London, Department of Health.

Department of Health (2000) *A plan for investment a plan for reform.* London, Department of Health.

Department of Health (2001) *Shifting the balance of power in the NHS. Securing Delivery.* London, Department of Health.

Donovan J (1991) Patient education and the consultation: the importance of lay beliefs. *Annals of the Rheumatic Diseases* 50:418–421.

Donovan J, Blake D (2000) Qualitative study of interpretation of reassurance among patients attending rheumatology clinics: 'just a touch of arthritis, doctor?' *British Medical Journal* 320:541–544.

Edwards J, Mulherin D, Ryan S *et al.* (2001) The experience of patients with rheumatoid arthritis admitted to hospital. *Arthritis Care & Research* 45:1–7.

Evers HK (1991) Care of the elderly sick in the United Kingdom. In: Redfern SJ (ed). *Nursing Elderly People* (2nd edn). Edinburgh, Churchill Livingstone 417–436.

Gibson C (1991) A concept analysis of empowerment. *Journal of Advanced Nursing* 16:354–361.

Guest D (2001) *A preliminary evaluation of the establishment of nurse, midwife and health visitor consultants: a report to the Department of Health.* London, Kings College.

Henderson V (1966) *The Nature of Nursing.* London, Collier-MacMillan.

Henderson A (1994) Power and knowledge in nursing practice. *Journal of Advanced Nursing* 20:935–939.

Hewlett S (1994) Patients views on changing disability. *Nursing Standard* 8(31): 25–29.

Hill J (1985) Nursing clinics for arthritics. *Nursing Times* 81:33–34.

Hill J (1986) Patient evaluation of a rheumatology nursing clinic. *Nursing Times* 82: 42–43.

Hill J (1992) A nurse practitioner rheumatology clinic. *Nursing Standard* 7(11): 35–37.

Hill J, Bird H, Lawton C *et al.* (1994) An evaluation of the effectiveness, safety and acceptability of a nurse practitioner in a rheumatology outpatient clinic. *British Journal of Rheumatology* 33:283–288.

Hill J, Thorpe R, Bird H (2003a) Outcomes for patients with RA – a rheumatology nurse practitioner clinic compared to standard outpatient care. *Musculoskeletal Care* 1(1):5–20.

Hill J, Hale C, Lightfoot K (2003b) The Academic and Clinical Unit for Musculoskeletal Nursing – a future direction? *Journal of Orthopaedic Nursing* 7(3):141–150.

Hill J, Pollard A (2004) Nurse clinics: not just assessing patients' joints. In: Oliver S (ed). *Chronic Disease Nursing: a Rheumatology Example.* London, Whurr Publishers.

Macleod Clarke J (1983) Nurse-patient communication – analysis of conversation from surgical works. In: Wilson-Barnett J (ed). *Nursing Research. Ten Studies in Patient Care*. Winchester, John Wiley.

MacMahon R, Peason A (1991) Nursing as Therapy. London, Chapham Hall.

Malin N, Teasdale K (1991) Caring versus empowerment. Considerations for nursing practice. *Journal of Advanced Nursing* 16:657–662.

May C (1991) Affective neutrality and involvement in nurse-patient relationships: perceptions of appropriate behaviours among nurses in acute medical and surgical wards. *Journal of Advanced Nursing* 16:552–558.

Newman S (1993) Coping with rheumatoid arthritis. *Annals of the Rheumatic Diseases* 52:553–554.

Nolan M, Nolan J (1995) Responding to the challenge of chronic illness. *British Journal of Nursing* 4(3):145–147.

Oliver S, Mooney J (2002) Targeted therapies for patients with rheumatoid arthritis. *Professional Nurse* 17:716–780.

Powell J (1991) Reflection and the evaluation of experience pre-requests for therapeutic practice. In: MacMahon R, Pearson A (eds) *Nursing as Therapy*. London, Chapman Hall.

Reed J, Bond S (1991) Nurse assessment of elderly patients in hospital. *Internal Journal of Nursing Studies* 28(1):55–64.

Reed J, Watson D (1994) The impact of the medical model on nursing practice. *Internal Journal of Nursing Studies* 31(1):57–66.

Royal College of Nursing (2001) *Standards for Effective Practice and Audit in Rheumatology Nursing*. London, Royal College of Nursing.

Ryan S (1996a) Living with rheumatoid arthritis: a phenomenological exploration. *Nursing Standard* 10(41):45–47.

Ryan S (1996b) Defining the role of the specialist nurse. *Nursing Standard* 10:27–29.

Ryan S (1998) The essence of rheumatology nursing. In: Hill J (ed). *Rheumatology Nursing – A Creative Approach*. Edinburgh, Churchill Livingstone.

Ryan S, Oliver S (2002) Rheumatoid arthritis. *Nursing Standard* 16(20):45–52.

Ryan S, Hill J (2004) A survey of practice in nurse led rheumatoid arthritis clinics. *Rheumatology* 43(suppl 2):411.

Salvage J (1990) The theory and practice of the 'new nursing'. *Nursing Times* 86(4):42–44.

Shaul M (1995) From early twinges to mastery: the process of adjustment in living with rheumatoid arthritis. *Arthritis Care & Research* 8(4):290–297.

Smith P (1992) The emotional labour of nursing. Worcester, Macmillan.

Temmink D, Hutten JBF, Francke AL et al. (2001) Rheumatology outpatient nurse clinics: a valuable edition? *Arthritis Care & Research*, 45:280–286.

Tijhuis GT, Zwinderman AH, Hazes JMW et al. (2002) A randomized comparison of care provided by a clinical nurse specialist, an inpatient team, and a day patient team in rheumatoid arthritis. *Arthritis Care & Research* 47:525–531.

Tones K (1991) Health promotion, empowerment and the psychology of control. *Journal of the Institute of Health Education* 29(1):17–25.

Wallerstein N, Bernstein E (1988) Empowerment education. Frere's ideas adapted to health education. *Health Education Quarterly* 4:379–394.

Wallston K (1995) Adaptation coping and perceived control in persons with rheumatoid arthritis. *Rheumatology in Europe* 2:291–304 (suppl), EULAR Publication.

Waterworth S, Luker K (1990) Reluctant collaborators: do patients want to be involved in decisions concerning care. *Journal of Advanced Nursing* 15:971–976.

Wilson-Barnett J (1984) *Key functions in nursing: the fourth Winifred Raphael memorial lecture.* London, Royal College of Nursing.

Wright S (1986) Building and Using a Model for Nursing. London, Edward Arnold.

Wright S (1991) Facilitating therapeutic nursing and independent practice. In: Mac-Mahon R, Pearson A (eds): *Nursing as Therapy.* London, Chapman Hall.

Yelin E, Callahan L (1995) The economic cost and social and psychological impact of musculoskeletal conditions. *Arthritis and Rheumatism* 38:1351–1362.

2 The Musculoskeletal System and the Rheumatic Diseases

V. ARTHUR
University Hospital, Birmingham, UK

J. HILL
University of Leeds, West Yorkshire, UK

The aim of this chapter is to provide a description of the anatomy and physiology of the musculoskeletal system, and provide a general overview of the diseases that relate to this system. After reading this chapter the reader should be able to:

- describe the structures that make up the musculoskeletal system;
- describe the anatomy and physiology of the musculoskeletal system in relation to the rheumatic diseases;
- discuss the current thinking on the aetiology and pathology of the common rheumatic diseases;
- differentiate between inflammatory, noninflammatory and soft tissue rheumatological conditions;
- describe the extra-articular manifestations of the rheumatic diseases;
- depict the problems that arise from these diseases and how they may affect patients and their families.

THE IMPACT OF RHEUMATIC DISEASE

There are over 200 rheumatic/musculoskeletal conditions which encompass an extensive range of severity and complexity. Although these diseases have been the subject of research for several decades, much remains to be learned (Symmons and Bankhead, 1994). Musculoskeletal diseases can cause great suffering and disability and can place a great social and economic burden on patients, their families and society. They account for 18.7% of all consultations in general practice; and it has been predicted that as the elderly popula-

Rheumatology Nursing: A Creative Approach, 2nd edn. Edited by Jackie Hill.
Copyright 2006 by John Wiley & Sons, Ltd.

tion increases so will the incidence of these complaints (Badley, 1991). Although rheumatic disease can affect any age group from babies to the very elderly, the greatest incidence in the UK is in females over the age of 65 years (Symmons *et al.*, 1994). With an ever-increasing elderly population of which the greater proportion will be women, the full impact of the consequences of these diseases has yet to be felt by health professionals, health authorities and society at large.

Nurses have an important role to play in the care of patients with rheumatic disease, as they are the members of the multidisciplinary team with whom patients are likely to have the most contact (Arthur, 1994). The reduction of junior doctors' hours and the advent of nurse-led clinics has increased the nursing component of care (Hill, 1992; Hill, 1997; Hill *et al.*, 2003). As the role of the nurse is extended and new therapies are being discovered, the nursing care of these patients will expand even further. An example is the introduction of the advent of biologic therapies and the evolution of the biologics nurse specialist. In order to practise at such a level, the nurse specialising in rheumatology must have a sound knowledge of:

- rheumatic diseases
- human anatomy
- physiology of the systems
- organs relating to the musculoskeletal system.

This knowledge will enable the nurse to assess and plan the appropriate nursing interventions necessary for the holistic care of patients and their families.

ANATOMY AND PHYSIOLOGY OF THE MUSCULOSKELETAL SYSTEM

COMPONENTS OF THE MUSCULOSKELETAL SYSTEM

The musculoskeletal system consists of:

- bones
- skeletal muscle
- connective tissue
- joints.

All these structures function as separate units within an interdependent system that allows a complex range of movement.

BONES

The skeleton is made up of various bones. Its functions are to:

- provide a framework to support the body,
- protect organs,
- store minerals,
- produce blood cells.

There are around 200 different bones in the body which are held together by cartilage and ligaments; and it is this complex structure, the skeleton, which supports the body (Figure 2.1).

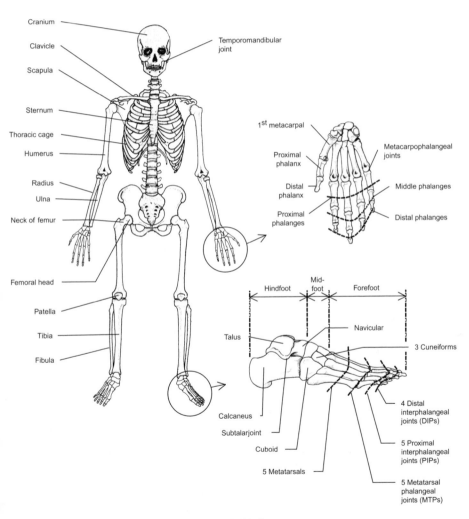

Figure 2.1 Skeleton.

The brain, heart, lungs and spinal cord are protected by the bony structures of the cranium, rib cage and vertebral spine. The pelvis and the muscles of the abdomen protect the vital abdominal organs.

Calcium is stored within the bones of the skeleton and is vital for bone formation, blood coagulation, nerve production and cardiac and skeletal muscle contraction. The musculoskeletal system contains 97% of the total bodily contents of calcium salts.

As well as storing calcium, the bones contain marrow that produces vital blood cells.

Structure of bone

Bone is the hardest tissue in the body and is made up of collagen fibres which consist of crystals of hydroxyapatites formed from phosphates of calcium. It is living tissue nourished by a system of blood and lymphatic vessels. Bone is composed of:

• Osteoblasts which deposit collagen fibres to form the matrix of the bone;
• Osteocytes which form the calcified matrix of the bone;
• Osteoclasts which reabsorb bone by phagocytic action.

Osteoblasts secrete collagen and once calcium deposition has occurred, become osteocytes. Osteocytes form the matrix or framework of bone and are connected to each other by a network of channels. Bone is reabsorbed by the phagocytic action of the osteoclasts.

There are two different types of bone: compact and trabecular.

The mature skeleton contains 80% compact bone and 20% trabecular bone.

Compact or dense bone is hard and white and makes up the shafts of the long bones and the surface of flat bones. Microscopic investigation reveals concentric plates of bone (lamella) interspersed by a system of Haversian canals. These provide access for blood and lymphatic vessels which nourish the osteocytes.

Trabecular or cancellous bone is spongy in appearance and is surrounded by compact bone. The strut-like arrangement of the cells can be seen under a microscope. This formation increases the strength of the bone. Haversian canals are also present in trabecular bone to supply the necessary nutrients.

Red bone marrow is a pulpy tissue found in the central cavity of the shaft of long bones and in the cancellous bone of the flat and irregular bones. The vertebrae, sternum, ribs, clavicles, scapulae, cranial bones and proximal ends of the femoral and humeral bones of adults all contain red bone marrow. Erythrocytes are produced in the red bone marrow. A good dietary intake of vitamin B12, folic acid and iron is necessary for this process.

Bones are covered by a tough, vasculitic outer covering known as the periosteum. In addition to blood supplied from the periosteum and the Haversian canals, long bones receive blood from an artery which enters the shaft through the nutrient foramen.

Foetal bone

Foetal bones are composed of fibrous or cartilaginous tissue. As the foetus develops, calcification of the bone occurs as calcium salts are deposited into the cartilage and osteoblasts lay down bone to replace the cartilage.

During childhood this process occurs mainly at the centres of ossification which enable the bone to grow. The centres of ossification are situated in the extremities of long bones and in the centre of bones. Each extremity or epiphysis of a long bone is separated from the shaft (diaphysis) by the epiphyseal line which is made of a layer of cartilage. Once adulthood is reached this layer becomes calcified and the epiphysis and diaphysis become fused and there is no further growth of the bone. Growth in the circumference of a bone occurs when osteoblasts lay down new bone under the periosteum which is the tough fibrous covering of the bone.

Requirements for bone formation

Bone formation and reabsorbtion is a continuous process which requires an adequate intake of calcium and Vitamin D. This process, known as bone turnover, is especially high during childhood, when an adequate dietary intake of calcium is necessary for the development of strong bones.

The growth of bones is affected by:

- pituitary growth hormone
- sex hormones (oestrogens and androgens)
- thyroid hormone.

Bones contain calcium salts. These are present in greater quantities in adults than in the bones of children which tend to be more elastic with a loose matrix. If trauma occurs, it may result in a partial fracture, instead of a complete break as would normally occur in mature, dense bones. In a freshly healed fracture, the bone matrix is less dense than normal.

Hormonal influence

Loss of bone density occurs as hormone levels decrease, as for example in menopausal women. This results in osteoporosis, a condition where the bones become less strong and are liable to fracture.

Specific bones

Bones come in all shapes and sizes depending on the size and function of the muscles which are attached to them.

Long bones

Long bones (Figure 2.2) consist of a shaft (diaphysis) with two extremities (epiphysis). The limbs are a made up of typical long bones such as the:

- femur
- tibia
- fibula
- humerus
- ulna
- radius.

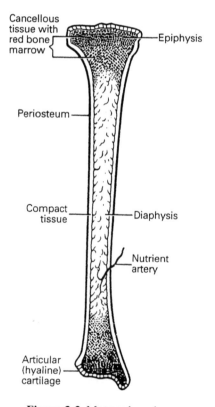

Figure 2.2 Mature long bone.

In mature bones the central shaft is made of compact bone which has a central channel filled with bone marrow. The extremities are made up of cancellous bone containing red bone marrow and are covered with a thin layer of compact bone.

Short bones

Short bones consist of cancellous bone covered by a layer of compact bone. They are box-like in shape such as the carpus of the wrist and tarsus of the ankle.

Flat bones

Flat bones are composed of a layer of cancellous bone between two layers of compact bone. Examples are the scapula, innominate bone and cranial bones.

Irregular bones

Irregular bones are formed from cancellous bone covered by an outer layer of compact bone. Examples are the vertebrae and facial bones.

Sesamoid bone

Sesamoid bones develop in the tendons of specific joints such as the sesamoid bone of the thumb. The most important sesamoid bone is the patella.

SKELETAL MUSCLES

Skeletal muscles provide force and power for the body to work and produce movement by working with other muscles.

Physical structure

Skeletal muscles are also known as striated or voluntary muscle and are made up of bundles of muscle fibres called fasciculi. The individual muscle fibres consist of thin filaments of contractile proteins that are covered by the sarcolemma. The endomysium is the fibrous tissue found in the spaces between the individual fibres. These lie parallel to each other and are grouped into fasciculi and covered by perimysium. The groups of fasciculi are in turn covered by a tough fibrous sheath or epimysium that covers the muscle itself.

Nutrition

Skeletal muscles are amply supplied by blood vessels and capillaries which provide the oxygen, calcium and chemical nutrients necessary for action and remove the waste materials incurred by such action.

Types of muscle

The titles of many muscles reflect their characteristics. For example:

- triceps (three heads) and formation
- flexor carpi ulnaris and movement
- sternomastoid and attachment
- occipitalis and position
- deltoid and shape.

The action of muscles

Striated muscle is supplied with motor nerves that enable it to contract in one direction. When action occurs the muscle fully contracts (shortens and thickens), and this is known as an isotonic state. They may also be stimulated to contract by electrical shock.

The upright posture of the body is maintained by muscle tone which provides the necessary amount of force to counteract the effects of gravity. Muscle tone means that the length of muscle does not change but that the muscle remains tense in an isometric state. This partial contraction of the muscle is absent during sleep or periods of unconsciousness.

Movement

Movement of the joints is produced by voluntary contraction of one or a group of muscles which pull the bones together.

Muscles are grouped in pairs, one muscle being the agonist or prime mover, and its partner being the antagonist. For example, the main agonist in the upper arm is the biceps, and the antagonist is the triceps. When the bicep contracts the tricep relaxes. Large muscles are often composed of several muscles. For example the quadriceps extensor is made up of four different muscles, the:

- rectus femoris
- vastus medialis
- vastus lateralis
- vastus intermedius.

Synergistic muscle groups act together to provide complicated actions at the wrists, shoulders, ankles and hips. They work as a group to perform one action that no one of them could perform alone. This synchronized action is called synergism.

Skeletal muscles are capable of a wide variety of movements. They range from powerful complicated actions as in the quadriceps, to the small, slight movements produced by the muscles of facial expression. Different muscles have individual functions as shown below:

- Flexors bend limbs.
- Extensors straighten limbs.
- Adductors move limbs from midline.
- Abductors move limbs towards midline.
- Rotators rotate a limb.
- Pronators turn palms downwards.
- Supinators turn palms upwards.
- Planatarflexors pull the foot up.
- Dorsiflexors push the foot down.
- Levators raise part of the body.
- Depressors lower part of the body.

CONNECTIVE TISSUE

The functions of connective tissue are to:

- attach bone to bone;
- attach muscle to bone;
- provide a point of anchorage for the action of muscles and bones;
- help to stabilise joints.

Tendons

Groups of muscles are attached to each other and surrounding tissue by tendons and fascia. Tendons are the connective tissue extensions of the perimysium and epimysium. They are strong, fibrous, inelastic cords which attach the muscle extremities to the bone at points of insertion or enthesis.

A flat expansion of tendonous tissue is known as an aponeurosis. For example, the lumbar fascia is an aponeurosis which attaches the latissimus dorsi muscle to the vertebral column. Where tendons pass under ligaments or through bony tunnels, as in the wrist and ankle, they are enclosed in a synovial membrane sheath that reduces friction and enables the tendons to glide smoothly.

Ligaments

Ligaments resemble tendons and are strong bundles of connective tissue attached from one bone to another bone around a joint. They are thickened and enlarged around many of the synovial joints and thus increase the strength of the joint capsule. They act as restraints and ensure that the joint movement is within an acceptable plane and range.

JOINTS

The functions of joints are to:

- stabilise the skeleton
- permit a range of movement.

Physical structure

Joints are where two or more bones meet. There are three different types of joints:

- Fixed joints, such as the squamous sutures of the skull interlock with each other. Whilst the brain is developing and growing these joints expand. As a child grows older they become fixed and immovable and so protect the soft tissue of the brain.
- Fibrocartilaginous joints are slightly moveable. Examples are the symphysis pubis, the costosternal joints and the vertebral bodies. In the case of the symphysis pubis the action of a hormone, relaxin, makes the joint more flexible and thus permits enlargement of the birth canal.
- Diarthroses or synovial joints (Figure 2.3) are the most common types of joint in the body. They are of particular interest in rheumatology as they are the joints most commonly affected by inflammatory joint diseases such as rheumatoid arthritis.

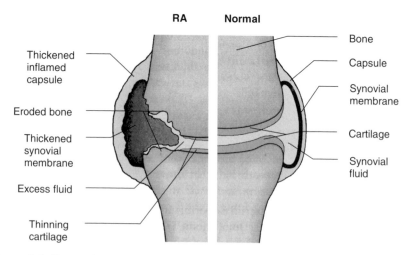

Figure 2.3 Comparison of a normal synovial joint versus an RA synovial joint (Reproduced with kind permission from Geoff Hill [2000] *Rheumatology – A Handbook for Community Nurses*).

Synovial joints are freely moveable and are surrounded by a joint capsule lined with synovium. This lining, also called the synovial membrane, covers all the intra-articular surfaces except the cartilage itself. It produces synovial fluid which lubricates the joint and feeds the cells of the articular cartilage.

The ends of the bones are covered and cushioned by hyaline cartilage. The joint capsule is made of fibrous tissue and strengthened by ligaments. It surrounds the whole joint and thus holds the bones together.

Cartilage

There are two types of cartilage:

- hyaline
- fibrocartilage.

Hyaline (articular) cartilage is a resilient structure that forms a firm cushion between the articulating or moveable surfaces of bone. It is not supplied with blood but gains all its necessary nutrients from the vasculature of surrounding tissues. These nutrients are carried to the cartilage by the synovial fluid which also removes the byproducts of metabolic activity within the cartilage.

Fibrocartilage has a definite matrix, is fibrous and compact. It is found at non-articulating joints such as the sternocostal, symphysis pubis and also between the intervertebral discs of the vertebrae.

Bursae

Bursae can be found close to joints where the skin moves directly over the bone. They are small synovial sacs acting as cushions to help relieve the pressure and friction over joints such as the knee, hip and ankle.

Movement of the joint

Movement of the joint is produced by the action of muscles and tendons and stabilised within a plane by ligaments. The different types of synovial joints permit a wide range and variety of movement. The planes of movement are:

- Flexion which is bending a joint.
- Extension which is straightening a joint.
- Abduction which is moving from the median or mid-line.
- Adduction which is moving towards the median or mid-line.
- Circumduction which is flexion, adduction, extension and abduction in sequence or in reverse order.
- Rotation which is movement around the long axis of a bone.

- Pronation which is rotation of the hand to face palm downwards.
- Supination which is rotation of the hand to face palm upwards.
- Opposition which is bringing the tip of the thumb to the tips of the fingers.
- Dorsiflexion which is pulling the foot up towards the leg.
- Plantar flexion which is pointing the foot down towards the ground.
- Inversion which is pointing the sole of the foot inwards.
- Eversion which is pointing the sole of the foot outwards.

Types of synovial joints

- Uniaxial (hinge) joints are capable of flexion and extension as in the elbow and interphalangeal joints.
- Polyaxial (ball and socket) joints can extend, abduct, adduct, rotate and circumduct as in the hips and shoulders.
- Ellipsoid joints permit flexion, extension, abduction and adduction but cannot rotate and combine the other movements to permit circumduction as in the wrist.
- Saddle joints flex, extend, circumduct and rotate as in the carpometacarpal joint of the thumb.
- Plane joints glide one across another as in the metatarsal joints.
- Bicondylar joints flex, extend and slightly rotate as in the knee and temporomandibular joints.
- Pivot joints only rotate, an example is the atlas vertebrae.
- Compound joints are capable of several movements which involve more than two bones articulating with each other, for example the elbow.

JOINTS COMMONLY AFFECTED BY RHEUMATIC DISEASE

The joints or groups of joints most commonly affected by rheumatic disease are the:

- shoulder girdle
- elbow
- wrist and hand
- pelvic girdle
- knee
- ankle and foot
- vertebral column
- jaw.

The shoulder girdle

The shoulder girdle is made up of the humerus, clavicle and scapula, which together provide a framework for the variety of movement found at this joint.

Movement is synchronized and therefore dependent on the joints, ligaments and muscles working in harmony. Failure of any of these structures results in restricted or deficient movement.

The four joints of the shoulder girdle are the:

* glenohumeral
* acromioclavicular
* sternoclavicular
* scapulothoracic.

The glenohumeral is multiaxial and the principle joint of the structure. The head of the humerus articulates within the glenoid fossa of the scapula, the diameter and depth of which is increased by a ring of fibrocartilage called the glenoid labrum. Free movement at this joint is allowed by the lax joint capsule which is strengthened by the glenohumeral, transverse humeral and coracoacriomial ligaments. The long head of the biceps muscle inserts into the capsule and stabilises the joint.

Further stability is given by the rotator cuff which provides a band around the anterior, superior and posterior aspects of the glenohumeral joint and thereby stabilises the head of the humerus within the glenoid fossa. The muscles that form the rotator cuff are the supraspinatus, infraspinatus, subscapularis, and teres major.

The acromioclavicular joint is a plane joint formed by the distal end of the clavicle and the acromion process of the scapula. It is surrounded by a joint capsule which is strengthened above by the acromioclavicular ligament. A fibrous pad permits some movement at this joint. It is stabilised by the coraclavicular ligaments that hold the scapula and clavicle together during movement.

The sternoclavicular joint is a saddle joint formed between the medial end of the clavicle and the manubrium sterni. This joint contains an intra-articular fibrous disc and is strengthened by anterior and posterior ligaments. The clavicle rotates during abduction and elevation of the shoulder.

The scapulothoracic joint is formed by the scapula articulating with the thoracic cage. The rotator cuff muscles, deltoid and trapezius insert around this articulation. Normal movement of the shoulder is dependent upon this joint.

The wide range of movement at the shoulder girdle depends upon the joints, muscles, tendons and ligaments working together.

Common disorders of the shoulder are:

* synovitis
* capsulitis (frozen shoulder)
* dislocation
* rotator cuff tears

- tendinitis
- biceptal tendinitis
- subacromial bursitis
- osteoarthritis.

The elbow joint

The elbow joint is a compound hinge joint formed by the articulation between the distal end of the humerus and the proximal ends of the ulna and radius. The radial and ulnar collateral ligaments provide support for the elbow and prevent varus or vagus instability.

The superior radioulnar joint is a fibrocartilaginous, uniaxial, pivotal joint at the articulation of the proximal ends of the radius and ulna. The joint capsule of the elbow joint also surrounds this joint. Several bursae can be found around the joint, the main one being the olecranon bursa.

The muscles responsible for the range of movement at the elbow are:

- biceps, brachialis, flexor carpi ulnaris which control flexion;
- triceps which control extension;
- pronator teres which control pronation;
- supinator which control supination.

Common disorders of the elbow are:

- synovitis
- lateral epicondylitis (tennis elbow)
- medial epicondylitis (golfer's elbow)
- olecranon bursitis
- entrapment neuropathy
- referred pain often from cervical or shoulder problems.

The wrist and hand

The wrist and hand form a complex structure, which together with the bones of the forearm permit complete manual dexterity. The range of movement is varied and is essential for all the complex movements necessary for self-care. Any problems within this structure will directly affect independent living.

The bones which make up the wrist are the distal ends of the radius and ulna and the eight carpal bones: trapeziod, trapezium, scaphoid, lunate hamate, pisiform, triquetrum and capitate. This structure provides a stable, strong support for the hand and its many functions (Figure 2.1).

The wrist is made up of the following joints:

- radiocarpal
- distal radioulnar
- intercarpal.

The radiocarpal joint of the wrist is an ellipsoid, compound joint between the distal end of the radius and the scaphoid, lunate and triquetrum. The radiocarpal and collateral ligaments strengthen the joint capsule.

The distal radioulnar joint is a pivot joint. The radius is attached to the ulna by an articular disc, which permits rotation of the ulna head around the radius thereby pronating and suppinating the hand.

The intercarpal joints are fibrocartilaginous, uniaxial, pivotal joints joined together by strong ligaments. One of the ligaments is the transverse carpal ligament (flexor retinaculum) on the volar aspect of the wrist. This forms the roof of the carpal tunnel by connecting the four bony prominences of the pisiform, hamate, scaphoid and trapezium. The flexor retinaculum prevents the flexor tendons from bowing out. Where tendons cross the wrist they are enclosed in tenosynovial sheaths. The flexor pollicis longus tendon sheath, the common flexor tendon sheath and the median nerve pass through the carpal tunnel to the hand. The ulnar nerve, artery and vein cross over the flexor retinaculum.

The extensor tendons are also enclosed in tendon sheaths and pass through fibro-osseous tunnels beneath the extensor retinaculum. This ligament binds deeply with the radius on the dorsum of the wrist and holds the extensor tendons to the wrist.

The muscles responsible for the range of movement at the wrist are:

- flexor carpi radialis and flexor carpi ulnaris which control flexion;
- extensor carpi radialis and extensor carpi ulnaris which control extension;
- flexor carpi radialis and extensor carpi radialis which control abduction;
- flexor carpi ulnaris and extensor carpi ulnaris which control adduction.

The anatomic snuffbox is the depression formed on the dorsum of the wrist by the extensor and abductor tendons of the thumb.

The carpometacarpal (CMC) joints are formed between the trapezium, trapeziod, capitate and hamate bones and the proximal ends of the metacarpal bones. They are capable of flexion and extension and are classed as ellipsoid joints with the exception of the thumb which is a saddle joint. This articulation between the distal end of the trapezium and the proximal end of the first metacarpal is capable of abduction, adduction and rotation as well as extension and flexion.

The metacarpophalangeal joints (MCPs) or knuckles are hinge joints capable of flexion and extension. They are formed by the articulation of the distal ends of the metacarpal bones with the proximal ends of the phalanges.

The proximal and distal interphalangeal joints (PIPs and DIPs) are hinge joints which permit flexion and extension of the fingers. Fibrous tenosynovial sheaths enclose the flexor tendons of the fingers.

Common disorders of the wrist and hand are

* synovitis
* carpal tunnel syndrome
* trigger finger
* De Quervain's tenosynovitis
* Dupuytren's contracture
* Raynaud's phenomenon.

The pelvic girdle

The pelvic girdle is composed of the innominate bone and the sacrum. There are three joints in the pelvis (Figure 2.4). They are the:

* hip joint
* sacroiliac joint
* symphysis pubis.

The hip is a multiaxial (ball and socket) joint. It is extremely strong, stable and capable of a variety of complex movements. The head of the femur articulates within the acetabulum of the innominate bone. The acetabulum is

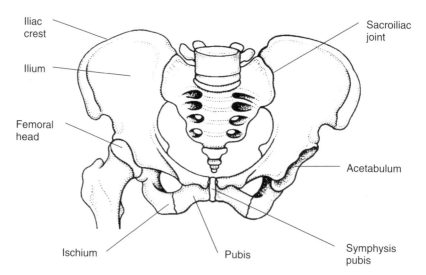

Figure 2.4 The pelvic girdle.

strengthened and made deeper by a ring of fibrocartilage. The stability of the joint is maintained by three large ligaments; the iliofemoral, the pubofemoral and the ischiofemoral. The trochanteric bursa is the most important of the bursae found around the hip joint.

The muscles responsible for the range of movement at the hip are:

- iliopsoas and sartorius which control flexion;
- gluteus maximus and hamstrings which control extension;
- gluteus medius and gluteus minimus which control abduction;
- adductors longus and brevis and magnus which control adduction;
- gluteus medius and gluteus minimus which control rotation (lateral);
- obturator and quadratus femoris which control rotation (medial).

The sacroiliac joint is a synovial joint with limited movement. It holds the sacrum firmly between the two ilium bones and thereby anchors the vertebral column to the lower limbs. The strong sacroiliac, sacroprial and sacrotubal ligaments help to stabilize and strengthen this joint and enable it to take some of the stress that occurs during the gait cycle.

The symphysis pubis is a fibrocartilaginous joint which holds the two pubic bones together. There is little or no movement at this joint except during late pregnancy and childbirth. Then hormonal changes alter the structure to allow more flexibility and permit enlargement of the birth canal.

Common disorders of the pelvic girdle are:

- trochanteric bursitis
- synovitis
- avascular necrosis
- congenital dislocation of the hip
- sacroiliitis.

The knee

The knee is a compound joint and is the largest joint in the body. It is supported by strong thigh muscles, which help to maintain its stability. Several ligaments strengthen the joint capsule. The patellar ligament supports the patella and the anterior part of the capsule. The anterior and lateral collateral ligaments, the anterior and posterior cruciate ligaments and the transverse ligament all increase the strength of the joint capsule. They are also vital in maintaining the strength and stability of the knee and in preventing valgus and varus deformities. Within the knee the semilunar cartilages or menisci help to deepen the articular surfaces at the proximal end of the tibia. Anteriorly the patella moves at the front of the knee between the lateral and medial condyles of the femur. There are many bursae around the knee, the main one being the prepatellar bursa (Figure 2.5).

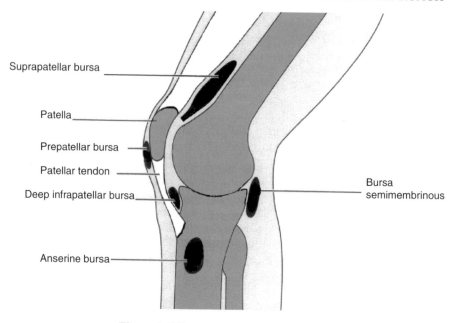

Suprapatellar bursa

Patella

Prepatellar bursa

Patellar tendon

Deep infrapatellar bursa

Bursa semimembrinous

Anserine bursa

Figure 2.5 Bursae surrounding the knee.

The muscles responsible for the range of movement at the knee are:

- quadriceps which control extension;
- hamstrings, gastrocnemius, sartorius and gracilis which control flexion;
- medial hamstrings, popliteus, sartorius and gracilis which control rotation (medial);
- biceps femoris which control rotation (lateral).

Common disorders of the knee are:

- synovitis
- bursitis
- tendinitis
- prepatellar bursitis (housemaid's knee)
- patellar bursitis (jumper's knee)
- popliteal cysts
- synovial chondromatosis
- chondromalacia patellae
- meniscal lesions
- ligamentous injuries.

The ankle and foot

The ankle and foot (Figure 2.1) are composed of many bones and several joints. The foot is divided into the hind, mid and forefoot.

The ankle, also known as the talocrural joint, is a compound hinge joint. The distal ends of the tibia and fibula articulate with the talus and form the ankle joint. The hind foot consists of the calcaneus and talus.

The talus also articulates inferiorly with the calcaneus at the subtalar joint and distally with the navicular bone at the midtarsal or talonavicular joint.

The distal tibiofibular joint is a fibrous joint that holds the distal ends of the tibia and fibula firmly together. Ligamentous bands strengthen the joint capsule medially and laterally.

Tenosynovial sheaths cover the tendons that run through this area. The extensor retinaculum, on the anterior aspect of the ankle is divided into two parts; the superior and inferior retinaculi. This strong ligament anchors the extensor tendons to the ankle and prevents them from bowing out. Medially, the flexor tendons are strapped down by the flexor retinaculum and the peroneal tendon is held down by the superior and inferior retinaculi. Posteriorly, the Achilles tendon inserts into the calcaneus. Numerous bursae can be found in the ankle especially around the Achilles tendon.

The muscles responsible for the range of movement at the ankle are:

- soleus and gastrocnemius which controls plantar flexion;
- anterior tibialis and extensor digitorum longus which controls dorsiflexion;
- peroneus longus, peroneus brevis and extensor digitorum longus which controls eversion;
- tibialis anterior, tibialis posterior and gastrocnemius which controls inversion.

Common disorders of the ankle are:

- sprains
- Achilles tendinitis
- Achilles tendon rupture
- Achilles bursitis
- plantar fasciitis
- abduction sprains of the medial ligament
- capsular ligament tears (sprained ankle)
- calcaneal spur (policeman's heel).

The midfoot is composed of the navicular, cuboid and the three cuneiform bones. It articulates with the hindfoot at the midtarsal joint and with the forefoot at the tarsometatarsal joints.

The midtarsal or transverse tarsal joint is the articulation of the talus with the navicular (talonavicular) and the calcaneus with the cuboid (calneocuboid). These are fibrous plane joints.

The forefoot is made up of the metatarsals and phalanges. The proximal ends of the metatarsals articulate with the distal ends of the three cuneiform bones and the cuboid at the tarsometatarsal joints.

The metatarsophalangeal joints (MTPs) are the articulations of the distal ends of the metatarsal bones with the proximal ends of the phalanges. These are ellipsoid joints and are surrounded by a joint capsule which is strengthened by collateral ligaments and the plantar aponeurosis. Small bursae lie between the metatarsal heads, which are held together by the transverse metatarsal ligament. An aponeurosis of the extensor tendons covers the dorsum of the foot.

Extension, flexion, abduction and adduction of the toes is achieved by the intrinsic muscles of the foot.

The proximal interphalangeal and distal interphalangeal joints are hinge joints capable of flexing and extending the toes.

The arches of the foot are formed by an arrangement of the bones, ligaments and muscles. Each foot has four arches; two transverse and two longitudinal which act as shock absorbers during weight bearing.

Common disorders of the mid and forefoot are:

• metatarsalgia
• metatarsal stress fractures
• hallux valgus (bunion)
• hallux rigidus (hammer toe)
• pes planus (flat foot)
• pes cavus (claw foot).

The vertebral column

The vertebral column forms a framework which supports the rest of the body and also encloses the spinal cord. It is constructed of several different types of bones or vertebrae, some of which are fused together. The vertebrae are separated by discs of fibrocartilage and attached to each other by strong ligaments and muscles, thus combining strength with a degree of flexibility. The spinal column is constructed and curved to permit walking in an upright posture. At birth the infant has two spinal curves. These primary curves are in the thoracic and sacral regions. The secondary spinal curves develop in the cervical and lumbar regions as an upright stance is assumed.

There are thirty-three vertebrae (Figure 2.6):

• Seven cervical vertebrae are moveable, convex forwards and are lordotic.
• Twelve thoracic vertebrae are moveable, convex backwards and are kyphotic.

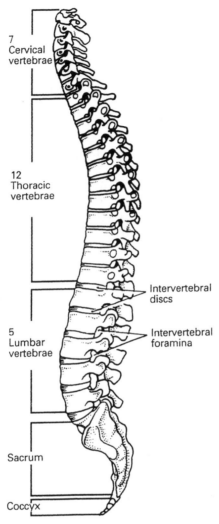

Figure 2.6 Lateral view of a vertebral column.

- Five lumbar vertebrae are moveable, convex forwards and are lordotic.
- Five sacral vertebrae are fused (sacrum), concave forwards and are kyphotic.
- Four coccygeal vertebrae are fused (coccyx) and concave forwards.

Although the vertebrae are of different shapes and sizes, with the exception of the atlas (the first cervical vertebra), they all have:

- spinous process (vertebral arch and a body)
- transverse processes (pedicles and laminae)
- articular processes.

All vertebrae are separated by intervertebral discs of fibrocartilage which are made up of a central ring-like structure called the annulus fibrosis surrounding the nucleus pulposus. The bodies of the vertebrae are held together by anterior and posterior longitudinal ligaments. The spinous processes are held together by the supraspinous ligaments. Spinal nerves pass from the spinal cord through the intervertebral foramen, a space between individual vertebrae.

Of the seven cervical vertebrae of the neck, the lower five are similar in shape. However, the upper two, the atlas and the axis, are different because they are specially adapted to carry the head and enable it to move in many directions. The atlas has no spinous process and no body. It supports the cranium at the atlanto-occipital joint and permits nodding of the head and lateral flexion of the neck. The axis has a peg, the odontoid process or dens, around which the atlas rotates at the atlanto-axial joint to enable movement of the head.

Common disorders of the cervical region are:

- atlanto-axial subluxation
- stenosis
- torticollis
- spondylitis
- whiplash injury
- osteoarthritis.

The twelve thoracic vertebrae have facets for the attachment of the heads of the ribs. This arrangement permits the expansion and contraction of the rib cage and therefore the lungs.

Common disorders of the thoracic region are:

- osteoporosis
- costocondritis
- ankylosing spondylitis
- osteoarthritis.

The five lumbar vertebrae are the largest and strongest. Their design enables them to carry the weight of the body and control its movements on the pelvis in the upright position.

Common disorders of the lumbar region are:

- sciatica
- prolapsed intervertebral disc

- low back pain
- spinal stenosis
- ankylosing spondylitis
- osteoarthritis.

The five sacral vertebrae are fused together to form the sacrum which makes up the posterior aspect of the pelvis. The sacrum is fused to the ilium at the sacroiliac joint. This strong structure enables the body to maintain an upright position and to take the stress of walking and running. It provides posterior protection for the abdominal organs. Females have a larger sacrum than males to allow for a larger pelvic cavity necessary for child bearing.

Common disorders of the sacral region are:

- low back pain
- sacroiliitis.

The coccyx is a triangular structure, formed by the fusion of the four coccygeal vertebrae, the base of which articulates with the apex of the sacrum above.

The spine controls a range of movement. Cervical vertebrae control:

- flexion (bending forwards)
- extension (bending backwards)
- rotation of the head
- lateral movement (bending from side to side).
  Thoracic vertebrae control lateral movement (bending from side to side).
  Lumbar vertebrae control flexion (bending forwards) and extension (bending backwards).
  The whole vertebral column controls rotation and twisting.

The muscles and ligaments of the vertebral column facilitate the range of movement in the back. These structures also support the vertebrae and thus the maintenance of an upright posture.

Jaw (temporomandibular joint)

The temporomandibular joint (TMJ) is formed between the condyle of the mandible (lower jaw) and the fossa of the temporal bone. It is the only articulating joint of the skull. It is lined by fibrous connective tissue rather than the normal hyaline cartilage and meniscii help to extend the range of movement. The joint itself is divided into two parts, the upper part enabling flexion and extension of the joint and the lower a gliding movement to permit lateral and protrusive movement of the lower jaw. It is the only joint in the body which works with a partner, for example both TMJs work as a pair and enable the mouth to be opened.

The muscles responsible for the range of movement of the jaw are:

• Temporal and masseter control chewing.
• Buccinator controls chewing and sucking.
• Pterygoid closes the mouth.

A common disorder of the jaw is synovitis.

THE COMMON RHEUMATIC DISEASES

The term rheumatic disease is used to describe the many conditions that affect the musculoskeletal system. They can affect the bones, joints, soft tissues and muscles. There are around two hundred such diseases (Symmons and Bankhead, 1994). The gamut of conditions ranges from the milder soft tissue rheumatism such as tennis elbow, to inflammation of joint linings, as in rheumatoid arthritis, and damage to the surface of the joints, as in osteoarthritis.

Many of the rheumatic diseases relate to each other and in some instances have overlapping signs and symptoms. The management of patients with rheumatic disease likewise has many common features whatever the disease. However, the course of each patient's disease will be different and therefore each patient must be treated as an individual with an individual plan of care. The common rheumatic diseases are shown in Table 2.1.

INFLAMMATORY JOINT DISEASE

Rheumatoid arthritis

Rheumatoid arthritis (RA) is a chronic inflammatory disease, mainly affecting the peripheral joints. It is characterised by exacerbation and remission of disease activity. Affected joints exhibit synovitis (inflammation of the synovial membrane), which is associated with pain, heat, stiffness, swelling and eventual joint destruction. The disease is systemic and may involve the organs.

Epidemiology

RA is found in approximately 1–3% of the population of western countries, although it appears to be less prevalent amongst oriental populations. It attacks all age groups and three times more women than men are affected (Arthritis Research Campaign, 2002). This female predominance may suggest that antibodies are important in pathogenesis (Edwards, 2002).

Table 2.1 Common rheumatic diseases

Category	Sub category
Inflammatory joint diseases	Rheumatoid arthritis
	Felty's syndrome
	Juvenile chronic arthritis
Spondyloarthropathies	Psoriatic Arthritis
	Ankylosing spondylitis
	Reiter's syndrome
	Behçet's syndrome
Crystal deposition diseases	Gout
	Pyrophosphate arthropathy
Joint failure	Osteoarthritis
Metabolic bone disease	Osteoporosis
Connective tissue diseases	Systemic lupus erythematosus
	Scleroderma
	Polymyositis
	Dermatomyositis
Nonarticular conditions	Polymyalgia rheumatica
	Giant cell arteritis
	Raynaud's phenomenon
	Sjögren's syndrome
Soft tissue rheumatism	Fibromyalgia
	Carpal tunnel syndrome
	Tennis and golfer's elbow

Aetiology

The aetiology is unknown but various factors such as infections, stress and trauma appear to act as a trigger in people with a genetic disposition. Smoking has now emerged as a clear external risk (Albano *et al.*, 2001). The body is unable to switch off the initial response to the disease and it becomes chronic. Criteria for the classification of rheumatoid arthritis were developed by the American Rheumatism Association in 1987 (Arnet *et al.*, 1988). Unfortunately, these criteria were not designed for the diagnosis of early RA and are not sensitive to patients with a disease duration of less than twelve months (Huizinga *et al.*, 2002).

Pathology

The synovial lining of the joint capsule becomes inflamed and congested with T lymphocytes, B cells, macrophages and plasma cells (Firestein, 1994). This lining gradually thickens and forms a pannus that invades the articular cartilage causing erosion of the cartilage and bone (Oliver and Mooney, 2002), visible on x-ray.

Increased disease activity produces an elevated erythrocyte sedimentation rate (ESR), positive rheumatoid factor and an elevated C-reactive protein (CRP). The platelet count may also be raised and anaemia can be present. Some patients have a normal ESR and CRP with a negative rheumatoid factor (Chapter 4). This type of disease is classed as seronegative RA and is usually less aggressive.

Presentation

The most common age of onset is the fourth and fifth decades (Hill and Ryan, 2000). Symmetrical swelling, pain and tenderness of the peripheral joints of the hands and feet are usually the predominant features. As the disease progresses, other joints such as the shoulders, elbows, wrists, hips, knees and ankles are affected (Hill and Reay, 2002). The approximate distribution of effected sites is shown in Figure 2.7. Eventually, damage and destruction cause the joints to become unstable and subluxation can occur. RA is a systemic disease that also causes general malaise, fatigue and depression.

Clinical features

Rheumatoid arthritis may be characterised by:

* pain and swelling of the affected joints;
* early morning stiffness which varies in duration from minutes to hours;
* inactivity stiffness which occurs after periods of rest;
* loss of mobility;
* fatigue;
* anxiety and depression.

Specific related problems

* Hand problems can arise even in early RA, including swelling around the proximal interphalangeal and metacarpal phalangeal joints, swelling of the extensor tendon sheath and the wasting of small muscles. Later problems include ulnar deviation, boutonnière and swan neck deformities. All cause loss of function. Tenosynovitis results in loss of flexion, triggering of the fingers and tendon rupture.
* Metatarsalgia, tendinitis of the plantar fascia and Achilles tendonitis cause pain and restrict mobility.
* Knee effusions can result in Baker's cysts which may be misdiagnosed as venous thrombosis.

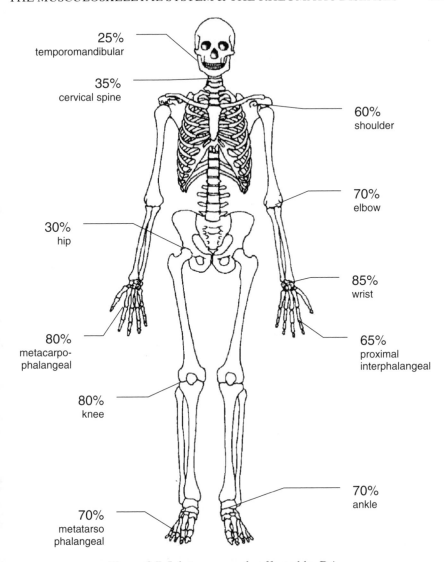

25%
temporomandibular

35%
cervical spine

60%
shoulder

70%
elbow

30%
hip

85%
wrist

80%
metacarpo-
phalangeal

65%
proximal
interphalangeal

80%
knee

70%
ankle

70%
metatarso
phalangeal

Figure 2.7 Joints commonly affected by RA.

- Bursitis of the greater trochanter, olecranon and knee can occur.
- Temporomandibular involvement can limit opening of the mouth.
- Cervical spine involvement causes pain and neurological symptoms in the arms and hands. Atlanto-axial subluxation results in paralysis or even death.

Extra-articular features

- anaemia which normally resolves as the disease remits
- muscular wasting around inflamed joints
- entrapment neuropathies such as median nerve involvement (carpal tunnel syndrome)
- rheumatoid nodules on the elbows, occiput, sacrum, scapulae, Achilles tendon, lungs and myocardium
- Sjögren's syndrome (dry eyes and mouth)
- lymphadenopathy resulting in diffuse pitting oedema of the ankles
- osteoporosis causing fractures of the spine, hip and wrist
- pericarditis, pericardial effusions and amyloidosis
- hepatomegaly caused by amyloid deposits
- fibrosing alveolitis and pleural effusions
- Felty's syndrome causing splenomegaly
- vasculitis causing nail fold infarcts and leg ulcers.

Management

The physical and psychological impact of RA can cause wide ranging problems that require holistic management and input from a multidisciplinary team. Daily living activities are greatly restricted by disease activity. Assessment of the problems, a plan of care and subsequent implementation and evaluation are important to enable the patient to lead as normal a life as possible within their own capabilities (Hill and Hale, 2004).

Therapies

Therapy may include:

- analgesia;
- nonsteroidal anti-inflammatory drugs (NSAIDs) to relieve pain, swelling and stiffness;
- glucocorticosteroids either orally or intramuscularly;
- second-line drug therapy to induce disease remission;
- biologic agents.

Multidisciplinary referrals

Referral to members of the multidisciplinary team should be considered for:

- education and information
- joint protection

- rest and relaxation
- physiotherapy
- advice about a healthy diet
- special shoes, wrist and ankle supports, collars.

Surgical intervention may be helpful for some patients (Chapter 14). Joint replacement of the hips, knees and shoulders may be indicated to give some measure of mobility, function and relief from pain. Other surgical procedures such as excision of metatarsal heads may also be undertaken to relieve pain and improve function. Cosmetic surgery is sometimes undertaken for deformities of the hand.

Felty's syndrome

Felty's syndrome occurs in 1% of the rheumatoid population (Campion and Maddison, 1986) and is characterised by splenomegaly, neutropaenia and deforming RA (Gornisiewicz and Moreland, 2001).

Aetiology

Little is known of the aetiology of this syndrome except that it affects both sexes equally, although men seem to develop the syndrome earlier in their rheumatoid disease. Patients are usually older than 50 years and have a high titre of rheumatoid factor in their blood. Morbidity and mortality are high and infection often leads to death.

Pathology

The production of neutrophils is decreased and the bone marrow reserve is suppressed. Raised levels of IgM, IgG and ANA are present in the blood serum (Chapter 4).

Presentation

Patients with long standing, seropositive, nodular, deforming RA may develop Felty's syndrome (Matteson *et al.*, 1994). Changes in the joints are usually mild with little clinical or radiological evidence. Splenomegaly, neutropenia and vasculitis may be present and weight loss is common. Frequent infections of the skin, lungs and kidneys occur but are not necessarily related to the neutropenia (Dieppe *et al.*, 1985). Liver involvement occurs in 65% of patients (Matteson *et al.*, 1994).

Clinical features

Felty's syndrome may have the following characteristics:

- Hyperpigmentation may occur on the shins.
- Chronic leg ulcers are more common than in rheumatoid arthritis.
- Raynaud's phenomenon and Sjögren's syndrome may be present.

Management

The problems are similar to those associated with RA and should be managed in a similar fashion. Spontaneous remission of the neutropenia occurs in some cases.

Therapies

Therapy may include:

- Second line drug therapy to suppress the rheumatoid disease (Chapter 12) may be given. This should induce neutrophilia and reduce the likelihood of infection.
- Splenectomy is sometimes undertaken but it is a controversial intervention. The benefit derived from the increase in neutrophils induced by the removal of the spleen, the site of neutrophil destruction, has to be balanced against the risks of operation and infection.

Juvenile chronic arthritis

Juvenile chronic arthritis (JCA) is defined as an inflammatory arthritis which presents before the sixteenth birthday. This condition is described in detail in Chapter 17.

THE SPONDYLOARTHROPATHIES

The rheumatological conditions grouped under this heading share many common features (Packham and Bowness, 2001) including:

- peripheral arthropathy
- seronegative rheumatoid factor
- positive HLA B27
- sacroiliitis evident on x-ray examination
- genetic predisposition.

Psoriatic arthritis

Psoriatic arthritis (PsA) is a chronic peripheral, polyarthritis similar to RA and is associated with a previous, ongoing psoriasis. It may progress to a severe form of PsA known as arthritis mutilans.

Epidemiology

PsA is a chronic inflammatory arthropathy with a prevalence between 0.1 and 1% and males and females are affected equally (Shbeeb *et al.*, 2000). A familial history of psoriasis is common. Psoriasis affects 1–3% of the population and of these about one-third develop PsA (Gladman, 1995).

Pathology

Blood tests show a normal ESR and negative rheumatoid factor. HLA B27 is positive especially in those patients with sacroiliitis and spondylitis. X-ray examinations reveal erosions of the joints, sclerosis of joint margins, cysts and ankylosis. Arthritis mutilans produces more severe changes such as the destruction of the ends of the distal bones making them impact and causing the fingers to telescope.

Presentation

The usual age of onset is between 20 and 50 years. Some patients have associated asymptomatic sacroiliitis and spondylitis. Psoriasis will be present in 75% of patients and one-third will have some eye involvement (Wright and Helliwell, 1992; Helliwell and Wright, 1994).

Clinical features

Psoriatic arthritis may be characterised by:

• inflammation of the DIPS and PIPs, dactylitis (sausage finger);
• hot, swollen and painful feet;
• enthesitis affecting Achilles tendons and plantar fascia;
• psoriasis affecting extensor surfaces of the knees, elbows and scalp;
• onycholysis (nail pitting).

Management

Patients with PsA experience similar problems to those with RA and management varies according their needs. However, patients with PsA are particularly unfortunate as they have to cope with the symptoms of two chronic, incurable diseases (Hill and Reay, 2002). This can have a tremendous psychological impact and if this is the case, counseling should be considered (Espinoza and Cuellar, 1994).

Therapies

Patients will need the services of the multidisciplinary team if all their requirements are to be met. The same types of drugs used for RA are useful in PsA. However, systemic corticosteroids are avoided if possible, as dose tapering can cause flares of psoriasis. Methotrexate works on both the arthritis and the skin problems of this disease and ultra-violet light is used for the psoriasis (Chapter 10). The biggest breakthrough has been the use of the biologic therapies which show very promising results in PsA (Chapter 12).

Ankylosing spondylitis

Ankylosing spondylitis (AS) is the most common of the spondyloarthritides and affects the axial skeleton (sacroiliac joints and the vertebral column). Initially, inflammation occurs at the sacroiliac joints and this is followed by the vertebral column (Rai and Struthers, 1994). This inflammation causes the bone to erode (enthesopathy), and as the bone repairs itself, it replaces the elastic tissue of the tendons and ligaments causing the bones to slowly fuse. It is this fusion of the vertebral column that results in the characteristic 'bamboo' spine (Sieper *et al.*, 2002). AS can occur in association with other diseases such as Reiter's syndrome, psoriasis, ulcerative colitis or Crohn's disease.

Epidemiology

AS has a prevalence of 0.2–0.86% in adult Caucasian populations (Packham and Bowness, 2001) and affects approximately three times more males than females (Khan, 2002). Geographical variation governs the frequency of ankylosing spondylitis as indicated by the racial incidence of the HLA B27 antigen.

Pathology

Blood tests show an elevated ESR (erythrocyte sedimentation rate) and CRP (C reactive protein) and a negative rheumatoid factor. More than 90% of patients are HLA B27 positive. Radiological examination eventually shows calcification of the spinal longitudinal ligaments, squaring of the vertebrae, spinal osteoporosis (bamboo spine) and the characteristic blurring of the sacroiliac joints.

Presentation

The average age of onset is 26 years (Khan, 1994). It starts in an insidious fashion with pain and stiffness in the lumbosacral region. Peripheral arthritis may be present but is uncommon and does not persist. Sleep disturbance due to pain and stiffness in the spine causes fatigue. Remissions and exacerbation of disease activity occur early in the disease, but eventually the spine stiffens and body posture changes as thoracic kyphosis develops and lumbar lordosis is lost. Cervical ankylosis with kyphosis leads to the loss of forward gaze. Although the majority of patients are able to remain in work and lead a reasonable life, in some patients, AS causes significant functional impairment that has a substantial economic effect on patients, their families and the healthcare system (Doran *et al.*, 2003). This is particularly so for those who develop hip and neck problems.

Clinical features

Ankylosing spondilitis may be characterized by:

- fatigue;
- low backache initially severe and later becoming dull;
- pain and stiffness particularly in the lower back after periods of inactivity but improved by exercise;
- unilateral or bilateral pain in the sacroiliac and gluteal regions;
- sciatica type pain radiating from the buttock into the leg;
- enthesopathy (costosternal, manubriosternal, Achilles tendinitis and plantar faciitis).

As the disease progresses there may be:

- restriction of spinal movement caused by ankylosis of the vertebrae;
- restricted range of movement in the hips and shoulders;
- flexion fractures of the hips;
- stiff neck resulting in torticollis;
- reduced chest expansion caused by fusion of the ribs to the transverse processes of the vertebrae.

Extra articular features include:

- iritis, conjunctivitis and uveitis;
- pulmonary fibrosis and aortic incompetence in severe cases.

Management

As AS is incurable, the focus of care is maintaining physical, psychological and social function (Cornell, 2004; Cornell and Oliver, 2004). Education is vital in order that patients and their families understand the value of daily exercises and prone lying which will ensure that spinal fusion is restricted and a straight spine is maintained. Regular physiotherapy and hydrotherapy are essential to maintain movement of the spine and hips.

Therapies

Therapy may include:

- Nonsteroidal anti-inflammatory drugs (NSAIDs) may be prescribed to relieve pain and stiffness.
- In contrast to RA, no disease-modifying antirheumatic drugs (DMARDs) are currently approved for the treatment of AS (Braun and Sieper, 2002). Of the few studies of DMARDs undertaken, none have shown efficacy in axial disease. Sulphasalazine has shown limited efficacy in peripheral arthritis (Clegg *et al.*, 1999); and methotrexate was shown to have limited efficacy in a few studies (Marshall and Kirwan, 2001).
- Two anti-TNFα drugs, infliximab and etanercept, are now licensed for AS and a third adalimumab is being studied. These drugs appear to be a break-through in the treatment of AS.

Psychological support is important for this group of patients who often experience anxiety, depression and problems with lack of self-worth and altered body image. Patients should be encouraged to join support groups such as the National Ankylosing Spondylitis Society which is known as NASS.

Reiter's syndrome and reactive arthritis

Reactive arthritis (Reiter's syndrome) is the triad of:

- arthritis
- urethritis
- conjunctivitis.

It usually occurs as a result of a reaction to a genital or gastrointestinal tract infection and the prospect of understanding the mechanism of linking infection and reactive arthritis remains a subject of intense research activity (Sieper *et al.*, 2000).

Epidemiology

Hans Reiter, a military doctor with the German army first described this syndrome. Reiter's syndrome is also termed a reactive arthritis, because the initial infection whether genital or gastrointestinal, causes a reaction elsewhere in the body. In one-third of patients no infectious cause is found. Men and women are affected equally (Toivanen, 1994).

Aetiology

A reactive arthritis which has been caused through sexual contact is termed SARA (sexually acquired reactive arthritis). Chlamydia trachomatis and gonococcal organisms are thought to be responsible. Shigella, salmonella, campylobacter and yersinia are the organisms associated with a reactive arthritis contracted through the gastrointestinal tract. The majority of patients (65–96%) are HLA B27 positive and often develop a more chronic type of disease (Toivanen, 1994).

Pathology

Blood tests reveal a negative rheumatoid factor and elevated ESR and CRP. Radiological examination shows osteopenia around the joints, calcaneal and plantar spurs and bilateral sacroiliitis.

Presentation

The peak age of onset is 16–35 years and it follows sexual contact or sometimes an attack of dysentery. A typical presentation is that of a young man with an acute, asymmetrical oligoarthritis affecting either the knees, ankles or feet. The affected joints are often severely inflamed with erythema, tenderness and large effusions. The lower limbs may be involved one at a time over several weeks. The elbows, wrists and fingers are occasionally affected. Sacroiliitis and spondylitis occur in the one third of those with recurrent disease. Symptoms may recur over a few years but they eventually resolve.

Clinical features

Reiter's syndrome may be characterised by:

- fever;
- synovitis of the knee or ankle;
- dactylitis or 'sausage toe';
- plantar fasciitis and Achilles tendonitis;
- conjunctivitis which may be bilateral but usually resolves;
- urethral discharge which may be mild, non purulent and is often missed;
- circinate balinitis and vulvitis;
- cystitis;
- keratoderma blenorrhagica (These skin lesions resemble pustular psoriasis and may appear on the palms of the hands and soles of the feet of patients with SARA.);

- onycholysis (nail pitting);
- ulcers on the tongue, palate, buccal mucosa and lips.

Management

Treatment should be symptomatic. Musculoskeletal symptoms may persist for several months and then resolve. Counselling and advice may be necessary especially where there is a worry about future sexual activity. In the case of SARA, sexual contacts should be traced so that they can be treated.

Therapies

Therapy may include:

- NSAIDs;
- tetracycline to treat urethritis;
- second-line drugs such as sulphasalazine and methotrexate for persistent disease;
- splinting or bed rest of the affected joints;
- aspiration and steroid injection of joint effusions;
- physiotherapy to regain muscle power and tone;
- local steroid injections to relieve pain caused by enthesopathies of the feet and ankles.

Behçet's syndrome

Behçet's syndrome is a systemic vasculitis associated with oral and genital ulceration and inflammatory eye disease.

Epidemiology

Behçet's syndrome is prevalent in Turkey, Iran, China, Japan and around the Mediterranean but is relatively unknown in Northern Europe and the Americas. Its distribution has suggested some link with the silk route from Europe to the Far East (Yazici, 1994). Both sexes are affected equally although the disease tends to be worse in males.

This syndrome was originally described as a triad of oral and genital ulcers and inflammatory eye disease. However, neurological, gastrointestinal and vasculitic clinical features are now recognised as part of the syndrome.

Aetiology

The aetiology remains unknown although streptococcal infections are thought to play a part and it has been suggested from Japan that there is a possible link with exposure to toxic chemicals (Barnes, 1991).

Pathology

Necrotising vasculitis is found in the vessels of skin, vulva, retina and brain. Blood tests may show a raised ESR, mild to moderate anaemia and hyperglobulinaemia.

Presentation

The peak age of onset is the third decade. The first symptom is usually recurring oral ulcers that are often very deep and cause scars. Genital ulcers occur in the majority of patients. They start as painful nodules in the groin, perineum, vulva and vagina of females and on the scrotum of males. Monoarticular or oligoarticular inflammatory arthritis affects 45% of patients (Barnes, 1991). Skin lesions such as erythema nodosum and acneiform nodules are typical features. Vasculitis occurs in a small number of patients and often leads to severe problems. The eyes can be affected and in some cases blindness may ensue. Gastrointestinal and neurological involvement may also occur.

Clinical features

Behçet's syndrome may be characterised by:

- oral ulcers (buccal mucosa, lips, tongue and pharynx);
- genital ulcers occur in both sexes;
- eye involvement (iritis is easily treated, but posterior uveitis may lead to blindness.);
- inflammatory arthritis of the knees, ankles, wrists and elbows which may be chronic or episodic;
- subcutaneous nodules and vasculitis similar to erythema nodusum may appear on the legs and feet;
- acne type pustules similar to those seen during adolescence;
- vascular symptoms (superficial thrombophlebitis, deep venous and arterial thromboses, aneurysms and occlusion of major vessels);
- central nervous system involvement (confused states and meningitis);
- colonic ulcers (pain, diarrhoea and haemorrhage);
- pathogenic reaction which may occur when the skin is hypersensitive to simple trauma (for example a needle prick causing a papule to form over the site of the injury).

Management

The aim of therapy is to treat symptoms and the ophthalmologist and dermatologist will need to be involved.

Therapies

Therapy may include:

- NSAIDs
- cyclophosphamide and corticosteroids to treat severe vasculitis.

CRYSTAL DEPOSITION DISEASE

These diseases occur when crystals are laid down in the joints and other organs. Gout is the most common of these conditions but they also include pseudogout or pyrophosphate arthropathy.

Gout

Gout is a disorder manifested by monosodium urate crystal deposition in articular tissues. Hyperuricaemia (high level of urate in the blood) predisposes to gout (Jordan, 2004). If left untreated it can progress through four clinical phases:

- asymptomatic hyperuricaemia
- acute gout
- intercritical gout
- chronic tophaceous gout.

Epidemiology

Gout is one of the oldest diseases known to man and has been described and catalogued since the time of Hippocrates. It is recognised world-wide and in males over 40-years-old is the most common inflammatory arthropathy. Life-style changes, drugs and an increasing elderly population are thought to be relevant factors leading to the increased incidence of gout (Cohen and Emmerson, 1994). In the elderly, it may be precipitated by the commencement of diuretic therapy (Jordan, 2004).

Aetiology

The common causes of hyperuricaemia are a high dietary intake of purines and under-excretion of urate. Thiazide diuretic therapy can decrease the excretion of urate thus raising the serum urate and precipitating gout (Gibson, 1988). There appears to be a genetic and familial association with the incidence of gout.

Pathology

Hyperuricaemia, defined as a serum uric acid level of more than 0.42 mmol/l (>7.0 mg/dl) in men and >0.36 mmol/l (>6.0 mg/dl) in women, predisposes to gout. Uric acid is retained in the synovial fluid and forms uric acid crystals. Occasionally uric acid calculi occur in the kidneys. Radiological examination reveals bony erosions related to tophi formation around the joints.

Presentation

The peak onset is in males between 40 and 50 years. Females are usually affected later in life. Acute attacks of gout present suddenly, usually in the early hours of the morning with severe pain in the big toe, heel or ankle. The pain builds up to a peak over several days. Usually only one joint is affected but further joints may be involved during subsequent attacks. Episodes of exacerbation and remission result in chronic gout particularly when hyperuricaemia is not controlled. Attacks of gout can be precipitated by acute illness, trauma, surgery, alcoholic excess and drugs which alter the plasma urate concentration (salicylates, thiazides, frusemide and pyrazinamide). If left untreated, the attack usually subsides in seven to ten days. The patient becomes asymptomatic and enters the intercritical period (the period between attacks).

Clinical features

Gout may be characterised by:

- swollen red joint often the big toe;
- severe and unremitting pain in the affected joint;
- fever may be present;
- tophi (nodular swellings) on the fingers, toes and ears which often produce a chalky exudates.

Management

Gout is the one rheumatic disease that can be fully controlled by drug therapy. Patient education and dietary advice enable patients to understand and control their disease (Hill, 1999).

Therapies

Therapy may include:

- NSAIDs (indomethacin in high doses to treat acute attacks);
- daily allopurinol or colchicine to reduce hyperuricaemia;
- probenecid when allopurinol is not tolerated;
- corticosteroids (oral, intra-articular or intramuscular steroids which are very useful if NSAIDs or colchicine is problematic).

Pseudogout (pyrophosphate arthropathy)

Pseudogout occurs when crystals of calcium pyrophosphate are deposited in the joints. The disease may be acute or chronic, the knee being the most commonly affected joint. Unlike gout, the big toe is rarely affected but the shoulders, elbows, wrists, hips and ankles may be involved. In acute disease, attacks last for months and usually recur. The chronic disease is progressive and can be similar to osteoarthritis.

Management

Management usually involves:

• aspiration and injection of the affected joints with corticosteroids;
• NSAIDs;
• rest.

JOINT FAILURE – OSTEOARTHRITIS

Osteoarthritis (OA) means inflammation of bone and joint. This disease causes destruction of the hyaline cartilage of the articular surfaces of the bone and varies in severity causing little inconvenience to some patients but chronic pain and disability in others. At one time, OA was considered to be an exclusively degenerative disorder which was simply the outcome of ageing and wear and tear. Current concepts emphasise the dynamic nature of the pathological processes in OA, with regeneration and increased turnover of cartilage matrix components, joint remodelling, incomplete repair and new bone formation as well as degeneration of articular tissues (Nuki, 2002).

Epidemiology

OA is recognised as the most common rheumatic disease in the UK. Radiographic evidence shows the disease to be present in 80% of the population over the age of 75 years (Cooper, 1994). More women than men are affected. A recent study demonstrated that in women aged 40 to 55 years, 6% had radiographic evidence of OA without pain and 31% had knee pain suggestive of OA in the absence of radiographic findings (Lachance *et al.*, 2001).

Aetiology

There is no known aetiology or cure for this chronic disease but OA may be related to a genetic factor, trauma or previous joint disease. Obesity, occupation and previous injury often determine which joints are affected and the severity of the disease. It can affect any joint but those most commonly affected are the DIPs, carpometacarpal of the thumb, knees, spine and hips.

Although efforts have been made to classify subsets, the term OA covers a range of heterogeneous diseases.

The disease is classified as primary, where there is no apparent cause, and secondary where the cause may be metabolic, anatomic, traumatic or inflammatory (Dieppe, 1994).

Secondary osteoarthritis may be caused by:

- metabolic diseases (acromegaly, calcium crystal deposition);
- structural disorders (Perthes' disease, congenital hip dislocation);
- trauma (surgical procedures such as menisectomy);
- previous inflammatory arthropathy such as rheumatoid arthritis;
- hypermobility causing a lax joint capsule leading to recurrent dislocation;
- fractures;
- occupational hazards.

Pathology

OA causes thinning, fibrillation (flaking) and destruction of the articular cartilage. The growth of fibrocartilage and bone at the joint margins produces osteophytes that are visible on X-ray. Other radiological changes are the loss of joint space, bony cysts and sclerosis in the subchondral bone. Loss of joint space affects the integrity of the joint causing pain, stiffness, deformity and disability.

Presentation

The peak age of onset is between 50 and 60 years and is usually gradual with an increase in pain and stiffness in the affected joints. Often, patients do not seek medical advice until their symptoms are severe and require surgical intervention.

Clinical features

Osteoarthritis may be characterised by:

- pain related to movement although it may be present at rest;
- pain that is severe and unremitting especially when the hip is affected;
- stiffness and gelling of joints that is relieved by movement;
- restricted range of movement that is crepitus and swollen joints;
- hands manifesting Heberden's nodes of the DIPs (Figure 2.8), squaring of the thumb (Z thumb) and Bouchard's nodes of the PIPs (Figure 2.8);
- knees manifesting crepitus or Baker's cyst;

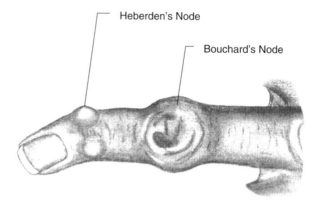

Figure 2.8 Heberden's and Bouchard's Nodes (Reproduced with kind permission from Geoff Hill [2000] *Rheumatology – A Handbook for Community Nurses*).

* hips and spine symptoms;
* feet manifesting hallux valgus (bunion).

The patient often experiences great pain, loss of mobility and an inability to perform everyday functions. In severe cases, loss of bone as well as cartilage affects the stability of the joints.

Management

The aim of treatment is to ensure that the patient remains as active and pain-free as possible. Education is a priority to enable the patient to understand the disease and use measures for symptomatic relief (Chapter 15).

Therapies

Therapy may include:

* exercise to maintain function and relieve stiffness;
* analgesia and NSAIDs to control pain and stiffness;
* weight reduction where obesity is a problem;
* education and information regarding pain and stiffness and the implications of obesity and lack of exercise;
* walking aids to relieve stress on weight bearing joints;
* major joint replacement – surgery of the hips, knees, shoulders and elbows to increase mobility and reduce pain in severely affected joints;
* surgical techniques include cartilage transplantation, cell and tissue engineering.

Many of these treatments are summarized in the proceedings of a Consensus Conference (NIH Conference, 2000).

METABOLIC BONE DISEASE – OSTEOPOROSIS

Osteoporosis is a systemic disease characterised by low bone mass, microarchitectural deterioration of bone tissue (Figure 2.9) and consequent skeletal fragility, with an increase in fracture risk (WHO, 1994). Loss of bone mass is one of the most common metabolic disorders of the skeleton and it leads to fractures.

Epidemiology

Osteoporosis is more prevalent in the Anglo-Saxon, Japanese and Indian races. Forearm fractures are often the first sign of skeletal fragility. Incidence rates in women increase linearly from the age of 40–65 years and then plateau, whereas in men it remains constant between 20 and 80 years. The age-adjusted female to male ratio for these fractures is 4:1 (Keen, 2000). The incidence of osteoporosis is increasing, possibly due to decreased physical activity in females and an increased life span (Badley, 1991). The socio-

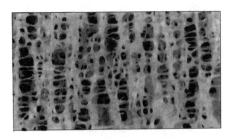

Normal Bone

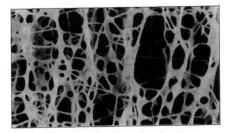

Osteoporotic Bone

Figure 2.9 Osteoporotic bone compared to normal bone.

economic implications of the increased disability and morbidity associated with fractures occurring as a result of osteoporosis cannot be ignored.

Aetiology

It is known that age, hormonal changes in women, lack of dietary calcium and lack of exercise all increase the risk of osteoporosis. Cardiac, respiratory, renal, neurological, gastrointestinal and rheumatic disease may lead to this condition. Data from twin- and family-based studies have demonstrated a strong genetic component (Smith *et al.*, 1973). Family history of fracture is a major clinical risk factor and there is evidence of site specificity in fracture risk (Keen, 2000).

Osteoporosis must always be considered in patients with rheumatic disease, particularly females who are predominately affected. Inflammatory joint diseases such as RA induce thin bones (osteopenia) and associated factors such as immobility and steroid therapy further increase the risk of osteoporosis. Risk factors in younger women are anorexia and exercise induced amenorrhoea. Alcoholism, hypogonadism and bone tumours are additional underlying causes of osteoporosis in men (Dixon, 1991).

Pathology

Loss of the bone mineral, hydroxyapatite, causes both cortical and trabecular bone to become osteopenic and susceptible to fracture. Bone turnover is reduced as the osteoclasts reabsorb bone more quickly than the osteoblasts can produce it. There is a negative calcium balance and breakdown of bone increases the urinary output of calcium.

Peak bone mass is reached in young adulthood, and is always higher in men than women. This level is consolidated from the age of twenty-five to thirty after which it slowly reduces. In the ten years following the menopause, bone loss accelerates in women and then levels out. Men start to lose bone mass after the age of sixty.

Presentation

Diagnosis does not usually occur until problems arise from fractures of the bones. Crush or wedge fractures of the vertebrae produce severe pain that usually resolves after a few months, although deformity of the spine may result. The most common fracture sites associated with osteoporosis are the proximal femur, distal radius and spine (Figure 2.10). When hospitalisation for fractured femur is necessary, the implications of surgical operation are serious, with the risk of venous thrombosis, pulmonary embolism and pneumonia in the elderly. Fracture of the distal radius (Colles' fracture) is also common and results in temporary loss of independence.

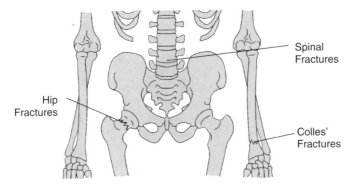

Figure 2.10 Common sites of osteoporotic fractures.

Clinical features

Osteoporosis may be characterised by:

- severe pain due to neurological compression as a result of a spontaneous fracture of the vertebrae;
- fracture of a long bone such as the femur or radius with resulting loss of independence;
- loss of height and thoracic kyphosis (Dowager's hump) especially in elderly women who may not have any other symptoms (Figure 2.11);
- breathing difficulties and symptoms of hiatus hernia often occur, caused by reduction of the space between the pelvis and rib cage due to spinal kyphosis.

Management

The management of osteoporosis should be directed at prevention. It is important for both health professionals and the public to be aware of the implications of this disease, risk factors and methods of prevention. An integral part of management is prevention through education.

Advice, including information and education, about risk factors related to osteoporosis include the following:

- Dietary requirements for calcium intake should be met.
- Excessive alcohol intake should be discouraged.
- Smoking should be discouraged due to the harmful effects of this habit.
- Benefits of exercise should be explained and exercise encouraged.
- Elderly patients should be reminded that the majority of falls and broken bones occur in the home often as a result of poorly fitting footwear, inadequate lighting, loose rugs, steep stairs, slippery floors and pets.

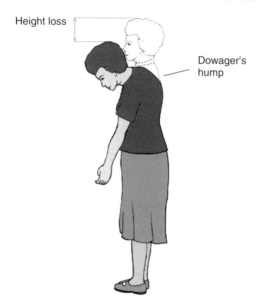

Height loss

Dowager's
hump

Figure 2.11 Dowager's hump in osteoporosis.

- Eyesight should be tested regularly and spectacles worn when prescribed.
- Patients with dizziness or unsteadiness due to conditions such as postural hypotension, transient ischaemic attacks, epilepsy, Meniere's disease and Parkinson's, should be advised to take care when standing up or mobilising. Some patients may need walking aids.
- Drugs, which cause dizziness, headache or drowsiness, should be prescribed only if really necessary; and patients should be advised to take care when mobilizing.
- Steroid therapy should be discussed with the patient and gradual withdrawal attempted.
- Thyroid therapy should be regularly monitored to ensure that the dosage of thyroxin is correct and does not need reduction.

Therapies

Drug therapy may include:

- hormone replacement therapy (HRT) for postmenopausal women and those who have undergone a hysterectomy or oophorectomy;
- supplemental calcium, didronel and Vitamin D which can be very helpful in preventing further loss of bone density.

CONNECTIVE TISSUE DISEASES

Although they are distinctive conditions, the diseases in this group have many common features, such as vasculitis. They are more common in women than men and there appears to be a genetic predisposition. Some of the diseases overlap, for instance progressive systemic scleroderma and systemic lupus erythematosus.

Systemic lupus erythematosus

Systemic lupus erythematosus (SLE) is the most common of the connective tissue diseases (Symmons and Bankhead, 1994). It is a chronic, inflammatory, systemic disorder of unknown aetiology which affects the joints and skin and may also involve the kidneys, lungs, heart, gastrointestinal tract and nervous system. Additional problems such as difficulties in fulfilling personal, social and financial responsibilities can lead to reduced quality of life for these patients (Khanna et al., 2004).

Epidemiology

Although it is found globally, it is most prevalent in the United States. Women are affected more than men at a ratio of 13:1. Afro-Caribbeans and Asians show the greatest incidence of this disease (Emery, 1994). For some patients with SLE, the prognosis is poor. However, survival rates have increased from less than 50% in 1955 to over 90% in 1990 (Gladman and Urowitz, 1994), possibly due to earlier diagnosis and treatment. Black patients fare worse than white patients due to an increased incidence of renal problems. Kidney and central nervous system involvement are associated with a poor prognosis.

Pathology

Skin biopsy reveals epidermal thinning and micro-infarcts due to deposits of immunoglobulin in the tissues. Evidence of an association with HLA B8, DR2 and DR3 antibodies and complement deficiency genes has been found. Blood tests may show an elevated ESR, positive antinuclear antibody (ANA) and antibodies to double stranded deoxyribonucleic acid (DNA), reduced neutrophils and platelets. Bone erosion and joint destruction do not normally occur.

Presentation

Patients present with a variety of symptoms ranging from fatigue, malaise and weight loss to rash and arthritis. Proteinurea, pleurisy and Raynaud's phenomenon may also be present at onset.

Clinical features

Systemic lupus erythematosus may be characterised by:

- butterfly rash of the face – raised, malar erythema lasting from days to weeks which may be puritic, painful and photosensitive;
- subacute cutaneous erythema;
- discoid lesions – erythematous plaques which become thick, adherent and scaly;
- alopecia – related to exacerbation of disease activity or due to scarring from discoid lesions (Hair growth normally resumes when the disease remits.);
- vasculitis – purpura, nail fold lesions, digital ulceration and subcutaneous nodules;
- polyarthritis of fingers, wrists, knees, ankles, elbows and shoulders which is usually flitting and rarely destructive;
- myalgia secondary to joint inflammation (SLE is often associated with polymyositis.);
- tenosynovitis leading to tendon ruptures;
- mucous membrane lesions on the mouth and vagina;
- renal involvement such as nephritis and proteinurea (The prognosis is worse if the kidneys are affected.);
- pulmonary involvement such as pleurisy, pleural effusions, pneumonitis and dyspnoea;
- cardiac involvement such as pericarditis, pericardial effusions, hypertension and myocarditis;
- gastrointestinal effects such as abdominal pain, loss of appetite, nausea, and vomiting caused by peritoneal inflammation;
- neurological effects such as migraine-like headaches, chorea, vascular accidents, peripheral neuropathy and cranial nerve lesions causing visual problems;
- psychiatric features such as severe depression, paranoia, anxiety, confusion, schizophrenia, dementia and fits.

Photosensitivity can produce exacerbation of skin lesions and systemic features of the disease. Patients run an increased risk of infection. Although SLE does not prevent conception, hormonal changes may result in spontaneous abortion. Certain drugs can induce a type of SLE in patients with a genetic predisposition to the disease. They include:

- procainamide
- hydralazine
- methyldopa
- phenytoin
- isoniazid

- oral contraceptives
- penicillin
- sulphonamides
- tetracycline
- streptomycin
- griseoflulvin
- penicillamine.

Once the drug is stopped, the symptoms usually disappear although evidence of the disease may be present in the blood for some years.

Management

Therapy depends on which organs are affected and patients may require referrals to the dermatologist, renal physician, neurologist, haematologist and psychiatrist. The disease needs to be treated as early as possible and the risk of infections and subsequent complications should always be considered. The monitoring of disease activity is important, as acute flares require immediate treatment.

Therapies

Therapy may include:

- steroid creams to heal skin lesions;
- NSAIDs to relieve arthralgia, arthritis and myalgia;
- antimalarial drugs for their anti-inflammatory and immunosuppressive effect;
- methotrexate as an alternative to antimalarials;
- corticosteroids in low doses to reduce disease activity and alleviate fatigue and loss of appetite;
- azathioprine as a steroid sparing agent once disease stability has been achieved;
- cyclophosphamide when patients have vasculitis, severe thrombocytopenia and renal disease.

Education

Patients need to understand their disease and they should be aware of the risks associated with unexplained weight loss, fatigue, fever and infections. The problems of photosensitivity should be discussed and ways of avoiding exposure to harmful solar radiation, such as covering up or the use of sunscreens should be encouraged. Birth control, the risks of pregnancy relating to the disease and the teratogenic effects of drug therapy need to be emphasised.

Scleroderma

Scleroderma is derived from the Greek meaning 'hard skin' and comprises a spectrum of autoimmune diseases that affects the connective tissue. Systemic sclerosis is the systemic form of scleroderma and although it is rare it is of concern because it has the highest case-specific mortality rate of all the rheumatic conditions (Denton and Black, 1999). Approximately 50% of diagnosed patients die in the first ten years (Silman, 1997). This is because systemic sclerosis does not just affect the skin, it also affects internal organs causing obliterative microvascular lesions in the kidney, lung, bowel and heart.

Epidemiology

The aetiology is unknown but there is some evidence that there may be a link with silica, vinyl chloride and silicone surgical implants. Women are affected more frequently than men at a ratio of 3:1. The peak age of onset is between the fourth and fifth decade (Siebold, 1994).

Pathology

Initially the small blood vessels of the body are affected, causing inflammation of the subcutaneous connective tissue which leads to atrophy and fibrosis of the skin and other organs. Blood tests show a raised ESR, positive rheumatoid factor and ANA. X-ray examination reveals soft tissue calcification, joint space narrowing and periarticular osteoporosis. Other tests may include ECG, Cardiac Echo, Chest x-ray, 24-hour creatinine clearance, pulmonary function tests and blood pressure.

Presentation

The initial presentation and course of the disease varies between individuals; but patients commonly present with fatigue, skin thickening, joints pains, altered facial appearance and depression. The inflamed joints tend to resolve as the disease progresses. These patients require careful monitoring to ensure that any complications due to involvement of the kidney, bowel, oesophagus, heart and lungs are treated as they arise.

Clinical features

Scleroderma can be characterised by:

• pain, swelling and stiffness of joints especially in the hands;
• flexion deformities of the fingers with reddened and ulcerated PIPs, DIPs and finger tips;

- nail fold capillary infarcts;
- oedema of the skin resulting in puffy fingers and hands;
- skin that is dry, tight, wasted, hard and tethered to underlying structures, especially on the hands and face;
- early morning stiffness;
- telangiectasia of the face and neck;
- arteritis of the renal vessels leading to renal failure with proteinurea and malignant hypertension;
- Raynaud's phenomenon;
- Sjögren's syndrome;
- dysphagia caused by fibrosis of the oesophagus;
- fibrosing alveolitis;
- microvascular lesions of the lung and heart.

Management

Symptomatic treatments are used as problems occur. However, the various complications of this disease call for integrated and empathetic care. Skin changes, especially to the face cause patients distress and loss of self-esteem (Chapter 10).

Therapies

Therapy may include:

- NSAIDs and analgesia for inflamed joints;
- immunosuppressants such as intravenous cyclophosphamide;
- bosentan or iloprost for pulmonary artery hypertension;
- angiotensin converting enzyme (ACE) inhibitors for prophylaxis of renal disease (Maddison, 2002);
- creams to relieve tight dry skin (Chapter 10);
- D-penicillamine for halting the progress of the fibrosis, though the risk of kidney involvement makes screening essential;
- steroid therapy;
- special makeup for patients with telangiectasia of the face.

CREST syndrome

CREST is an acronym for:

calcinosis
Raynaud's
esophageal dysmotility (using the American spelling)
sclerodactyly;
telangiectasia.

This condition is similar to scleroderma, but systemic involvement, apart from oesophageal disturbance, is not apparent until later in the disease. The initial presenting symptom is Raynaud's phenomenon with swollen fingers and hands.

Polymyositis and dermatomyositis

Two major forms of inflammatory myopathy are recognised. They are polymyositis and dermatomyositis.

Polymyositis is a connective tissue disorder that causes weakness of the proximal musculature due to inflammation. When a characteristic skin rash is present with polymyositis, the condition is known as dermatomyositis. The aetiology of these diseases is unknown.

Pathology

Muscle biopsy is mandatory for diagnosis (Behan, 2004). Blood tests show an elevated ESR and creatinine phosphokinase (CPK), and rheumatoid factor and ANA may be positive. Monitoring the level of CPK is a useful indicator of disease activity and the efficacy of drug therapy.

Presentation

The peak age of onset is between 30 and 60 years. Patients may present with arthritis of the hands, wrists, elbows, shoulders, knees and ankles. Symmetrical wasting and weakness of limb girdle muscles is common, as is restriction of movement. Some patients develop joint contractures. Respiratory failure is common and 15% of those affected die from this cause (Huskisson and Dudley Hart, 1987).

Clinical features

Polymyositis may be characterized by:

- swollen, warm and tender joints with effusions;
- early morning stiffness;
- malaise and weight loss;
- muscular weakness with muscular pain or tenderness;
- Sjögren's syndrome;
- dysphagia with oesophageal involvement;
- Raynaud's phenomenon;
- skin lesions such as malar, lilac rash which may be photosensitive.

Management

High dose prednisolone (60 mgs daily) is used initially and the dose gradually reduced once the arthritis has remitted and the muscle weakness has resolved. Therapy with immunosuppressive drugs such as azathioprine or cyclophosphamide is used where remission does not occur. Alternative drugs such as tacrolimus and mycophenolate may be used in those with a poor response. Monthly intravenous immunoglobulin infusions have shown modest clinical benefit and can be useful in patients who relapse on standard therapy or when prolonged cytotoxic therapy is contraindicated. There are anecdotal reports based on small numbers of patients, that anti-TNF blocking agents may be of benefit (Behan, 2004).

Physiotherapy exercises help to improve muscle weakness and function.

NONARTICULAR CONDITIONS

Nonarticular conditions are those rheumatic diseases associated with muscle weakness and pain rather than joint involvement.

Polymyalgia rheumatica and giant cell arteritis

Polymyalgia rheumatica (PMR) is a common disorder of the middle-aged and elderly which causes symmetrical pain and stiffness in the neck, shoulder and pelvic girdle (Dasgupta and Kalke, 2000). It is associated with giant cell arteritis that can affect the temporal artery and result in blindness (Hazelman, 1992; Hazelman, 1994).

Epidemiology

Both PMR and giant cell arteritis are diseases of the elderly and are rarely diagnosed in persons younger than 50 years. Giant cell arteritis mostly affects whites of European background although some cases have been reported in the American black population. The incidence of PMR increases with age and there is a male:female ratio of 1:2 (Hosie, 2003).

Pathology

Blood tests show an extremely elevated ESR and raised alkaline phosphatase levels. Thyroid and liver function abnormalities may also be apparent from blood tests. Temporal artery biopsy often shows the temporal artery to be inflamed, enlarged, nodular and with a narrow lumen (temporal arteritis). Thromboses may develop at sites of inflammation.

Presentation

The onset is usually acute with patients complaining of extreme pain and stiffness in the shoulder, hips and thighs. The shoulder girdle is more commonly affected than the pelvic girdle. Early diagnosis may be hindered by initial symptoms of fever, fatigue, weight loss, anorexia and depression. Arteritis of the temporal artery can occur and needs immediate treatment with oral steroids to prevent blindness.

Clinical features

Polymyalgia rheumatica and giant cell arteritis may be characterised by:

- early morning stiffness in the shoulders, neck and pelvis which is usually symmetrical and worse after rest;
- myalgic pain in the neck, shoulders and pelvic girdle which is aggravated by movement and is often worse at night;
- limited range of movement of shoulders and hips;
- synovitis which is usually mild and resolves quickly;
- malaise, low grade fever and weight loss;
- temporal headache radiating into the occiput;
- sleep disturbance caused by scalp tenderness around the temporal and occipital arteries;
- pain in the mouth and throat when chewing;
- tingling of the tongue and loss of taste;
- visual disturbances or even loss of vision if untreated (Blindness occurs suddenly and painlessly and is permanent.).

Management

Corticosteroids are always used to reduce the risk of arteritis and subsequent blindness. Pain and stiffness are relieved quickly within a few days by this treatment. High doses of steroids are used initially and then decreased slowly as symptoms subside. The reduction of steroids is often seen as too slow by some patients who want to stop the treatment as soon as they feel better. Because of this, patient education is important to ensure that patients understand the need for the slow reduction of steroid treatment as symptoms can recur. Most patients will remain on steroid therapy for at least two years, but for some it may be longer. Monitoring of ESR levels should be carried out once therapy has ceased, to detect any relapse. Patients should be warned to seek advice should their symptoms return.

Raynaud's phenomenon

Raynaud's phenomenon was first described by Maurice Raynaud over 120 years ago. It is defined as vasospasm of arteries or arterioles causing pallor and at least one other colour change upon reperfusion, such as cyanosis or redness (Thompson and Pope, 2005). The usual episode occurs with the fingers going white, cyanosed and then red.

Aetiology

It is thought that cold, emotion, trauma, hormones and chemicals such as nicotine produce this effect. Raynaud's phenomenon is often associated with scleroderma, SLE, RA, dermatomyositis and polymyositis. Occupation plays a part in the incidence of this condition, especially manual work and work involving the packing of frozen food, the use of vinyl chloride, ammunition and nitrates.

Pathology

Systemic vasospasm restricts the blood flow to the hands, fingers and in some cases the nose, tip of the tongue and ear lobes. Raynaud's phenomenon is present in 5–10% of the population in varying degrees of severity (Blech, 1987). It affects nine times more women than men and may be a precursor of systemic illness.

Presentation

This varies from mild to severe disease and usually presents as pallor and cyanosis of the fingers as the digital blood vessels go into spasm. This is then followed by rubor (redness) as the circulation returns to normal. Pain may be present depending on the amount of vasospasm. In more severe cases, digital ulceration and gangrene can occur.

Management

The management of this condition is predominately educational and may include the following.

• Information about cold avoidance measures such as thermal socks and gloves, electrically heated gloves, chemical hand warmers and padded or fleece-lined shoes should be given.
• Patients should be strongly advised to stop smoking.
• Nifedipine may be used to increase the peripheral blood supply.
• The Raynaud's Association is a support group that provides useful patient information.

Sjögren's syndrome

Primary Sjögren's syndrome is a chronic inflammatory autoimmune disease characterised by symptoms of dry eyes and mouth, various extraglandular symptoms, hypergammaglobulinaemia and abundant autoantibody production (Petrovaara *et al.*, 2004).

Epidemiology

Sjögren's syndrome is the second most common rheumatic disease and affects more women than men.
There are three classifications:

- primary Sjögren's syndrome
- Sjögren's associated overlap syndromes
- secondary Sjögren's syndrome with rheumatoid arthritis.

Primary Sjögren's syndrome This condition mainly affects the exocrine glands and is usually so mild that medical advice is rarely sought. Other conditions such as nonerosive arthritis, Raynaud's phenomenon and purpuric rash of the lower legs may be associated.

Sjogren's associated overlap syndromes Besides affecting the exocrine glands, this condition often has features associated with SLE and other autoimmune rheumatic diseases such as scleroderma and polymyositis.

Secondary Sjogren's syndrome with rheumatoid arthritis The features of this classification are dry eyes, dry mouth, vasculitic changes such as nailfold infarcts, ulcers and rheumatoid nodules.

Pathology

Investigations have shown that the disease seems to start as a persistent viral infection of the salivary glands, which results in an attack on the salivary epithelium. The Epstein-Barr virus is often present on biopsy of the salivary epithelium. Schirmer's tear test can confirm the diagnosis of dry eyes (keratoconjunctivitis sicca). Dry mouth (xerostomia) can be detected by tests that reveal a reduced salivary flow rate. Blood tests often show a raised ESR, raised rheumatoid factor and hypergammaglobulinaemia.

Presentation

Onset can be between 15 and 65 years and patients complain of dry, gritty, sore eyes and a dry mouth that causes difficulty in swallowing food.

Management

Dry eyes can be treated with artificial tears (hypermellose eye drops).
   Sucking sweets and chewing gum increases the salivary flow and eases a dry mouth. In more severe cases artificial saliva may be prescribed.

SOFT TISSUE RHEUMATISM

Soft tissue rheumatism describes those conditions that affect the muscles, tendons, tendon sheaths and nerves.

Fibromyalgia syndrome

Fibromyalgia (FM) gained official recognition when the American College of Rheumatology published their still-accepted criteria (Wolfe *et al.*, 1990). The diagnosis of FM is based on a history of chronic widespread pain and the presence of at least eleven out of eighteen specified 'tender points' (Bergman, 2003). Fatigue is common and headache, abdominal pain and bowel disturbance may also be present. Investigations are undertaken to exclude other conditions such as systemic lupus erythematosus, hypothyroidism, polymyalgia rheumatica and carcinoma. In the past, patients with these symptoms were often classed as having psychological rather than physical problems.

Aetiology

The aetiology remains unknown but is likely to involve more than one factor. The condition occurs mainly in women aged between 25 and 45 years. A recent study has indicated that it affects 3.4% of women and 0.5% of men (Wolfe *et al.*, 1995).

Presentation

The patient complains of fatigue and tenderness in the upper and lower limbs, base of the skull, lower cervical spine, shoulders and hips. These hyperalgesic or tender sites are distributed symmetrically and firm digital pressure upon them causes the patient to wince and withdraw (Figure 2.12).

Clinical features

Fibromyalgia may be characterized by:

- pain at tender sites or sometimes more widespread;
- morning stiffness which is generalised;
- fatigue, inability to sleep properly, tiredness on waking;
- irritability, weepiness;
- headache, forgetfulness, poor concentration;

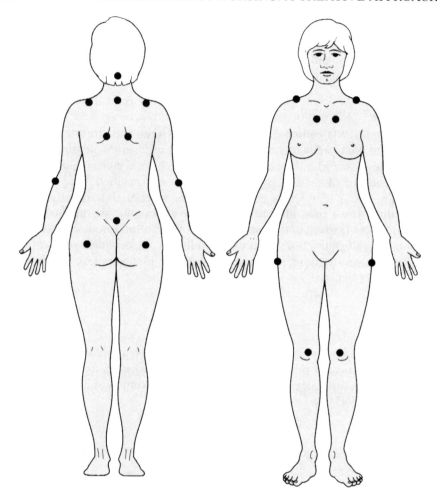

Figure 2.12 Tender points used to assess fibromyalgia.

- numbness, pins and needles of hands and feet;
- inability to perform daily living activities.

Management

The prognosis of fibromyalgia is poor and some patients experience their symptoms for many years with little or no relief. Education of the patient and family enables most patients to cope with their condition. Some patients may benefit from counselling. Low dose amitriptyline (25–75 mgs) taken at night helps to induce sleep. Although it may be initially painful, patients should be encouraged to undertake a personal exercise programme to improve fitness and enable them to take control of their condition.

Carpal tunnel syndrome

Carpal tunnel syndrome is caused by elevated pressure in the carpal tunnel resulting in ischaemia of the median nerve at the wrist, and consequent impaired nerve conduction (Barnado, 2004). This results in tingling, paraesthesia and pain in the fingers.

Pathology

The median nerve runs through the carpal tunnel and compression of the nerve produces tingling and sometimes loss of sensation to the thumb, index, second and half of the third finger. It usually occurs in middle aged women and may be due to synovitis of the wrist, bony lesions, obesity or fluid retention. The prevalence is 2% in men and 3% in women.

Presentation

A numb, tingling sensation in one or both hands, which occurs initially at night and then during the day. Patients may subsequently experience weakness, particularly with the thumb grip, clumsiness of fine finger function and a history of dropping things.

Clinical features

Carpal tunnel syndrome may be characterised by:

- pain spreading up the forearm;
- tingling and numbness in the thumb, index, second and half of the third fingers, which is usually present at night but may occur during the day;
- wasting of the thenar eminence, due to motor involvement with a resultant loss of power and muscle wasting.

Management

A nerve conduction study often helps to verify the diagnosis.
  Therapy may include:

- diuretics if caused by fluid retention;
- wrist splints to relieve symptoms in mild cases;
- local steroid injection and the use of wrist splints for 48 hours;

- surgical decompression when other more conservative measures have failed to bring relief. Surgery is usually successful and involves division of the flexor retinaculum.

Lateral and medial epicondylitis (tennis and golfer's elbow)

These common rheumatic conditions cause pain and tenderness around the lateral epicondyle (tennis elbow) and medial epicondyle (golfer's elbow). The condition occurs in individuals whose occupation involves repeated gripping and twisting movements of the forearm.

Pathology

Inflammation or damage is present at the enthesis of the carpi radialis component of the extensor tendon (tennis elbow) or the flexor tendon (golfer's elbow).

Presentation

The peak age of onset is between 40 and 60 years. The affected epicondyle is tender and varying degrees of pain are present. Gripping and twisting movements exacerbate the pain that varies from mild discomfort to severe pain.

Clinical features

Lateral and medial epicondylitis may be characterised by:

- pain which may be bilateral and radiates down the posterior aspect of the forearm (tennis elbow) or down the flexor aspect of the forearm (golfer's elbow);
- pain on palpation of the lateral or medial epicondyle;
- soft tissue swelling around the area.

Management

These conditions can persist for a year or more. Conservative measures such as elbow splints and ultrasound therapy are used initially. Where the condition persists, a local corticosteroid injection into the affected area followed by a few days' rest usually brings relief. In more chronic cases, manipulation of the elbow under general anaesthetic helps to break down fibrous adhesions and restore mobility. Surgical intervention to divide the tendon (tenotomy) may help when the condition is severe.

OTHER CONDITIONS

AMYLOIDOSIS

Amyloidosis often occurs in patients with long standing RA. Males and females are affected equally with the peak age of onset being between 50 and 60 years. Amyloid deposits are found in the liver, spleen, kidneys, gastro-intestinal tract, heart, tongue, nervous system and joints. These deposits are made up of an insoluble protein-like substance. Peripheral neuropathies and heart failure often result. The prognosis for this condition is poor.

BAKER'S CYST

A Baker's cyst is a swelling that develops at the back of an inflamed knee. This may rupture allowing synovial fluid to track down into the back of the calf. Patients presenting with such a rupture may be misdiagnosed as having a deep vein thrombosis.

BURSITIS

Bursitis is inflammation of a bursa that may be due to rheumatic disease or trauma. Pain and swelling is present around the site, the most common being the knee (housemaid's knee), shoulder, elbow (olecranon bursitis), hip (trochanteric bursitis) and ankle.

Treatment with analgesia and rest may help, but in persistent cases aspiration and injection of corticosteroid is necessary.

CALCANEAL SPUR

A calcaneal spur is a bony growth protruding from the calcaneus, which causes great pain and discomfort on walking. Relief can be obtained through protective heel pads inserted into the shoe and injection of corticosteroid.

CHONDROMALACIA PATELLAE

Chondromalacia patellae refers to softening of the articular cartilage of the patella, causing anterior pain in the knee. Isometric quadriceps exercises and hamstring stretching will help to build up the surrounding musculature and strengthen the joint.

ERYTHEMA NODOSUM

Erythema nodosum presents as tender nodules in the skin of the lower leg. It is commonly seen in sarcoidosis but may occur with Behçet's syndrome,

Crohn's disease, infections, malignant disease and drug reactions. Arthritis is often present with this complaint and usually presents a few weeks before the nodules appear.

FASCIITIS

Fasciitis is inflammation of the enthesis of the fascia. In particular, plantar fasciitis is associated with rheumatic disease especially the spondoarthropathies. A heel pad in the shoe may help to relieve the pain associated with this condition.

HYPERMOBILITY SYNDROME

Hypermobility is caused by ligamentous laxity that may be inherited and is common in many dancers, gymnasts and athletes. Patients with this syndrome are able to overextend the range of movement in their joints. The knees and hands are commonly affected. Hypermobility often leads to OA in later life. Treatment is centered on advice about the benefits of exercise, joint protection and the use of analgesia.

REPETITIVE STRAIN SYNDROME

This refers to inflammation of joints or tendons, usually of the hands, caused by repetition of the same action. Typists, till operators and machinists are prone to this condition. Rest and the use of non steroidal anti-inflammatory drugs can obtain relief. When inflammation is persistent a steroid injection into the tendon sheath may also help.

RHEUMATOID NODULES

Rheumatoid nodules are small growths that are characteristic features of destructive RA. They occur subcutaneously over bony prominences and tendons, for example elbows, Achilles tendons, shoulder blades, and fingers. They may also be present inside organs such as the heart and lungs. At the center of these nodules is an inner core of necrotised collagen, fibrin and cell debris. In some instances subcutaneous nodules discharge and care must be taken to ensure that they do not become infected.

SARCOIDOSIS

Sarcoidosis is a systemic disease in which epithelial cell granuloma can be found in the lungs, lymph glands, spleen, joints and skin. It often presents as a polyarthritis with erythema nodosum and may be acute and transient, or chronic and persistent.

SEPTIC ARTHRITIS

Septic arthritis may be due to diabetes, RA, joint trauma, steroid therapy or an infection elsewhere in the body. The affected joint is infected with a pyogenic bacterium and will show the typical signs of inflammation. The joint rapidly becomes swollen and painful and fever is usually present. Treatment should be started immediately and comprises aspiration of the affected joint, rest, and antibiotic cover. Culture of synovial fluid and blood is usually positive. If left untreated, this condition leads to destruction of the joint, septicaemia and death.

TELANGIECTASIA

Telangiectasia is often found in patients with progressive systemic scleroderma or the CREST syndrome. Dilated capillaries and venules, which blanch on pressure, can be seen on the hands, lips, tongue and mucous membranes.

TENOSYNOVITIS

Tenosynovitis is inflammation of the synovial lining of the tendons and is common in inflammatory joint diseases such as RA. Rupture of the extensor tendon or tendon slip often occurs in patients with inflammatory joint disease especially in the hands.

TRIGGER FINGER

In trigger finger, the flexor tendon sheaths of the fingers become inflamed and rough. Crepitus and nodules are common, inhibiting the smooth movement of the tendon within the sheath and causing the finger to stick. A steroid injection into the sheath usually relieves this condition.

ACTION POINTS FOR PRACTICE

- Mr. Partridge is a 76-year-old man who is experiencing great difficulty in doing up his shirt buttons. He has tingling and loss of sensation in the thumb and first three fingers of both hands.
  What do you think is wrong with him?
  How might the multidisciplinary team help him?
- Doreen is a 60-year-old lady who was seen in clinic complaining of pain in her shoulders and upper arms. A blood test revealed an ESR of 100 mm/hr.
  What is her probable diagnosis?
  What action should be taken to help this lady?

What problems may ensue?
How should she be managed in the future?

• Peter is 28 years old and has ankylosing spondylitis. He has found difficulty in coping with his disease, especially as he has increasing stiffness and restriction in his spine.
What measures should be taken to help him?
Write a care plan.

REFERENCES

Albano SA, Santana-Sahagun E, Weisman MH (2001) Cigarette smoking and rheumatoid arthritis. *Arthritis and Rheumatism* 31:146–159.
Arthritis Research Campaign (2002) *Arthritis – The Big Picture*. Chesterfield, Arthritis Research Campaign.
Arnet FC, Edworthy SM, Bloch DA *et al.* (1988) The American rheumatism association 1987 revised criteria for the classification of rheumatoid arthritis. *Arthritis Rheumatism* 31:315–324.
Arthur V (1994) Nursing care of patients with rheumatoid arthritis. *British Journal of Nursing* 3(7):325–331.
Badley EM (1991) Population projections and the effect on rheumatology. *Annals of Rheumatic Disease* 50:3–6.
Barnardo J (2004) *Carpal tunnel syndrome*. Chesterfield, Arthritis Research Campaign.
Barnes CG (1991) Behçet's syndrome. In: *Collected reports on the rheumatic diseases*. Chesterfield, Arthritis and Rheumatism Council, 109–114.
Behan WMH (2004) *Idiopathic inflammatory myopathies*. Chesterfield, Arthritis Research Campaign.
Bergman S (2003) *The general practice approach to management of chronic widespread musculoskeletal pain and fibromyalgia*. Chesterfield, Arthritis Research Campaign.
Blech JJF (1987) Raynaud's phenomenon. In: *Collected reports on the rheumatic diseases*. Chesterfield, Arthritis and Rheumatism Council, 101–104.
Braun J, Sieper J (2002) Therapy of ankylosing spondylitis and other spondyloarthritides: established medical treatment, anti-TNF-alpha therapy and other novel approaches. *Arthritis Research* 4:307–321.
Campion G, Maddison PJ (1986) Felty's syndrome. In: *Collected reports on the rheumatic diseases*. Chesterfield, Arthritis and Rheumatism Council, 52–55.
Clegg DO, Reda DJ, Abdellatif M (1999) Comparison of sulphasalazine and placebo in the treatment of axial and peripheral articular manifestations of the seronegative spondyloarthropathies. A Department of Veterans Affairs Cooperative Study. *Arthritis and Rheumatism* 42:2325–2329.
Cohen MG, Emmerson BT (1994) Gout. In: Klippel JH, Dieppe PA (ed) *Rheumatology*. St Louis, Mosby 7.12:1–15.
Cooper C (1994) Osteoarthritis epidemiology. In: Klippel JH, Dieppe PA (ed) *Rheumatology*. St Louis, Mosby 7.3:1–4.

Cornell P (2004) Clinical update on ankylosing spondylitis. *Professional Nurse* 19(8):431–432.

Cornell P, Oliver SM (2004) Ankylosing spondylitis: clinical update. *Musculoskeletal Care* 2(3):187–193.

Dasgupta B, Kalke S (2000) *Polymyalgia rheumatica and giant cell arteritis.* Chesterfield, Arthritis Research Campaign.

Denton C, Black C (1999) Systemic sclerosis: an overview of pathogenesis and treatment. *CPD Rheumatology* 1(1):33–39.

Dieppe PA (1994) Osteoarthritis. In: Klippel JH, Dieppe PA (ed) *Rheumatology.* St Louis, Mosby 7.2:1–6

Dieppe PA, Doherty M, Macfarlane DG *et al.* (1985) *Rheumatological medicine.* Edinburgh, Churchill Livingstone 4, p 56–57.

Dixon A St.J (1991) Osteoporosis and the family doctor. In: *Collected reports on the rheumatic diseases.* Chesterfield, Arthritis and Rheumatism Council, 122–125.

Doran MF, Brophy S, Mackay K *et al.* (2003) Predictors of long-term outcome in ankylosing spondylitis. *Journal of Rheumatology* 203(30):316–320.

Edwards JCW (2002) *Pathogenesis of rheumatoid arthritis.* Topical Reviews, Chesterfield, Arthritis Research Campaign.

Emery P (1994) Systemic lupus erythematosus. In: *Collected reports on the rheumatic diseases.* Chesterfield, Arthritis and Rheumatism Council, 87–92.

Espinoza LR, Cuellar ML (1994) Psoriatic arthritis: management. In: Klippel JH, Dieppe PA (ed) *Rheumatology.* St Louis, Mosby 3.33:1–6.

Firestein GS (1994) Rheumatoid arthritis and spondyloarthropathy, rheumatoid synovitis and pannus. In: Klippel JH, Dieppe PA (ed) *Rheumatology.* St Louis, Mosby 3:12.1–12.30.

Gibson T (1988) The treatment of gout: a personal view. In: *Collected reports on the rheumatic diseases.* Chesterfield, Arthritis and Rheumatism Council, 69–71.

Gladman DD (1995) Psoriatic Arthritis. *Baillieres Clinical Rheumatology* 9:319–329.

Gladman DD, Urowitz MB (1994) Systemic lupus erythematosus – clinical features. In: Klippel JH, Dieppe PA (ed) *Rheumatology.* St Louis, Mosby 6:2.1–2.20.

Gornisiewicz M, Moreland LW (2001) *Rheumatoid arthritis.* In: Robbins L (ed) Clinical Care in the Rheumatic Diseases. Atlanta, American College of Rheumatology, p 92.

Hazelman BL (1992) Polymyalgia rheumatica and giant cell arteritis. In: *Collected reports on the rheumatic diseases.* Chesterfield, Arthritis and Rheumatism Council, 97–100.

Hazelman BL (1994) Polymyalgia rheumatica and giant cell arteritis. In: Klippel JH, Dieppe PA (ed) *Rheumatology.* St Louis, Mosby 6:18.1–18. 8.

Helliwell PS, Wright V (1994) Psoriatic arthritis: clinical features. In: Klippel JH, Dieppe PA (ed) *Rheumatology.* St Louis, Mosby 3:31.1–31.8.

Hill J (1999) Gout, its causes, symptoms and treatment. *Nursing Times* 95(47): 48–50.

Hill J (1997) The expanding role of the nurse in rheumatology. *British Journal of Rheumatology* 36(4):410–412.

Hill J (1992) A nurse practitioner rheumatology clinic. *Nursing Standard* 7(11): 35–37.

Hill J, Hale C (2004) Clinical skills: evidence-based nursing care of people with rheumatoid arthritis. *British Journal of Nursing* 13(14):852–857.

Hill J, Reay N (2002) The diagnosis, assessment and management of complex rheumatic diseases. *Nursing Times* 98(9):41–44.

Hill J, Ryan S (2000) *Rheumatology – A Handbook for Community Nurses.* London, Whurr Publishing.

Hill J, Thorpe R, Bird H (2003) Outcomes from patients with RA: a rheumatology nurse practitioner clinic compared to standard outpatient care. *Musculoskeletal Care* 1(1):5–20.

Hosie G (2003) *Polymyalgia Rheumatica.* Chesterfield, Arthritis Research Campaign.

Huizinga TW, Machold KP, Breedveldd FC *et al.* (2002) Criteria for early rheumatoid arthritis. *Arthritis and Rheumatism* 46:1155–1159.

Huskisson EC, Dudley Hart F (1987) *Joint disease and all the arthropathies.* Bristol, Wright.

Jordan KM (2004) *An update on gout.* Chesterfield, Arthritis Rhesearch Campaign.

Keen R (2000) *Osteoporosis and metabolic bone disease.* Chesterfield, Arthritis Research Campaign.

Khan MA (1994) Ankylosing spondylitis. In: Klippel JA, Dieppe PA (ed) *Rheumatology.* St Louis, Mosby 3:25.1–25.10.

Khan MA (2002) *Ankylosing Spondylitis – The Facts.* Oxford, Oxford University Press.

Khanna S, Pal H, Pandey M (2004) The relationship between disease activity and quality of life in systemic lupus erythematosus. *Rheumatology* 43:1536–1540.

Lachance I, Sowers MF, Jamadar D *et al.* (2001) The experience of pain and emergent osteoarthritis of the knee. *Osteoarthritis Cartilage* 9:527–532.

Maddison P (2002) Prevention of vascular damage in scleroderma with angiotensin converting enzyme (ACE) inhibition. *Rheumatology* 41:965–971.

Matteson EL, Cohen MD, Conn DL (1994) Rheumatoid arthritis. Clinical features – systemic involvement. In: Klippel JH, Dieppe PA (ed) *Rheumatology.* St Louis, Mosby 3:5.1–5.8.

Marshall R, Kirwan J (2001) Methotrexate in the treatment of ankylosing spondylitis. *Scandinavian Journal of Rheumatology.* 30:313–314.

NIH Conference (2000) Osteoarthritis: new insights. Part 2: Treatment approaches. *Annals of Internal Medicine* 133:726–737.

Nuki G (2002) *Osteoarthritis: risk factors and pathogenesis.* Chesterfield, Arthritis Research Campaign.

Oliver S, Mooney J (2002) Targeted therapies for patients with rheumatoid arthritis. *Professional Nurse* 17(12):716–729.

Packham JC, Bowness P (2001) *Seronegative spondyloarthropathies.* Chesterfield, Arthritis Research Campaign.

Pertovaara M, Lehtimäki T, Rontu R *et al.* (2004) Presence of apolipoprotein E ε4 allele predisposes to early onset of primary Sjögren's syndrome. *Rheumatology* 43:1484–1487.

Rai A, Struthers G (1994) Ankylosing Spondylitis. In: *Collected reports on the rheumatic diseases.* Chesterfield, Arthritis and Rheumatism Council, 65–68.

Seibold JR (1994) Systemic sclerosis: clinical features. In: Klippel JH, Dieppe PA (ed) *Rheumatology*. St Louis, Mosby 6:8.1–8.14.

Shbeeb M, Uramoto KM, Gibson LE *et al.* (2000) The epidemiology of psoriatic arthritis in Olmsted County, Minnesota, USA, 1982–1991. *Journal of Rheumatology* 27:1247–1250.

Sieper J, Braun J, Kingsley GH (2000) Report on the fourth international workshop on reactive arthritis. *Arthritis and Rheumatism* 43:720–734.

Sieper J, Braun J, Rudwaleit M *et al.* (2002) Ankylosing spondylitis: an overview. *Annals of the Rheumatic Diseases* 61(supl 3):8–18.

Silman AJ (1997) Scleroderma – demographic and survival. *Journal of Rheumatology* 48:58–61.

Smith DM, Nance WE, Kang KW *et al.* (1973) Genetic factors in determining bone mass. *Journal of Clinical Investigation* 52:2800–2808.

Symmons D, Bankhead C (1994) *Health care needs assessment for musculoskeletal diseases*. Chesterfield, Arthritis and Rheumatism Council.

Symmons DPM, Barrett EM, Bankhead C (1994) The incidence of rheumatoid arthritis in the United Kingdom; results from the Norfolk arthritis register. *British Journal of Rheumatology* 33:735–739.

Thompson AE, Pope JE (2005) Calcium channel blockers for primary Raynaud's phenomenon: a meta-analysis. *Rheumatology* 44:145–150.

Toivanen A (1994) Reactive arthritis. In: Klippel JH, Dieppe PA (ed) *Rheumatology*. St Louis, Mosby 4:9.1–9.8.

Wolfe F, Ross K, Anderson J *et al.* (1995) The prevalence and characteristics of fibromyalgia in the general population. *Arthritis Rheumatism* 38:19–28.

Wolfe F, Smythe HA, Yunus MB *et al.* (1990) The American College of Rheumatology 1990 criteria for the classification of fibromyalgia. Report of the Multicenter Criteria Committee. *Arthritis and Rheumatism* 33:160–172.

World Health Organisation (1994) *Assessment of fracture risk and its application to screening for postmenopausal osteoporosis*. Geneva, WHO Technical Report series.

Wright V, Helliwell PS (1992) Psoriatic arthritis. In: *Collected reports on the rheumatic diseases*. Chesterfeld, Arthritis and Rheumatism Council, 56–58.

Yazici H (1994) Behçet's syndrome. In: Klippel JH, Dieppe PA (ed) *Rheumatology*. St Louis, Mosby 6:20.1–20.6.

3 The Immune System and Rheumatic Disease

S. OLIVER
Litchdon Medical Centre, North Devon, UK

The aim of this chapter is to provide an overview of the immune system and autoimmunity related to inflammatory joint diseases in the context of new therapies. After reading this chapter, nurses caring for people with an auto-immune disease should be able to:

- describe the immune system;
- discuss the consequences of autoimmunity;
- relate the mechanisms of action of therapies to the immune response;
- ensure that patients are appropriately informed, assessed and managed during treatment.

THE IMMUNE SYSTEM

A SIMPLIFIED MODEL

Immunology is the study of the body's protective mechanisms used to guard against foreign molecules or invading antigens. Immunity relies upon:

- the immune system's ability to recognise itself (self-tolerance);
- the ability of the body to recognise molecules which are foreign to itself and adequately respond to the insult using various defences.

To understand immunity it is useful to think of the immune system as a highly trained army with T and B cells being the two key regiments and the lymphoid organs as base camps stationed throughout the body (Isenberg and Morrow, 1995; Oliver, 2003). An antigen is a foreign substance that invades the body. The body's response to antigens or foreign invaders is to launch a response from lymphocytes, specific white blood cells that start as stem cells originating in bone marrow. These stem cells are similar to new young soldiers and

Rheumatology Nursing: A Creative Approach, 2nd edn. Edited by Jackie Hill.
Copyright 2006 by John Wiley & Sons, Ltd.

the bone marrow can be thought of as a major development and recruitment centre. The general soldiers developed in the bone marrow are called B lymphocyte cells and may migrate to base camps (lymphoid organs) around the body. Other lymphocytes may migrate to the thymus and become T lymphocyte cells. The defensive (immune) system is very efficient with good communications between lymphoid tissues (base camps) and other areas of lymphoid tissue using the lymphatic system as an efficient means of travel (Figure 3.1).

AUTOIMMUNE DISEASE

Autoimmune disease is the failure of the immune system to tolerate or recognise endogenous cells. This failure of self-tolerance results in an immune response that is launched against those tissues of the body that are incorrectly identified as foreign. The predisposition to develop an autoimmune disease can be revealed in an individual's genetic make-up.

The signs and symptoms that develop as a result of specific tissues being targeted are the characteristics of the disease and ultimately aid the diagnosis. For instance, in rheumatoid arthritis (RA), the key signs are synovitis, bone loss, erosions and ultimately joint deformities; whereas scleroderma is characterised by fibrotic arteriosclerosis of peripheral and visceral vasculature

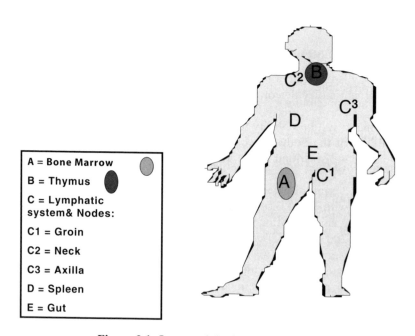

A = Bone Marrow

B = Thymus

C = Lymphatic system& Nodes:

C1 = Groin

C2 = Neck

C3 = Axilla

D = Spleen

E = Gut

Figure 3.1 Organs of the immune system.

identified by the accumulation of collagen in skin and viscera (Seibold, 1995).

Chronic inflammatory rheumatic diseases that have an autoimmune component include:

- RA
- ankylosing spondylitis (AS)
- psoriatic arthritis (PsA)
- systemic lupus erythematosus (SLE)
- scleroderma.

IMMUNE SYSTEM ORGANS

The immune system is designed to protect the body from damage caused by any micro-organisms such as bacteria, virus, fungi and parasites. The organs of the immune system are stationed throughout the body and are concerned with the development and deployment of lymphocytes and are generally referred to as lymphoid organs. They comprise:

1. primary lymphoid tissues
   - bone marrow
   - thymus
2. secondary lymphoid tissues
   - lymph nodes
   - spleen
   - tonsils and adenoids
   - appendix
   - Peyer's patches (clumps of lymphoid tissue in the small intestine)
3. additional contributors
   - blood
   - lymphatic vessels

The integrity of the immune system relies upon:

- recognition of the infectious agent/micro-organism;
- discrimination between self and nonself;
- specificity of response required;
- immunological memory.

TYPES OF IMMUNITY

The immune system can be discussed in the context of the type of response and whether it is specific or nonspecific; innate (active/nonspecific) or adaptive (acquired/specific) immunity. There are also terms to describe whether the immune response is based upon a cellular or humoral immune response (Figure 3.2).

INNATE ACTIVE IMMUNITY

The innate immune system is able to distinguish foreign tissues and organisms, but is nonspecific for any infectious agent and is not improved by repeated encounters with the same agent. Innate active immunity can act in conjunction with both the complement system and phagocytosis (the ingestion and killing of micro-organisms by specialist cells called phagocytes).

The complement system supports the immune responses by providing innate immunity, coating targets so they are marked and quickly identified for elimination. The system comprises approximately thirty inactive protein cells found in blood plasma and on cell membranes which activate when antibodies and antigens form. A key component of the system is a plasma protein called C3 (Hoffbrand and Pettit, 1993). There are three ways in which complement is activated:

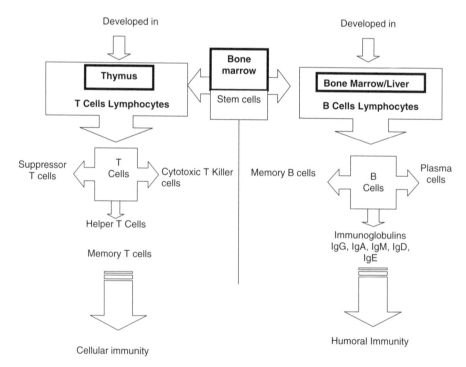

Figure 3.2 Lymphocyte development and the immune system.

- The classical pathway is activated when Immunoglobulin IgM and IgG antibodies bind to antigens.
- The alternative pathway uses opsonisation in which C3 fragments bind to the surface of the antigen, which then adheres directly to receptors on phagocytes to promote phagocytosis.
- The lectin pathway is similar to the classic pathway but complement activation does not require the presence of specific antibodies in this case.

Several complement proteins can clump together to form a membrane attack complex that destroys the membrane of the microbe causing cell death (cytolysis).

In some diseases such as Lupus, C3 and C4 levels can be measured to provide information on disease activity.

ADAPTIVE ACQUIRED IMMUNITY

The key features of adaptive immunity are those of memory and specificity (Male, 1998). This means that the body has the ability to recognise micro-organisms that have previously invaded resulting in a specific and targeted response to the invader. Lymphocytes are the only cells capable of recognising antigens (Abbas and Lichtman, 2003). Adaptive acquired immunity is specific to the infectious agent and is enhanced by repeated encounters. Following recovery, immunity will have developed against that specific infective agent.

Acquired immunity can be defined as either active or passive.

Active immunity

Active immunity can result from either having the infection or receiving an inoculation with a vaccine containing a killed or modified antigen. This stimulates the body's own immune system to develop antibodies or sensitised lymphocytes to the inoculated antigen. An effective immune response to the vaccine usually takes a few days and the immunity may last a few months or many years. However, in many cases a course of the vaccines may be required for sufficient antibodies to provide optimum protection.

In individuals who are immunosuppressed, the appropriate immune response may be insufficient to result in immunity.

It should be noted that individuals who are immunosuppressed may fail to gain an appropriate immune response to live vaccines and caution should be observed in individuals who are receiving steroids or immunosuppressant therapies including disease-modifying drugs and biologics.

Passive immunity

Passive immunity is gained when an individual is inoculated with serum containing antibodies and lymphocytes that have already acquired immunity and have a memory that can be used to launch a specific response against the inoculated infectious agent in the future. The effect of passive immunity is immediate but short-lived and is not sustained. However, if a second attack of the infectious agent occurs, the body's T and B cells recognise the antigen and respond by launching an immune response (Betts and Langelaan, 1996).

CELLULAR IMMUNITY

Lymphocytes transported from the bone marrow to the thymus gland become T cells and produce cellular immunity. As well as responding to viruses, fungi and bacteria, cellular immunity is responsible for delayed allergic reactions, rejections of transplant or foreign tissues and the body's defence against tumours (Ganong, 1995).

HUMORAL IMMUNITY

Humoral immunity is mediated by B lymphocytes that migrate from the bone marrow and can be found circulating in the blood and lymphatic system. They secrete antibodies to defend against extracellular microbes and toxins and play a major role in the defences against bacterial infections. This form of immunity can be transferred from immune-naïve individuals using serum (Abbas and Lichtman, 2003).

COMPONENTS OF THE IMMUNE SYSTEM

White blood cells (WBCs) work closely with soluble proteins (immunoglobulins) and complement to guard against infection. The lymphocyte cells communicate with other cells, in part, via chemical messengers called cytokines. WBCs can be considered in two groups, phagocytes and immunocytes.

PHAGOCYTES

Phagocytes engulf and digest cell debris and foreign materials. They comprise:

• granulocytes (which are of three main types: neutrophils, eosinophils and basophils)
• monocytes
• macrophages.

Granulocytes

Neutrophils are professional phagocytes and form approximately 70% of leucocytes (Male, 1998).

Eosinophils have an important role in allergic reactions and parasitic diseases. They are capable of engulfing antigen-antibody complexes and can release enzymes that disarm histamine. They have receptors for IgE, IgG, C3 and C5 complement (Panayi, 1994). Levels are commonly raised in patients with allergic disease such as asthma.

Basophils and mast cells are involved in host defence against parasites but also play an important role in immediate hypersensitivity reactions when allergens bind to their receptors. Basophils are found in circulating body fluids whereas mast cells are tissue bound. Basophils and mast cells have receptors for C3 and C5 complement proteins. The interaction between IgE and basophils results in the release of inflammatory mediators into the circulation whereas mast cells have a more localised response (Panayi, 1994).

Monocytes

Monocytes enter the blood from the bone marrow and have a life of about 72 hours. They can enter the tissues and mature to tissue macrophages. They are also capable of phagocytosis and ingesting cell debris and foreign materials.

Macrophages

Macrophages work principally as antigen presenting cells (APC) although they play numerous roles as part of the immune army, secreting cytokines, responding to cytotoxic killer T cells and engulfing bacteria. Macrophages migrate from the tissues when activated by cytokines from T lymphocytes and work throughout the immune system.

IMMUNOCYTES – T CELLS AND B CELLS

A number of blood cells are produced in the bone marrow, all starting life as stem cells. There are two major classes of lymphocytes, B cells and T cells.

This classification is dependent on their place of maturation and ultimately their role in immunity.

After birth a small proportion of lymphocytes are formed in the bone marrow but most are developed in the lymph nodes, thymus and spleen. Lymphocytes enter the bloodstream via the lymphatic system and normally only about 2% of lymphocytes circulate in the peripheral blood, the remainder residing in the lymphoid organs. There are many subsets of lymphocytes, which differ in function and protein products. Lymphocytes are the only cells capable of specifically recognising different antigens and have the characteristics of the adaptive immune response, specificity and memory (Abbas and Lichtman, 2003).

Lymphocytes developed in the thymus become T cells and those developed in the bone marrow become B cells (Figure 3.2). T cells and B cells are classified as naïve when they migrate from the primary lymphoid tissues and enter the blood and then into secondary lymphoid tissues. T and B cells share some common characteristics (Figure 3.3).

Both are capable of clonal expansion and have the ability to reproduce themselves rapidly when needed. They have receptors that enable good communication and contact with antigens and they secrete chemical messengers called cytokines.

B cells mature in a sequence (Figure 3.4). The immature B cells (stem cells) leave the bone marrow and enter the spleen where only ten percent will undergo maturation. These naïve B cells can become plasma cells or memory B cells residing in the tissues or secondary lymphatic tissue and producing antibodies (immunoglobulins). Memory B cells are the principal memory of the immune system. They are smaller than plasma cells and wait to be activated by previously identified antigen (Abbas and Lichtman, 2003). When immature B cells are activated as a result of primary immune response, they undergo clonal expansion in which some of the B cells become memory cells allowing a specific secondary immune response on subsequent antigen exposure. They ensure a rapid production of immunoglobulins to match the antigen. Plasma cells secrete immunoglobulins that match the structure of the parent B cell.

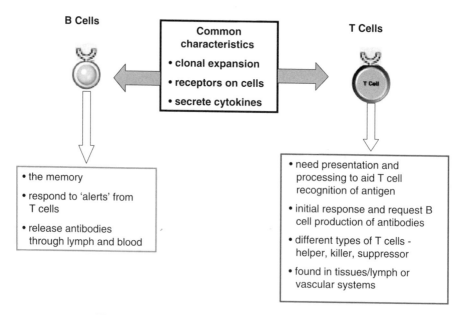

Figure 3.3 Common characteristics of T and B cells.

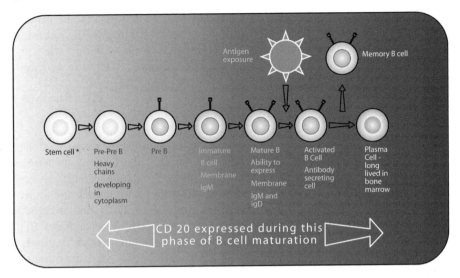

Figure 3.4 B cell maturation. (Reproduced with kind permission from Susan Oliver [2004] *Immunology*, and thanks to Roche Products Ltd.)

CELL DIFFERENTIATION (CD) CD4 AND CD8 T CELLS

Cell differentiation (CD) markers are important surface protein markers. T cells express markers CD4 or CD8 (Male, 1998). CD4 T lymphocytes require an antigen to be presented to them in the major histocompatibility cell (MHC) of a class II antigen. It is the CD4 T cells that are recognised as being integral to the pathogenesis of RA (Panayi, 1994).

The majority of T helper cells have CD4 markers and are a key communicator, producing essential messengers called cytokines. T cytotoxic cells express CD8. T cells can be subdivided into TH1 and TH2 cells. TH1 cells are concerned primarily with cellular immunity. They are the focus of immunological responses related to inflammatory arthritis, secreting cytokines which are pro-inflammatory mediators. TH2 cells interact primarily with B cells in humoral immunity and are thought to be involved in promoting IgE and IgG production (Male, 1998). However, this clear delineation between TH1 and TH2 cells may be too simplistic to explain all aspects of responses to cytokine therapies (Mpofu *et al.*, 2004).

In order to recognise a protein antigen B cells require CD4 helper T lymphocytes to activate their response. The B cells will respond quickly to requests from T cells when they recognise the initial attack from an antigen. Linked recognition is the mechanism that causes B cells to communicate with CD4 T helper cells primed to the same antigen and results in enhanced B cell expansion (Silverman and Carson, 2003). B cells remember the antigen. In subsequent attacks by the same antigen, they initiate a tailor-made antibody, through the lymphatic or blood system, in order to destroy it. In general, B cells respond to natural antigens on T cell activation, although in some circumstances B cells can respond to antigens without activation from T cells (Merck Manual, 2004).

ANTIGEN PRESENTING CELLS (APCS)

In order for the lymphocytes to recognise the foreign invader, antigens need to be presented to the T cell by antigen presenting cells. The role of APC is to capture, process and present the antigen to the T cell. The T cell can then identify the specific markers on the antigen and therefore launch the appropriate immune response. This process is essential for CD4 T helper cells. B cells may also prime APC to interact with T helper cells. Macrophages, dendritic cells and B cells can all act as highly specialized and tightly regulated APCs and are constantly sampling the environment to identify potential antigens.

MAJOR HISTOCOMPITABILITY CELLS AND HUMAN LEUCOCYTE ANTIGENS

A series of molecules that are the products of a cluster of genes are known as major histocompatibility complex (MHC) and in a human they are also referred to as human leucocyte antigens (HLA). MHC and HLA are essential to immunity and the interactions with T cells that ensure tolerance of endogenous cells. HLA antigens are present on the surface membrane of most cells with a nucleus and play a major role in immune recognition and reaction. Antigens are transported within a specific binding groove of a MHC molecule that is transported on the surface of the APC. MHC has two class types:

• MHC I expressed on all nucleated cells. CD8 (Cell Differentiation) T cytolytic T cells respond to antigens with type I MHC.
• MHC Type II are closely associated to the cells of the immune system. CD4 T cells only recognise antigens with a type II MHC (Male, 1998).

HLA may be distinguished by one of a variety of antigen markers on their cell membrane or surface and a number of these antigens have been linked to specific immunological susceptibility (Hoffbrand and Pettit, 1993). There are many cell membrane markers and their subsets have been given different names to aid classification, for example HLA-DRB4 or CW6.

Rheumatoid arthritis is strongly linked to the HLA-DRB4 and/or HLA-DRB1 markers, ankylosing spondylitis (AS) to HLA B27 and psoriasis to CW6 (Hoffbrand and Pettit, 1993).

IMMUNOGLOBULINS (ANTIBODIES)

Immunoglobulins belong to a family of large protein molecules also known as antibodies. Immunoglobulins are produced by B cells in response to a challenge to the immune system. B cells that have had no antigen/antibody reaction (naïve B cells) produce a good, but not highly specific, immunoglobulin response on first contact or prior to clonal expansion. Immunoglobulins can become more specific and able to recognise an antigen following an initial interaction, resulting in a more rapid and effective response in subsequent immune challenges. When an immunoglobulin develops a specific targeted response, it is said to have a shared epitope. This is a state of match between immunoglobulin and antigen, so that the key of the antigen is a perfect fit in the lock of the immunoglobulin (Figure 3.5).

There are nine distinct classes of human immunoglobulins that are expressed on the surface membrane of the B lymphocyte:

- IgGs (Immunoglobulin Gamma), including four subclasses of IgG
- IgA, including two subclasses of IgA
- one IgM
- one IgE
- one IgD.

The IgG immunoglobulins comprise up to 85% of circulating immunoglobulins (Rote, 2000). IgG enters the tissue spaces and responds promptly to invasions by coating the antigen/micro-organisms and speeding up the rapid response of other immune processes.

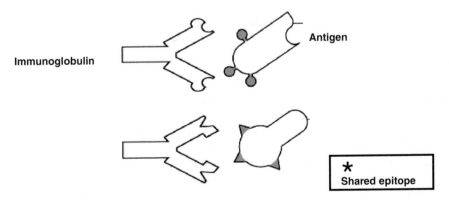

Figure 3.5 Shared epitope.

How an immunoglobulin works

Many different potential antibody-producing B cells pre-exist in the body and each has the ability to make antibody of a different specificity. When a B cell recognises an antigen it sends out an immunoglobin specifically made to match that antigen. Matching is achieved by an arrangement of tiny jigsaw-like sections on the V portion of the immunoglobulin being an exact match to the antigen. This ensures that the immunoglobulin and antigen fit together like a lock and a key or like jigsaw pieces (Figure 3.5). The region of the antigen recognised by the immunoglobulin is called an epitope. If an immunoglobulin and antigen are perfectly matched they are said to have a shared epitope. This is an effective immune response. On binding antigen, the cell is activated to divide and produce identical cells (clonal expansion) producing identical antibodies to the specific antigen. If the antigen is a new antigen, the B cell will need to develop identical cells, producing identical immunoglobulin (antibody) to the specific antigen for an optimal immune response.

Significance of immunoglobulin in the control of autoimmune disease

Immunoglobulin is Y-shaped, which is a significant factor in some of the new treatments in controlling auto-immune disease. The stem of the Y is constant whereas the V-shaped part is flexible or changeable. The V can be manipulated in the laboratory and is where the antigen sticks when it is trapped by the immunoglobulin (Figure 3.6).

CYTOKINES

Cytokines are proteins or glycoproteins that deliver important intercellular messages into the blood or lymphatic systems. Monocytes, macrophages, fibroblasts, T and B cells are capable of releasing cytokines on stimulation. Cytokines can be grouped into families and are also classified according to the pro- or anti-inflammatory actions and often have a synergistic effect with other cytokines or groups of cytokines.

Cytokines implicated in musculoskeletal diseases

Some cytokines families are of particular interest because of their pro-inflammatory effects in chronic inflammation. Interleukins, tumour necrosis factor alpha (TNFα) and granulocyte macrophage colony stimulating factor (GM-CSF) are abundant in inflamed joints and are implicated in activating (inducing) an acute phase response, increasing cell adhesion, cell growth and increasing production of destructive enzymes in the inflammatory process.

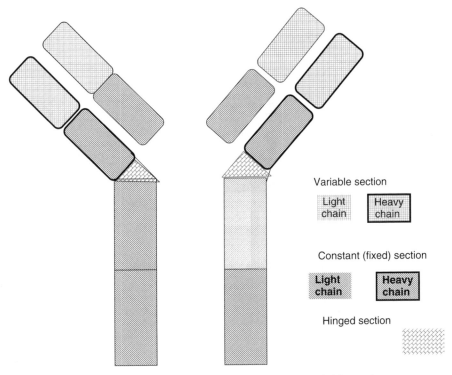

Variable section

| Light chain | Heavy chain |

Constant (fixed) section

| Light chain | Heavy chain |

Hinged section

Figure 3.6 Immunoglobulin showing fixed and variable sections.

Inflammatory cascade – pro- and anti-inflammatory cytokines

An inflammatory cascade is the activation of cytokines responsible for producing the classic immunological responses that result in the key signs of inflammation (Figure 3.7). Tumour necrosis factor alpha (TNFα) appears to have a pivotal role in the inflammatory cascade having a synergistic effect with other cytokines such as interleukins, GM-CSF.

The normal immune response is a return to a state of equilibrium, once resolution from infection is achieved. However, in autoimmune disease this process fails because the body loses the important self-tolerance mechanism and continues to recognise the body's own tissues as foreign antigen; and therefore continues the immune response.

Cytokine activation

To activate or induce an effect, the cytokine must be released (or cleaved) and lock into a T cell receptor (TCR) (Figure 3.8).

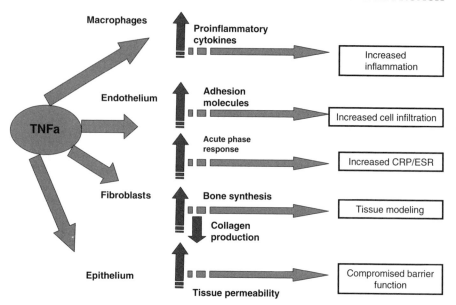

Figure 3.7 Inflammatory cascade. (Reproduced with kind permission from Schering Plough Ltd.)

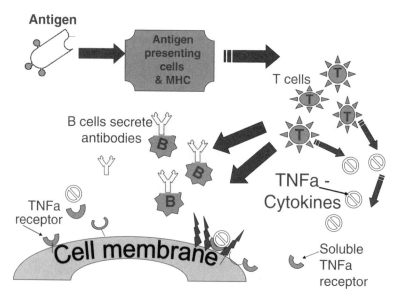

Figure 3.8 T cells and receptors.

The response that is activated as a result of the cytokine locking in will vary according to the role of the cytokine, for example pro- or anti-inflammatory. In a normal immune response, following the release of a cytokine and when a subsequent effective response has been achieved, a suppressor T cell will release a cytokine that in effect advises the army to stand down, signalling that the immune response has been effective and should stop. This is when the antigen has been rendered inactive and is no longer functioning or has been adequately disarmed.

T CELL RECEPTORS (TCR)

Receptors play an essential role in cell to cell activation and interactions for a wide range of biological responses. TCRs are essential to achieve effective immune responses. TCRs can be either:

- circulating in soluble form in the blood or lymphatic system
- tissue bound in cells such as synovial tissue.

TCRs for cytokines can also be classed into families depending upon their structural make-up. Two types of TCR for tumour necrosis factor alpha (TNFα) are p55 and p75 (Maini and Feldmann, 2000).

The cytokine activation or locking in to a receptor results in a burst of activity with the release of cytokines and other inflammatory mediators causing various processes in the body to respond to the attack. This response is called the inflammatory cascade (Figure 3.7).

DISEASE-MODIFYING ANTIRHEUMATIC DRUGS

TRADITIONAL

In the past many of the traditional DMARDs were found to have beneficial effects on disease activity, sometimes without a clear understanding of their mechanism of action. Recent research into the pathophysiology of the immune system has provided a greater understanding of the mechanisms of actions of traditional DMARDs. Three mechanisms have been suggested:

- Reducing key metabolites necessary for immune cells to proliferate and replicate, compromising the ability of the immune and autoimmune responses
- Direct or indirect inhibition of pro-inflammatory cytokines
- Modifying effect on the arachidonic acid and prostaglandins

Greater detail is provided in Table 3.1

Table 3.1 Mechanisms of action of DMARDs

DMARD	Mechanism of Action
Azathioprine	While the precise mode of action remains unclear it has been proposed that azathioprine has an effect on cell synthesis preventing proliferation of cells involved in determination and amplification of the immune response this may be as a result of damage to deoxyribonucleic acid (DNA) through incorporation of purine thio-analogues (Glaxo Smith Kline, 2003).
Cyclosporin	Cyclosporin has been shown to reduce synthesis of lymphocytes by reducing the transcription of IL-2 by binding to cyclophilins required in gene transcription and expression by messenger ribonucleic acid (mRNA). There is also some evidence that cyclosporin inhibits bone resorbing activities in vitro (Dinnarello and Moldawer, 2000).
Gold Injections (auranofin)	Gold has been shown to reduce the steady state of mRNA of IL-1 beta (IL-1β) and TNF-α and as a result inhibits synthesis of these cytokines in mouse macrophages these results were also demonstrated in human endothelial cells (Dinnarello and Moldawer, 2000).
Cloroquine & Hydroxy-chloroquine	Antimalarial agents interfere with enzyme activities necessary for cell replication, inhibit prostaglandin formation and possibly interfere with Interleukin 1 production (Sanofi Synthelaboratories, 2003).
Leflunomide	Leflunomide inhibits dihydro-orotate dehydrogenase, which inhibits pyrimidine biosynthesis, resulting in similar anti-proliferative properties to methotrexate. Leflunomide also has secondary actions by inhibition of interleukin 2 (IL-2) synthesis and transforming growth factor alpha (TGF-a) and inhibiting T and B cell lymphocyte proliferation and antibody production (Furst, 1999; Aventis Pharma, 2004).

Methotrexate	Studies with a parent folic acid antagonist compound (Aminopterin) led to the development of methotrexate, initially for the treatment of psoriatic arthritis (Furst, 1995). Further studies have clearly highlighted the role methotrexate plays in diminishing cell replication by influencing several metabolic pathways including inhibiting dihydrofolate reducatese (Black *et al.*, 1964, cited in Weinblatt, 1995). A recent study demonstrated an inhibitory effect of methotrexate on T cell activated cytokine production (Slot, 2001, Gerards *et al.*, 2003).
Penicillamine	Penicillamine is strongly plasma-protein bound. Most penicillamine is bound to albumin but some is bound to α-globulins or ceruloplasmin (Alliance Pharmaceuticals, 2003).
Sulphasalazine	Sulphasalazine appears to have an overall action with some anti-bacterial effects but more importantly appears to exert immunimodulatory effects on the arachidonic acid inflammatory cascade and altering the activity of some enzymes (Sanofi Synthelaboratories, 2003).
Newer DMARDS	
Mycophenolic Acid (Mycophenolate)	Mycophenolate inhibits the proliferation of B and T lymphocytes by inhibition of purine biosynthesis resulting in an anti-proliferative effect on lymphocytes. Mycophenolate has less of an effect on other rapidly dividing cells (Dinarello and Moldawer, 2000).
Tacrolimus	Tacrolimus is a drug traditionally used for immunosuppression in transplant surgery to prevent rejection of donor organ tissues. Its mechanism of action is to inhibit calcineurin. Calcineurin plays an essential role in the T cell activation pathway as it is a key component of the nuclear element of message transduction in activated T cells. In cell cultures tacrolimus demonstrated an inhibition of spontaneous IL-5 production. (Dinnarello and Moldawer, 2000; Fujisawa Ltd., 2002).

NEW THERAPIES

The development of therapies designed to disarm the action of pro-inflammatory cytokines is the result of biological technology (Oliver and Mooney, 2002). Many of the new biologic therapies act by mimicking the normal immune processes and prevent or displace a cytokine from locking into its defined receptor. This prevents the activation of pro-inflammatory cytokines responsible for ensuring an inflammatory cascade. The characteristics of licensed biologics are shown in Figure 3.9.

The management of those receiving biologic therapies and the detailed risks and benefits of treatment are discussed in Chapter 12.

Biotechnology

The use of recombinant biotechnology enables the manipulation and redesign of key aspects of the body's cell-to-cell communications and interactions. Biotechnology enables immunoglobulins to be designed to trap key inflammatory cytokines, preventing their ability to lock into their receptors (Figure 3.8).

Biotechnology research into inflammatory joint diseases has so far resulted in therapeutic targets for interleukin 1 (IL-1) and TNFα and more recently depleting CD20 B cells. However, as research continues to reveal the more

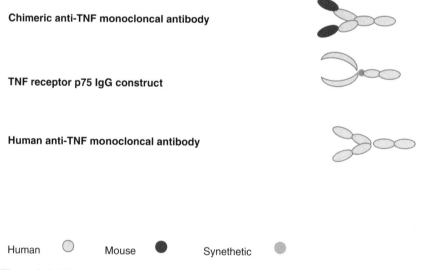

Figure 3.9 Characteristics of biologic therapies. (Adapted with kind permission from Abbott Laboratories Ltd.)

detailed aspects of cell development and the cell-to-cell interactions in immunity there are numerous new pathways to be explored in the modification mechanisms that drive auto-immune diseases.

Compared to DMARDs and corticosteroids, biologics have a more specific and targeted effect at cell level. Traditional therapies have the ability to suppress the normal immune response but are not so specifically targeted on cell-to-cell interactions. Additionally, biologics have a direct or indirect effect on other key cells in the immune responses resulting from this effective blocking of the inflammatory cascade. As a consequence, practitioners need to ensure a rigorous approach to assessing patients for all forms of opportunistic infection.

Trials of anti-TNα therapies have shown some side effects that are only partially explained including possible risks related to exacerbations of cardiac and demyelinating diseases. However, research needs to continue to explore the significance of these side effects in relation to biologic therapies.

All biologic therapies have been developed using proteins that allow the effective blocking of cytokine activation. As with all injected foreign proteins, such as blood transfusion, there is the potential for the body to develop antibodies to the protein and/or hypersensitivity reactions.

New biologic treatments

The identification of key cytokines and a greater understanding of cell-to-cell interaction have enabled the development of therapies that are having a significant impact in the treatment of auto-immune diseases. It is likely that many more therapeutic targets will be identified in the immune pathway. A number of new drug therapies have already been developed:

- Interleukin-1 receptor antagonists (IL-1Ra) – anakinra;
- Anti-tumour necrosis factor alpha (anti-TNFα) – adalimumab, etanercept and infliximab;
- CD20 B cell – rituximab.

IL-1Ra

In normal joints IL-1Ra modifies the activity of Interleukin 1, a pro-inflammatory cytokine. IL-1Ra binds to IL-1R1 receptors, and prevents IL-1 binding into its receptors. This reduces the number of receptors available for IL-1 to lock into and cause an inflammatory response. This is the body's normal response to maintain equilibrium and ensure an appropriate level of inflammatory response. There is only one IL-1Ra therapy licensed for RA – anakinra, which is discussed in Chapter 12.

Anti-TNFα

TNFα is a significant cytokine in the inflammatory response. This response is activated when the TNFα cytokine is released and locks into a TCR for TNFα, resulting in a cascade of responses from other pro-inflammatory cytokines. There are two types of receptor for TNF that bind with comparable affinity, p55 and p75. Some anti-TNFα therapies can block both receptors, others block only one and may also block lymphotoxin α. The full significance of these differences is not completely understood. However there are variations in the structure and composition of the anti-TNFα therapies, as well as differences in plasma half-lives and routes of administration. These may be relevant to understanding the differences in each therapy. The minor variations between therapies may also explain differing benefits to specific diseases. For example the ability of etanercept to block lymphotoxin α may explain the benefits achieved in juvenile idiopathic arthritis (JIA) as lymphotoxin α is identified in inflamed joints of JIA patients (Pisetsky, 2000).

CD20 B Cell

B cells may have additional stimulatory effects in inflammatory arthritis and a number of studies have focussed on their role in the immunopathogenesis of RA (Shaw et al., 2003). There are a number of theories to explain the way in which they work, including that they:

• act as antigen presenting cells and as a costimulator of T cells;
• secrete pro-inflammatory cytokines and chemokines (small cytokines);
• produce rheumatoid factor (RF), and since positive RF is linked to aggressive disease, they may be implicated in enhancing stimulus to T cells.

The pre B and mature B lymphocytes with cell surface markers of CD20 have been identified as a therapeutic target enabling the depletion of B cells and ultimately removal of pre B (naïve) and mature B cells (Edwards et al., 2004). Rituximab focuses specifically on these pre B and mature B lymphocytes, binding to the cell surface marker CD20. CD20 is expressed on both normal and malignant B cells but does not circulate freely in the plasma and is not shed from the surface of the B cells. CD is not found on normal plasma cells in other tissues.

Rituximab binds to the CD20 antigen on the B lymphocytes and it is suggested that it:

• induces cell death (apoptosis) of CD20 positive B cells;
• sensitises cells to the action of conventional cytotoxic drugs (NICE, 2002).

Rituximab is currently licensed for the treatment of non-Hodgkin's lymphomas (NHL); but appears from early research to be a therapeutic option in the treatment of inflammatory joint diseases. Following completion of treatment for NHL B cell levels return to normal within nine to twelve months (Roche, 2002).

IMMUNE RESPONSES – HYPERSENSITIVITY AND ANAPHYLAXIS

Hypersensitivity is characterised by an immune mechanism that triggers inflammation and subsequent destruction of healthy tissues (Rote *et al.*, 2000). All foreign agents, either injected or absorbed, have the potential to induce immune response. All current biologic therapies are derived from foreign proteins that have the potential to cause a hypersensitivity reaction and possible anaphylaxis. Anaphylaxis is an allergic response mediated by IgE and causes the release of mast cells, basophils and complement components, C3a, C4a and C5a (Rote *et al.*, 2000). The introduction of any foreign protein can promote this response in the same ways that a blood transfusion may promote reactions. Parenteral routes have a higher incidence of anaphylactic reactions (O'Dowd, 2004) and if exposure has been uninterrupted are less likely to result in a severe reaction than intermittent dosing. However, individuals with a history of hypersensitivity are at an increased risk of subsequent anaphylaxis. The individual's history is relevant to their risk of subsequent response to treatment to the same or similar agents or foreign proteins, notably:

• prior exposure
• route of exposure
• previous anaphylactic episodes.

Hypersensitivity reactions can vary from mild atopic symptoms such as rhinitis to more severe and rapid symptoms seen in anaphylaxis. Individuals that are sensitised may respond to exogenous stimuli such as allergens (for example dust mite) or foreign proteins (blood transfusions or biologic therapies) with a hypersensitivity reaction (O'Dowd, 2004). There are a number of causes of hypersensitivity reactions and some of the most common include:

• therapeutic compounds
• insect bites
• contrast medium used for radiographic investigations
• blood products
• foods, such as eggs, nuts and seafood
• latex and rubber products.

IMMUNOLOGICAL INVESTIGATIONS

A number of blood tests can provide information on immune system and specific immunological responses. These include:

- rheumatoid factor
- anticyclic citrullinated peptide
- complement levels
- antinuclear antibodies and double-stranded DNA
- antineutrophil cytoplasmic antibodies
- antibodies to biologic therapies.

RHEUMATOID FACTOR (RF)

RF is a human antibody against portions of the IgG molecules. RF is approximately 50% sensitive in early disease although for the diagnosis of RA in patients with established disease, sensitivity rises to 70–80%. High RF titres are an important prognostic indicator, identifying individuals who are more likely to have more severe erosive sero-positive RA (Vittecoq et al., 2003). However caution is required in interpreting results, as false positive RF can be detected in a number of diseases.

ANTI-CYCLIC CITRULLINATED PEPTIDE (CCP)

Amino acids are the building blocks of proteins that form genetic codes for DNA. Citrulline is an immune protein linked to Arginine, an important protein required for DNA. Research has shown that T cells can stimulate B cells in peripheral blood and synovial fluid to produce antibodies to CCP. Antibodies to CCP have been found in bone marrow and at the site of inflammation within the inflamed joints in RA (Reparon-Schuijt et al., 2001).

Early research suggests that in RA, measuring antibodies to CCP may be more effective than measuring RF (Bas et al., 2003). Anti-CCP has been detected in people several years before they develop RA (Jansen et al., 2003).

COMPLEMENT

The consumption of complement during an accelerated immune response results in depleted levels within the body. C3 and 4 are the two most clinically relevant complement assays in SLE. They support the clinical diagnosis and help in the assessment of disease activity.

ANTI-NUCLEAR ANTIBODY (ANA) AND DOUBLE-STRANDED DNA (DSDNA)

ANA are antibodies against large cellular complexes containing protein and nucleic acid. Research suggests that ANA antibodies are T cell dependent and driven by the autoimmune processes (Maddison, 2002). A positive ANA can be seen in a variety of infections and auto-immune diseases as well as being induced by drugs such as hydralazine. ANA are defined by their target antigen including dsDNA, RNA-protein complexes and nonhistone nuclear proteins. Some of these tests are specific for certain diseases. Staining patterns identified in ANA tests reflect the presence of antibodies against one or more nuclear antigens, for example, speckled patterns. However, the titre is more clinically relevant than the staining patterns and positive results are commonly found in the normal population (Barland and Wach, 2002). A detailed description of ANA and dsDNA tests is provided by Maddison (2002).

ANTINEUTROPHIL CYTOPLASMIC ANTIBODIES (ANCA)

ANCA are antibodies directed against neutrophils granule. This causes changes to the cell which are characterised by the changes seen on staining, and the distribution of the granular patterning may help to establish a definitive diagnosis. The two forms of staining are:

- pANCA – perinuclear ANCA
- cANCA – circulating ANCA.

The presence of ANCA is linked to diseases such as primary systemic vasculitis (PSV) (Watts and Scott, 2003). Examples of PSV include:

- polyarteritis nodosa
- Wegener's granulomatosis
- Churg-Strauss syndrome.

HUMAN ANTI-CHIMERIC ANTIBODIES (HACA) OR ANTIBODIES TO BIOLOGIC AGENTS

Anti-TNFα therapies consist of foreign proteins and antibodies to these agents have been identified in all clinical trials but at present it is not clear whether they significantly impair the therapeutic benefit of treatment (Mpofu et al., 2004). HACA are the specific antibodies related to the protein (mouse/murine) portion of a monoclonal antibody, for example, as seen in the composition of infliximab. When infliximab is co-prescribed with methotrexate it improves clinical response and appears to reduce levels of HACA. However, it is unclear if this effect is independent of reducing HACAs (Mpofu *et al.*, 2004). One side effect, infusion site reactions, may be related to HACA.

Raised antibody levels to foreign proteins such as the monoclonal antibodies, have been identified in all biologic therapies. The significance of these raised levels remains unclear. Recent research suggests that 10% of patients treated with etanercept and methotrexate experienced less injection site reactions compared to 21% who had etanercept alone (Klareskog *et al.*, 2004). This combination also shows an improved response to treatment (Weinblatt *et al.*, 1999). Adalimumab has also shown a reduction in anti-adalimumab antibody (ANA) and greater therapeutic benefit when coprescribed with methotrexate (Machold and Smolen, 2003).

INFECTIONS IN RELATION TO IMMUNOSUPPRESSION AND CYTOKINE BLOCKING

GENERAL INFECTIONS

The body's ability to resolve infection relies upon a competent immune system with an ability to launch an appropriate response to an infecting agent. A wide range of therapies have the potential to dampen the full immune response to infection including:

• corticosteroids
• cytotoxic agents
• DMARDs
• biologic therapies.

The more specific and targeted suppression of the specific key cells, such as T or B cell suppression, the greater the vigilance required to manage potential opportunistic infections, particularly as the symptoms of infection and subsequent fevers may be masked (Schering Plough, 2003). All types of infections can present in these circumstances but some documented infections include:

• tuberculosis and pneumocystis carnii
• histoplasmosis
• aspergillosis
• listeria
• new or re-emergence of previous septic arthritis/osteomyelitis/wound infections.

Serious infections remain a significant life-threatening risk to immunocompromised patients.

TUBERCULOSIS

Tuberculosis (TB) is typically a disease of the lung (World Health Organisation, 2003) and is a growing world-wide health problem with two million deaths and eight million new cases annually (Kaufmann, 2002). An additional problem is that of multidrug resistant strains of Mycobacterium TB (M.TB). One-third of the world population is infected with M.TB, fortunately fewer than 10% will ever develop the disease (Jasmer et al., 2002). The usual route for infection is via droplets inhaled and engulfed by alveolar macrophages which then transport the organisms to the lymph nodes. This is where M.TB is first contained and where the initial immune response occurs. T cells and macrophages target the site and engulf the invading organism before granuloma lesions appear. This containment is reliant upon an effective immune system and the work of the CD 4 T helper cells and supporting cytokine networks.

Interferon gamma (IFNγ), tumour necrosis factor alpha (TNFα) and lymphotoxin alpha (LTα) are central agents in protection against TB (Kaufman, 2002). However, research shows that IFNγ is also a potent mediator and plays a key role in protection. This is achieved by a combination of TNFα and IFNγ inducing optimum macrophage activation and ultimately leading to containment of the TB (Kaufmann, 2002).

It is important to note that the suppression of TNFα activation with antiTNFα therapies prevents the normal containment of tuberculosis bacterium within organised granuloma lesions.

CARDIAC DISEASE

A growing body of evidence has demonstrated that individuals with high inflammatory indices in musculoskeletal diseases such as RA having an increased risk of cardiovascular disease (McEntegart et al., 2001; Kitas and Erb, 2003). Two major classes of cytokines have been identified in heart failure:

- vasoconstrictor cytokines such as endothelin
- vasodepressor proinflammatory cytokines such as TNFα or Interleukin 6 (IL-6).

TNFα receptors p55 and 75, have been identified in cardiac myocytes. TNFα also appears to be increased in class III–IV congestive heart failure with higher levels of TNFα correlating with the deterioration in heart failure (Bozkurt, 2000). TNFα is not found in healthy myocardium (Torre-Amione et al., 1999). These findings have not been as consistent in the case of IL-6.

Research suggests that heart failure progresses after activation of the inflammatory cascade following myocardial injury. Individuals with predisposing heart failure experience a deterioration following over expression of cytokines such as TNFα (Torre-Amione *et al.*, 1999). Further research is required to clarify whether there is a class effect, confined to specific therapies or there are some additional predisposing factors.

MULTIPLE SCLEROSIS (MS)

MS is an autoimmune disease with multiple plaques inflammation and demyelination and sclerosis or scarring of the myelin sheath of the central nervous system (Robinson *et al.*, 2001). Lymphotoxin and TNFα are key elements in multiple sclerosis (Lock *et al.*, 1999) and studies have demonstrated that increased levels of TNFα exacerbate the disease. However results of studies to block TNFα have been disappointing as this treatment appeared to make the disease worse (Lock *et al.*, 1999).

THE FUTURE FOR TARGETED THERAPIES

A greater understanding of the immune system and the cell-to-cell interactions has enabled advances in more specific targeted therapies for many autoimmune-driven diseases and revealed other potential therapeutic targets. This knowledge fuels further research studies exploring alternative therapeutic options. One particular area of research is in the quest for the greater understanding of the human genome and identification of key factors that may identify an individual's risk of developing a disease and the particular features of their disease, for instance understanding more about seropositive or seronegative RA.

It is important that traditional bench-to-bedside research continues with the support of sophisticated new research methods exploring the human genome to ensure that studies continue to explore the spectrum of immunity and immune responses enabling epidemiologist, geneticists and clinicians to complete the fascinating and as yet, partly complete puzzle of autoimmune disease (Dayer, 2004).

ACTION POINTS FOR PRACTICE

- Consider the issues related to immunisation and the immunocompromised patient. Discuss how a patient's immunological status should be considered prior to commencing treatment with a DMARD or biologic therapy.
- Based upon what you have read in this chapter, explore options in accessing or producing relevant literature that can help individuals understand the relative risks and benefits of treatments for inflammatory joint diseases.

• Review Chapter 12 and describe the relevant points for the nursing assessment and management of a patient eligible for a biologic therapy.

REFERENCES

Abbas A, Lichtman A (2003) *Cellular and Molecular* Immunology 5th Edition. Philadelphia, Saunders.

Alliance Pharmaceuticals (2003) Alliance Pharmaceuticals: Penicillamine: *Summary of Product Characteristics*. www.medicines.org.uk (16 October 2004).

Aventis Pharma (2004) Aventis Pharma Limited: Leflunomide: *Summary of Product Characteristics*. www.medicines.org.uk (16 October 2004).

Barland P, Wach J (2002) *Measurement and clinical significance of antinuclear antibodies*. www.Uptodate.com (7 June 2004).

Bas S, Genevay S, Meyer O *et al.* (2003) Anti-cyclic citrullinated peoptide antibodies, IgM and IgA rheumatoid factors in the diagnosis and prognosis of rheumatoid arthritis. *Rheumatology* 42(5):677–680.

Betts A, Langelaan G (1996) Acquired defences. In: Hinchuff SM (ed), *Physiology for Nursing Practice*, 2nd edn. London, Balliere Tindall.

Black RL, O'Brien WM, Van Scott E *et al.* (1964) Methotrexate therapy in psoriatic arthritis. Double blind study on 21 patients. *Journal of American Medical Association* 189:743–747.

Bozkurt B (2000) Activation of cytokines as a mechanism of disease progression in heart failure. *Annals of the Rheumatic Diseases* 59:suppl I, i90–i93.

Dayer JM (2004) The process of identifying and understanding cytokines: from basic studies to treating rheumatic diseases. In: *Clinical Rheumatology: Scientific basis of rheumatology.* 18:31–45.

Dinarello CA, Moldawer LL (2000) *Proinflammatory and anti-inflammatory cytokines in Rheumatoid Arthritis.* Amgen. California.

Edwards JCW, Szcsepanski L, Sxechinski J *et al.* (2004). Efficacy of B cell targeted therapy with rituximab in patients with rheumatoid arthritis. *The New England Journal of Medicine* (35):2572–2581.

Fujisawa Ltd (2002) Fujisawa Ltd: Tacrolimus: *Summary of Product Characteristics.* www.medicines.org.uk (3 June 2004).

Furst DE (1999) Practical clinical pharmacology and drug interactions of low dose methotrexate therapy in rheumatoid arthritis. *British Journal of Rheumatology* 34(suppl 2):20–25.

Ganong WF (1995) *Circulating Body Fluids. Review of Medical Physiology* 17th ed. 473:489. McGraw Hill, Appleton and Lange.

Gerards AH, de Lathouder S, de Groot *et al.* (2003) Inhibition of cytokine production by methotrexate. Studies in healthy volunteers and patients with rheumatoid arthritis. *Rheumatology* 42(10):1189–1196.

GlaxoSmithKline UK (2003) Azathioprine: *Summary of Product Characteristics.* www.medicines.org.uk (3 June 2004).

Hoffbrand AV, Pettit JE (1993) *Essential Haematology* 3rd edn. Oxford, Blackwell Scientific Publications.

Isenberg D, Morrow J (1995) *Friendly Fire: Explaining Auto-immune Disease*. Oxford, Oxford University Press.

Jansen LM, van Schaardenbury D, Van der Horsrt Bruinsma *et al*. (2003) The predictive value of anti-cyclic citrullinated peoptide antibodies in early arthritis. *Journal of Rheumatology* 30(8):1691–1691.

Jasmer RM, Nahid P, Hopewell PC (2002).Clinical practice. Latent tuberculosis infection. *New England Journal of Medicine* 34(23):1860–1866.

Kaufmann SEH (2002) Protection against tuberculosis: cytokines, T cells and macrophages. *Annals of the Rheumatic Diseases* 61(suppl II):ii54–ii58.

Kitas GD, Erb N (2003) Tackling ischaemic heart disease in rheumatoid arthritis. *Rheumatology* 42(5):607–613.

Klareskog L, van der Heijde D, Jager JP *et al*. (2004) Therapeutic effect of the combination of etanercept and methotrexate compared with each treatment alone in patients with rheumatoid arthritis; double blind randomised controlled trial. *The Lancet* 363:675–681.

Lock C, Oksenberg J, Steinman L (1999) The role of TNFa and lymphotoxin in demyelinating disease. *Annals of the Rheumatic Diseases* 58(suppl I):1121–1128.

Machold KP, Smolen JS (2003) Adalimumab – a new TNF-a antibody for treatment of inflammatory joint disease. *Expert Opinion Biological Therapy* 3(2):351–360.

Maddison PJ (2002) *Rheumatic diseases associated with antinuclear antibodies*. Topical Reviews, Chesterfield, Arthritis Research Campaign.

Maini RN, Feldmann M (2000) *TNFa antagonism and Rheumatoid Arthritis*. London, Science Press.

Male D (1998) *Immunology*: An Illustrated Outline 3rd Ed. London, Mosby.

McEntegart A, Capell HA, Creran D *et al*. (2001) Cardiovascular risk factors, including thrombotic variables in a population with rheumatoid arthritis. *Rheumatology* 40(6):640–644.

Merck Manual (2004) The Merck Manual: *Immunology and Therapies* Chapter 146: Section 12. www.merck.com (9 May 2004).

Mpofu S, Fatima F, Moots RJ (2004) Anti-TNFa therapies: they are all the same (aren't they?) *Rheumatology*. www.rheumatology.org (23 November 2004).

National Institute of Clinical Excellence (2002) *Rituximab for aggressive non-hodgkins lymphoma*. London, NICE. www.nice.org.uk (7 June 2004).

O'Dowd LC (2004) *Anaphylaxis*. www.UpToDate.com

Oliver S, Mooney J (2002) Targeted therapies for patients with rheumatoid arthritis. *Professional Nurse* 17(12):716–780.

Oliver S (2003) The immune system and new therapies for inflammatory joint disease. *Musculoskeletal Care* 1(1):44–57.

Panayi G (1994) *Basic science of immunology* 1:1–12. Medical Imprint, London.

Pisetsky DS (2000) Tumour necrosis factor blockers in rheumatoid arthritis. *New England Journal of Medicine* 342(11):808–811.

Reparon-Schuijt CC, van Esch WJ, van Kooten C *et al*. (2001) Secretion of anti-citrulline-containing peptide antibody by B lymphocytes in rheumatoid arthritis. *Arthritis and Rheumatism* 44(1):41–47.

Robinson WH, Genovese MC, Moreland LW (2001) Demyelinating and neurologic events reported in association with tumour necrosis factor alpha antagonism. *Arthritis and Rheumatism* 44(9):1977–1983.

Roche Pharmaceuticals (2002) Roche Pharmaceutical: Rituximab: *Summary of Product Characteristics*. www.medicines.org.uk (7 June 2004).

Rote NS (2000) Immunity. In: Huether SE, McCance KL (eds); *Understanding Pathophysiology*. St Louis, Mosby.

Rote NS, Huether SE, McCance KL (2000) Hypersensitivities, infection and immunodeficiencies. In: Huether SE, McCance KL (eds); *Understanding Pathophysiology* 2nd edn. St Louis, Mosby, 180–220.

Sanofi Synthelab (2003) Sanofi Synthelabo: *Sulphasalazine (Salazopyrin) Summary of Product Characteristics*. www.medicines.org.uk (7 June 2004).

Sanofi Synthelab (2003) Sanofi Synthelabo: Hydroxychloroquine (Plaquenil) *Summary of Product Characteristics*. www.medicines.org.uk (7 June 2004).

Schering Plough (2003) *Summary of Product Characteristics*: Infliximab 30th May. Schering Plough.www.medicines.org.uk (7 June 2004).

Seibold JR (1995) Clinical features of systemic sclerosis. In: Klippel JH, Dieppe PA (eds). *Practical Rheumatology*. London, Mosby.

Shaw T, Quan J, Totoritis MC (2003) B cell therapy for rheumatoid arthritis; the rituximab (anti-CD20) experience. *Annals of the Rheumatic Diseases* 62(suppl II): ii55–ii59.

Silverman GJ, Carson DA (2003). Roles of B cells in Rheumatoid Arthritis. *Arthritis Research Therapy* 5(supply 4):S1–S6. www.arthritis-research.com (3 June 2004).

Slot O (2001) Changes in plasma homocysteine in arthritis patients starting treatment with low-dose methotrexate subsequently supplemented with folic acid. *Scandanavian Journal of Rheumatology* 30:305–307.

Torre-Amione G, Stetson SS, Farmer JA (1999) Clinical implications of tumour necrosis factor alpha antagonism in patients with congestive heart failure. *Annals of the Rheumatic Diseases* 58(suppl I):1103–1106.

Vittecoq O, Pouplin S, Krazanowska K *et al.* (2003). Rheumatoid factor is the strongest predictor of radiological progression of rheumatoid arthritis in a three year prospective study in community recruited patients. *Rheumatology* 42(8):939–946.

Watts R, Scott DGI (2003) Primary Systemic Vasculitis. Rheumatic Diseases: *Topical Reviews* (11), Chesterfield, Arthritis Research Campaign. www.arc.org.uk (22 October 2004).

Weinblatt ME (1995) Efficacy of methotrexate in rheumatoid arthritis. *British Journal of Rheumatology* 34(suppl 2):43–48.

Weinblatt M, Kremer JM, Bankhurst AD *et al.*.(1999) A trial of etanercept, a recombinant tumour necrosis factor receptor Fc fusion protein, in patients with rheumatoid arthritis receiving methotrexate. *New England Journal of Medicine* (340)4:253–259.

World Health Organisation (2003) *1st International review meeting; practical approaches to lung health strategy*. Rabat Morocco. Geneva, World Health Organisation. www.who.int (May 2004).

4 Biochemical, Haematological and Clinical Assessments in the Rheumatic Diseases

J. HILL
University of Leeds, West Yorkshire, UK

The aim of this chapter is to describe the most commonly used biochemical and clinical methods of assessment used in the rheumatic diseases. After reading this chapter the reader should be able to:

- understand the meaning of common haematological and biochemical tests used in rheumatology;
- describe a variety of standard clinical assessment tools in current use;
- discuss their value in following the course of disease and efficacy of treatment;
- demonstrate understanding of how such tools can be used to monitor and audit delivery of care.

The most obvious need for assessment is to monitor the progress of disease and assess the efficacy of treatment, but this is only one part of the requirement. The development of generalist and biologics nurse-led rheumatology clinics, compounded with financial restraints, makes it imperative that nurses evaluate their effectiveness. It is also important that we know how the patient actually feels, rather than how health professionals think they should feel on the basis of clinical and biochemical tests. This means that measurement should not focus only on assessing disease process by biochemical means, but should incorporate areas such as anxiety, depression and all the facets of the quality of a person's life.

HAEMATOLOGICAL AND BIOCHEMICAL TESTS AND INVESTIGATIONS

There are many tests and investigations used in rheumatology and some of those used most frequently are described here. It is important to appreciate that ranges of values that are considered normal may differ between hospitals and from consultant to consultant.

HAEMOGLOBIN (HB)

This test measures the concentration of oxygen-carrying protein in blood cells and so provides a measure of the oxygen-carrying capacity of blood (Kee, 1987). The normal ranges are 13.5–18g/dl in males and 11.5–16.5g/dl in females (McGhee, 1993). Patients with rheumatoid arthritis often suffer from normocytic, normochromic anaemia, the more severe the disease activity the more severe the anaemia. If the disease comes under control, the anaemia disappears. Other problems associated with arthritis include blood loss from taking nonsteroidal anti-inflammatory drugs and in some cases poor nutrition (Chapter 10).

WHITE BLOOD COUNT (LEUCOCYTES)

Leucocytes can be divided into two groups:

* polymorphonuclear leucocytes, comprising neutrophils, eosinophils and basophils;
* mononuclear leucocytes, comprising monocytes and lymphocytes.

The role that leucocytes play in immunity is discussed in Chapter 3.

The normal range of the total white blood cell count is $4.9–10.0 \times 10^9/l$. A decrease in the count can be caused by drug therapy and a low level is found in systemic lupus erythematosus and Felty's syndrome. Conversely, an elevated white cell count can be present in rheumatoid arthritis, gout, fever and acute infections (Kee, 1987; McGhee, 1993).

PLATELET COUNT

The main function of platelets is in the process of blood clotting. When the level is low it is known as thrombocytopenia. This can occur in autoimmune diseases, with platelet antibody formation, for example in systemic lupus erythematosus. In some inflammatory conditions such as rheumatoid arthritis, the level can be found to be high, when it is known as thrombocytosis (Weller, 1989). The normal range is $150–400 \times 10^9/l$ (McGhee, 1993).

ERYTHROCYTE SEDIMENTATION RATE (ESR)

The erythrocyte sedimentation rate is an indirect measurement of acute phase reactants and so is commonly used to assess disease activity in rheumatic disease (Maclean et al., 1991). Unfortunately, the ESR is nonspecific and can be affected by age, sex and physiological factors. It can produce positive findings in people who are healthy or have illnesses such as anaemia (Wener, 2001).

The test is undertaken by placing blood in a 100 mm capillary tube and leaving it to settle for an hour. The sedimentation of the red cells is related to the quantity of acute phase proteins synthesized by the liver. When the acute phase response is high, the ESR reading will be high and this helps to distinguish an inflammatory from a degenerative disease (Ryan S, 1999). The normal ranges are 4–20 mm/hr in males and 10–25 mm/hr in females (Bird et al., 1985). The ESR is elevated in diseases such as:

- rheumatoid arthritis
- ankylosing spondylitis
- polymyalgia rheumatica
- systemic connective tissue disorders
- acute gout
- psoriatic arthritis
- reactive and infective arthritis.

C REACTIVE PROTEIN (CRP)

When inflammation occurs, the liver and other protein synthesizing tissues increase the production of acute phase reactants including C reactive protein. In the presence of inflammation the concentration of CRP rises rapidly and may increase by a factor of 100 or more, and importantly, these changes can be measured in the serum. CRP also returns to normal more quickly than the ESR and is not affected by anaemia. This makes CRP a useful measurement to monitor disease activity and the effectiveness of drug therapy in inflammatory rheumatic diseases. In systemic lupus erythematosus and Sjögren's syndrome, the CRP can be normal even when the ESR is raised and the disease is active (Kee, 1987; Maclean, 1991). The normal range is 0–8 (mg/l) (McGhee, 1993).

PLASMA VISCOSITY (PV)

Plasma viscosity is often used in preference to the erythrocyte sedimentation rate. It is raised when the erythrocyte sedimentation rate is raised due to an increased concentration of proteins. Plasma viscosity is found to be raised in inflammatory conditions and in paraproteinuraemias such as myeloma (Evans, 1981). The normal range is 1.50–1.72 cp (Weller, 1989).

RHEUMATOID FACTOR

Rheumatoid factor is an IgM/IgG complex. It is found in the blood of 40% of people with early rheumatoid arthritis and eventually 70%–80% will become rheumatoid factor positive. Those who have rheumatoid arthritis and remain rheumatoid-factor negative are said to have seronegative rheumatoid arthritis. These patients tend to have a better outcome in terms of disease severity and disability than those with a high titre of rheumatoid factor.

There are a number of techniques used to test for rheumatoid factor. Some laboratories use an agglutination test using sheep's red blood cells or latex particles coated with IgG. This is reacted with the patient's serum. The particles or cells will agglutinate or clump together if IgM rheumatoid factor is positive. The test result is provided as a titre as the serum is diluted until visible agglutination occurs; the higher the titre the more active the disease. For instance, a typical Rose Waaler agglutination test result is expressed as 1:32, 1:64, 1:128 and so on. The first result is probably not significant but the latter are, and as the numbers increase, more severe disease is indicated.

A more up-to-date technique has been developed using a machine called a nephelometer. This instrument measures the amount of light scattered by a beam passing through a solution. A typical significant positive result using nephelometric techniques is 50 IU/ml (Wener, 2001).

It should be remembered that being rheumatoid-factor positive is not diagnostic of rheumatoid arthritis. About 4% of the health population produce false positives and other rheumatic diseases and diseases such as tuberculosis and bacterial endocarditis may all produce positive results (Wener, 2001).

ANTINUCLEAR ANTIBODIES (ANA)

Antinuclear antibodies are commonly seen in autoimmune rheumatic diseases and the test is regularly used in the diagnosis of the autoimmune collagen disease, systemic lupus erythematosus. However, ANA can occur in systemic sclerosis, Sjögren's syndrome, polymyositis and in low titre in rheumatoid arthritis.

The immunoglobulins IgM, IgG and IgA are the antinuclear antibodies that react with the nuclear part of leucocytes forming antibodies to deoxyribonucleic acid (DNA) and ribonucleic acid (RNA) and others (Kee, 1987). A technique known as immunofluoresence is used to detect their presence. ANA titres of less than 1:80 are considered to be less clinically significant than those of higher titre (Wener, 2001). Values of 1:200 or more in the presence of antiDNA antibodies are likely to confirm the diagnosis of lupus (Ryan, 1999).

This test is useful in the diagnosis of systemic lupus erythematosus where it is found to be positive in approximately 95% of patients. It is also positive in 40%–50% of patients with rheumatoid arthritis, 70%–90% of those with Sjögren's syndrome and 80% of people with systemic sclerosis. Antinuclear antibodies can also occur in patients with:

- mixed connective tissue disease
- myositis
- juvenile chronic arthritis.

ANA has also been detected in the relatives of patients with systemic lupus erythematosus. In the healthy population, the incidence of ANA increases in older adults and can be affected by certain drugs (Kee, 1987; Maclean *et al.*, 1991; McGhee, 1993).

COMPLEMENT

The complement system plays an important part in boosting the inflammatory process and fighting infection, and raised complement levels are found in many inflammatory rheumatic diseases. Three common measurements of serum complement are C3, C4 and CH_{50}. The latter is a biologic measure of the entire complementary pathways. A raised C3 and normal C4 indicate an acute phase response. A raised or normal C4 occurs in rheumatoid arthritis. Low C3 and/or C4 can suggest systemic lupus erythematosus, rheumatoid arthritis and other connective tissue disorders or a glomerulonephritis caused by immune complex disease (Bird *et al.*, 1985; Kee, 1987; Maclean *et al.*, 1991; Weller, 1989). Normal values are: C3, 0.63–1.70g/l; and C4, 0.11–0.45g/l (McGhee, 1993).

SERUM URIC ACID

Hyperuricaemia is the term generally used to describe an elevated serum uric acid level. In the body, uric acid is produced as a by-product of purine metabolism or oxidation. Gout is the most common condition caused by hyperuricaemia. As well as elevated levels in the patient's blood, urates or salts may crystallise to form deposits (Tophi) in joints and tissues. They also form insoluble stones in the urinary tract (Kee, 1987; Weller, 1989).

Hyperuricaemia is defined as a serum uric acid level of more than 0.42mmol/l (>7mg/dl) in men, and 0.36mmol/l (>6g/dl) in women (Jordan, 2004).

HUMAN LEUCOCYTE ANTIGEN (HLA B27)

Human leucocyte antigens play an important role in determining the genetic predisposition to autoimmune diseases. HLA B27 is found to be positive in 95% of patients with ankylosing spondylitis, 80% of those with Reiter's syndrome and in juvenile chronic polyarthritis. It is also positive in 5% of the normal population (Arnett, 1994).

ALKALINE PHOSPHATASE

Alkaline phosphatase is an enzyme found localised on cell membranes that hydrolyses phosphate esters liberating inorganic phosphate. It is produced mostly in bone and in the liver and is therefore a useful test in diagnosing liver and bone diseases. In bone disorders, abnormal osteoblastic activity or bone cell production causes elevated levels. It is elevated in Paget's disease, osteitis deformans, osteomalacia and active rheumatoid arthritis (Bird *et al.*, 1985). Normal range is 100–300IU/l.

BENCE-JONES PROTEIN

This protein is of low molecular weight and can be found in the urine of patients with multiple myeloma, other bone tumours, hyperparathyroidism, amyloidosis, leukaemia and metastatic carcinoma. This test requires a specimen of urine for laboratory analysis (Bird *et al.*, 1985).

CLINICAL ASSESSMENTS

Nurses undertake many clinical assessments during the course of their care, and so it is important that they understand the usefulness and reason for undertaking this activity. The most important point to remember is to choose the right assessment tool for the job! The choice of tool for use in rheumatology nursing clinics has been well-described by Hewlett (2004).

Hill (1991) has stated that a good clinical assessment should fulfill a number of criteria including:

- accurate detection of small changes
- demonstrate the trends of change
- be quick and easy to use
- not involve expensive equipment
- be scientifically sound and well-validated.

In addition to measuring the activity and progress of the disease and the efficacy or nonefficacy of treatment, it is necessary to assess the effect that the disease actually has on the patient. Therefore a number of different assessment tools are described that assess all aspects of a patients life.

ASSESSING PAIN

Pain is a complex and individual response, making it extremely difficult to assess. Seers (1989) considers that its complexity should be seen as a challenge, not an obstacle. The nurse's perception of pain may differ from that of the patient and several studies have demonstrated that nurses underestimate the degree of pain experienced by the patient (Seers, 1989; Bondestam *et al.*, 1987). In order to treat pain effectively, it is essential to assess it accurately.

A detailed discussion of pain is included in Chapter 8, but the following are some examples of pain assessment measures that can be used both for judging the need for intervention and monitoring the efficacy of those interventions.

Visual analogue scale (VAS)

A visual analogue scale is shown in Figures 4.1a and b. It comprises a 10 cm long horizontal line. It is marked at each end with a marker and a descriptor. For example, for the measurement of pain it could read 'no pain' at one end, and 'pain as severe as it could be' or 'intolerable pain' at the other. The patient is asked to place a mark on the line to illustrate the level of pain experienced over a given period of time, for example during the past seven days. The distance of the mark from the end of the scale is then measured in centimetres to provide a measure of pain experienced.

Patients often find the concept of the visual analogue scale difficult to grasp initially, and they tend to place their marks towards either end of the scale, particularly to the left (Hill, 1991). Their understanding can be assisted by adding such indications as 'slight', 'moderate' and 'severe' along the 10 cm line, as shown in Figure 4.1b.

Bird *et al.* (1985) have stated that patients appear to relate more easily to a descriptive scale, such as that shown in Figure 4.1c. This one-to-five scale is graded from 'no pain' through to 'unbearable pain'.

Body map

A body map is shown in Figure 4.2. A 10 cm visual analogue scale or five-point descriptive scale can be combined with a body map to indicate the area and severity of pain. Many pain assessment charts and questionnaires have been developed combining the above tools with descriptive words and records of interventions, both pharmaceutical and nonpharmaceutical. Examples of these include the London Hospital Pain Observations chart (cited by Raiman, 1986) and the McGill Pain Questionnaire (Melzack, 1975). The latter was revisited by Jamieson (1988). Although not specifically designed for patients with rheumatoid disease, they are useful and well-validated tools, and have been used unmodified in rheumatic diseases. They could form a basis from which to develop more specific questionnaires and assessments.

Daily diary cards

A simple daily diary card as seen in Figure 4.3 can be filled in by the patient at home or hospital. It has several advantages including that it:

- provides necessary data for the management of the disease;
- serves as a basis for discussion and planning future interventions;
- enables the patient to be an active participant in treatment and decision making;
- forms an invaluable educational tool, allowing the patient to identify those factors which influence their symptoms.

A diary card should include:

- a simple pain scale;
- a record of analgesia required, in addition to regular medication;
- space to record what made the pain worse and what reduced it;
- space to record duration of morning stiffness.

a. 10 cm visual analogue scale

No Pain I---I Intolerable Pain

b. 10 cm visual analogue scale (with added indications)

No Pain I---I Intolerable Pain

          Slight   Moderate   Severe

c. descriptive scale

    [1]   No Pain

    [2]   Mild Pain

    [3]   Moderate Pain

    [4]   Severe Pain

    [5]   Unbearable Pain

Figure 4.1 Pain scales.

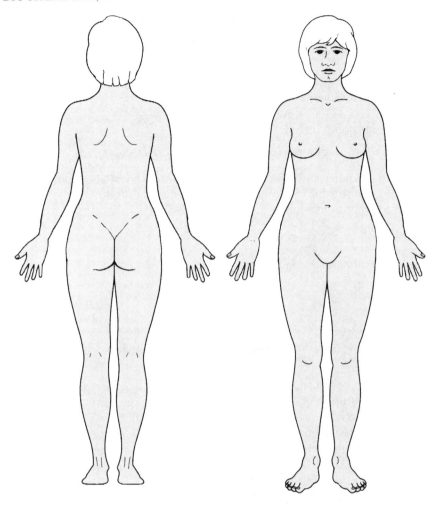

Instructions:
Please put an 'X' on the obove body outline where you feel pain.
Put 'O' after the 'X' if you feel the pain is on the outside of your body.
Put 'I' after the 'X' if it is an internal pain.

Figure 4.2 Body map.

EARLY MORNING STIFFNESS

A daily diary card can also be used to assess early morning stiffness as can a simple question such as 'How long does your morning stiffness last?' The latter has the advantage of speed. However, it can be misleading if the patient is having an exceptionally good or bad day.

Instructions: Please fill in the diary each day. Record the worst pain that you feel by circling one of the numbers.

1 = no pain
2 = mild pain
3 = moderate pain
4 = severe pain
5 = very severe pain

Please write down any activity that causes or increases your pain and anything that relieves it.

Please write down the number of painkillers that you take every day.

DATE	PAIN Circle one of these numbers	WHAT CAUSES YOUR PAIN? WHAT RELIEVES YOUR PAIN?	NUMBER OF PAIN KILLERS
	1 2 3 4 5		
	1 2 3 4 5		
	1 2 3 4 5		
	1 2 3 4 5		
	1 2 3 4 5		
	1 2 3 4 5		
	1 2 3 4 5		
	1 2 3 4 5		
	1 2 3 4 5		

Figure 4.3 Pain diary.

Stiffness has been used as an assessment of disease activity for many years and it is the duration of the stiffness rather than its intensity that correlates with disease activity (Hill, 1991). Steinberg (1978) defines stiffness as 'the discomfort or restriction perceived by the patient when attempting the first part of an easy movement of a joint, after a period of inactivity. For some patients, stiffness is a sensation of no greater discomfort than the sensation that the fingers contain too much fluid.'

Morning stiffness can create many difficulties for the patient; some report having to get up much earlier than the rest of the family in order to prepare for the day; washing, dressing and breakfasting can all take longer. Because of this, the implications of early morning stiffness must be considered during a hospital admission, particularly when planning such activities as physiotherapy and occupational therapy assessments. A slow release anti-inflammatory medication taken late in the previous evening, a warm shower first thing in the morning, as well as gentle massage can all be helpful.

Initially patients may find the duration of early morning stiffness difficult to judge and some find it difficult to differentiate between pain and stiffness. Consequently, some patients may require encouragement when first using a diary card, until they gain the confidence that they can record consistent data.

A more detailed discussion of stiffness is given in Chapter 8.

GRIP STRENGTH

The appearance of the hand is not always a true indicator of functional ability. The patient with a hand that is devastated and disorganised by disease activity has often learned strategies of maintaining some grip, whereas an apparently normal hand can have its grip weakened by painful joints. This can lead not only to difficulties with activities of living, but can also have safety implications.

Grip strength is measured using a dynamo-sphygmomanometer. A small bag, similar to a sphygmomanometer cuff is attached to a mercury manometer graduated from 20–300 mm Hg. The bag is inflated to a pre-determined pressure, usually 20 or 30 mm Hg, to ensure that it is comfortable for the patient to grip. The patient is then asked to squeeze the bag with one hand whilst holding the elbow away from the body. The peak pressure is recorded. Peak pressure is used in preference to sustained pressure, as the latter would possibly cause the patient more discomfort. The exercise is repeated with the other hand.

It is advised that three readings are taken from each hand and the mean pressure is recorded. Ideally, to avoid discrepancies, the recordings should be taken at approximately the same time of day, as diurnal variations can occur. To avoid observer variations, the same assessor should perform the test each time, using the same equipment.

There is no normal range of grip strength, although a healthy adult has no problem obtaining readings of over 300 mm Hg. A person with hands affected by rheumatoid disease may record readings as low as 30–40 mm Hg during periods of high disease activity.

Once a baseline for a particular patient is established, serial improvement can be demonstrated when treatment is effective.

ARTICULAR INDICES

Articular indices are used to assess inflammatory activity, usually in rheumatoid arthritis. The earliest index was the Ritchie Articular Index (Ritchie *et al.*, 1968), but this has been largely superseded by the 28 joint count (Fuchs *et al.*, 1989).

Ritchie Articular Index

The Ritchie Articular Index can be a valuable tool as it incorporates so many joints that it can highlight specific problem areas throughout the body. On the down side, it takes much longer to perform than the 28-joint count. Unfortunately, extra pain may be inflicted when this assessment is carried out, so it is essential that a full explanation is given to the patient.

The assessment of tenderness is undertaken by applying firm pressure over the joint margin. In the cervical spine, the hips, the talo-calcaneal joints and the midtarsal joints, the application of firm pressure is impracticable, and so passive movement is used. The patient's response to pressure on the joint margin is scored as follows:

- No pain or tenderness is reported – 0.
- The patient says that pain is felt – 1.
- The patient feels pain and winces – 2.
- The patient feels pain, winces and withdraws the joint – 3.

The following joints are treated as single units for scoring purposes:

- temporomandibular joints
- cervical spine
- sternoclavicular joints
- acromioclavicular joints
- metacarpophalangeal joints of each hand
- proximal interphalangeal joints of each hand
- metatarsophalangeal joints of each foot.

The highest scoring joint from each unit is taken as the score for the whole of that unit. The maximum possible is 78. However a score of 30 or more is considered high, and indicates that reassessment of all therapies is required.

Disease activity score (DAS 28)

The DAS 28 is a measurement of disease activity and comprises both objective and subjective indices (Prevoo *et al.*, 1995). This composite score includes:

- the number of tender joints (subjective);
- the number of swollen joints (objective);
- the patient's global assessment of their well-being (subjective);
- erythrocyte sedimentation rate (objective).

It is assessed by the application of firm pressure around the margin of the following joints:

- shoulders
- elbows
- wrists
- metacarpophalangeal joints
- proximal interphalangeal joints
- knees.

Swelling is also assessed separately. Both swelling and tenderness are scored as being either absent (0) or present (1). The score (0–28) for each symptom is then totalled.

This DAS 28 is calculated in the following way:

$$DAS\ 28 = 0.555\sqrt{(28\ \text{tender joint count})} + 0.284\sqrt{(28\ \text{swollen joint count})}$$
$$+ 0.70\ln(ESR) + 0.0142(\text{patient global assessment})$$

This is obviously not a straightforward equation and there are handheld calculators and computer programmes available to make the task easier. Scores can range from 0–9.07, assuming that an ESR of 100 is taken as the upper limit.

Levels of disease activity are defined as:

- mild disease activity – DAS 28 ≤3.2
- moderate disease activity – DAS 28 >3.2 and ≤5.1
- severe disease activity – DAS 28 >5.1.

The DAS 28 is an important assessment as it can be used in large studies and in clinical practice (Van Riel and Schumacher, 2001). It can also be used to assess change longitudinally, by comparing scores over two or more time points (Harth and Pope, 2004). However, the DAS 28 really came to prominence with the introduction of biologic therapies. These new drugs are tenfold more expensive than the previous most expensive agents, £10–£12,000 per patient per year. In 2000, the British Society for Rheumatology produced clinical guidelines (BSR, 2000) recommending thresholds for starting therapy and, for those who responded, continuing their therapy (Griffiths *et al.*, 2004). The DAS 28 was the index used to assess disease activity and response. In 2002, the National Institute for Clinical Excellence (NICE) approved the use of etanercept and infliximab, recommending the use of the BSR guidelines.

To be eligible for a biologic agent the patient must have:

- failed to respond to two disease-modifying anti-rheumatic drugs;
- one of the drugs must be methotrexate;
- treatment should have been at a sufficient dose for a sufficient period of time for it to become efficacious, except when severe side effects had prevented this happening;
- a DAS 28 score >5.1 taken on two consecutive occasions and assessed one month apart.

Response to antiTNFα therapy is known to be rapid and efficacy should be seen within three months. The criteria for improvement are either:

- the DAS 28 score should have decreased by at least 1.2 points compared to the last score; or
- the DAS 28 score should be >3.2.

If this has not occurred, the drug is deemed to have failed and the biologic discontinued.

THE STANFORD HEALTH ASSESSMENT
QUESTIONNAIRE (HAQ)

The HAQ measures function by assessment of the activities of daily living. It was devised and evaluated by Fries *et al.* (1980). It includes five categories of measures:

- death
- disability
- discomfort (pain)
- drug toxicity
- dollar cost.

It has been modified for use in other countries, including Britain (Kirwan and Reeback, 1986). It contains twenty questions and includes a 15 cm visual analogue pain scale. It provides a format for assessment of current disability, progress of disability and improvement in ability.

The twenty questions are divided into eight categories:

- dressing/grooming
- arising
- eating
- walking
- hygiene
- reach
- grip
- activities.

The patient is asked to tick the answer which best describes their usual ability over the past week, and to indicate if any aids are used or help required from another person.

The replies are scored as follows:

- without difficulty – 0
- with some difficulty – 1
- with much difficulty – 2
- unable to do – 3.

The score for an individual item is adjusted when assistive devices or help from another person is required. For example, if the answer to the question 'Can you dress yourself?' is 'with some difficulty' the score is 1. However, if the use of dressing devices is indicated, this score is increased to 2. The highest score within any category determines the score for that category. The total functional ability index is calculated by adding the scores of each category and dividing by the total number of categories answered. This gives a final score in the 0–3 range with higher scores indicating higher levels of disability. The 15 cm Visual Analogue Scale is measured from the left-hand side, and the result divided by 5, to give a score in the 0–3 range.

The information gained from the responses to individual sections on this questionnaire enables the care team to plan which are the most appropriate treatments to introduce. The need for occupational therapist and physiotherapist input may be indicated, as may intervention from other agencies. It is also a useful tool when supporting patients applying for social, domestic and financial assistance and benefits. When used at initial diagnosis, it provides a baseline, and the efficacy or otherwise of a period of inpatient treatment can be demonstrated by comparing scores on admission and discharge or subsequent follow-up appointments.

As well as being a practical outcome measure and an evaluation tool, the health assessment questionnaire is widely accepted as a research tool.

THE ARTHRITIS IMPACT MEASUREMENT SCALES (AIMS)

The AIMS combine function, pain and psychological assessments within one questionnaire (Meenan *et al.*, 1980) and has been used in many countries worldwide. Hill *et al.* (1990) modified it for use in the UK. Forty-five questions form the basic scales, measuring:

- mobility
- physical activity
- activities of daily living
- pain
- anxiety
- depression.

An additional three items are useful for obtaining general estimates of health status and there are further questions to assist in assessing general health perceptions. The final item is a Visual Analogue Scale to estimate the overall impact of arthritis on the patient. This makes a total of 53 items on the questionnaire, but if required, further items can be added concerning use of medication, comorbidity and demographic data.

The questionnaire is self-administered and takes 10–15 minutes to complete. Scoring also takes 10–15 minutes. The range of possible scores in a given scale depends on the number of items included in that scale, so a normalisation procedure is performed, so that all scores are expressed in the 0–10 range, with 0 representing good health status, and 10 representing poor status.

Each of the basic scales can be used alone or in combination, depending on which are most appropriate to the user's needs.

There is a short form AIMS 2 also available (Meenan *et al.*, 1992), but this has not been validated for use in the UK.

HOSPITAL ANXIETY AND DEPRESSION SCALE (HAD)

Psychological well-being is an important dimension when looking at quality of life. (Chapter 5). Studies indicate that people with rheumatoid disease have a higher incidence of depression than the general population (DeVellis, 1993). The Hospital Anxiety and Depression Scale is an instrument developed in the UK to examine states of depression in a general medical outpatient setting (Zigmond and Snaithe, 1983). It contains seven items on anxiety and seven on depression, with higher scores indicating higher levels of anxiety or depression.

Each question has four response options, in order to discourage the patient from opting for the midpoint. As anxiety may be increased by a clinic visit or hospital admission, the patient is asked to indicate the response that relates most accurately to feelings over the past week. The score is added up using the scoring grid. Anxiety and depression are scored separately.

The Hospital Anxiety and Depression Scale can be used as a tool to assess clinical effectiveness, as a research tool, and also for audit purposes. Although self-report questionnaires are not adequate for diagnosing clinical depression (Rodin *et al.*, 1991), some authors believe that this tool can be useful in guiding treatment, and for giving an indication of when to refer to a clinical psychologist or to seek psychiatric assistance. A score of 8–10 is suggested as borderline, with a score of over 11 indicating the necessity for further intervention.

SELF-EFFICACY

Increasing a patient's self-efficacy is one of the most important outcomes of rheumatology nursing. The reason for this is that patient education is the foundation on which self-care activities are based, and patient education has been shown to be one of the priorities of many clinical nurse specialists (Carr, 2001). The underlying theory supporting patient education is self-efficacy, that is a person's confidence in his/her ability to perform a certain task or achieve a particular objective (Hill and Hale, 2004). The Arthritis Self-Efficacy Scale (ASES) was designed by Lorig (1989) to assess the patient's belief that they can manage their pain, function and other symptoms. It is scored by visual analogue scales anchored at each end with 'very uncertain' or 'very certain'. The visual analogue scales are then measured and the results (1–10) are simply totalled and then averaged. A high score indicates high self-efficacy.

The ASES was designed to be used in patients with any form of arthritis. However, Hewlett *et al.* (2001) has developed a tool specifically for British patients who have RA.

QUALITY OF LIFE (QOL) MEASURES

In the absence of cure, the overall aim of management of chronic, rheumatic diseases must be to improve the quality of the patient's life. At present there is no tool specifically designed to assess the outcome from rheumatology nursing, care but QOL is a reasonable substitute. The RAQOL was developed specifically for use with RA patients. The first stage of the development was undertaken by Whalley *et al.*, (1997); and De Jong *et al.*, (1997) then undertook sensitivity testing. The instrument comprises 30 questions and is completed by yes/no answers (yes = 1 point; no = 0 points). The range is therefore 0–30. The higher the score the worse the patients QoL is deemed to be.

Other well-developed and validated QOL scales are available for people with psoriatic arthritis (McKenna *et al.*, 2004) and ankylosing spondylitis (Doward *et al.*, 2003).

CLINICAL ASSESSMENTS USED FOR SPECIFIC RHEUMATOLOGICAL CONDITIONS

ANKYLOSING SPONDYLITIS

Several assessment strategies are employed when caring for patients with ankylosing spondylitis. A visual analogue scale may be used to assess pain and stiffness.

One of the characteristics of ankylosing spondylitis is chronic enthesitis and the pain this causes. An enthesis index has been developed (Mander *et al.*, 1987) and is a convenient and non-invasive measure of disease severity.

The scoring is based on the patient's response to firm palpation over the enthesis points. Some of the sites are scored as a group, the highest scoring site within that group being the score recorded for the group as a whole. These groups are:

- nuchal crests
- costochondral joints
- sacroiliac joints
- cervical spinal processes
- thoracic spinal processes
- lumbar spinal processes.

The remaining sites are scored individually left and right.

The scoring is as follows:

- no pain – 0
- mild pain – 1
- moderate tenderness – 2
- wince or withdraw – 3.

The total possible score is 90.

To enable the patient to differentiate between the sensation of firm palpation and the discomfort or pain caused by enthesitis, it is suggested that a control point is selected where enthesitis does not occur. The midpoint of the clavicle is an example. The pressure on this point is demonstrated to the patient at the start of the procedure.

The Enthesis Index has been found to correlate with severity of pain and stiffness, and reductions in scores have been demonstrated when the patient is taking nonsteroidal anti-inflammatory medication.

The effects of ankylosing spondylitis on posture can be difficult to quantify. Measurements used include the distance between the wall and the patient's tragus or occiput. Forward flexion of the lumbar spine can be measured by the use of the modification of Schober's technique (McRae, 1969). The lumbar-sacral junction is identified between the dimples of Venus, and with the patient upright, a point is taken 5 cm below this and 10 cm above. The patient is then asked to flex as far forward as possible, and the difference above initial 15 cm separation is noted. This technique measures skin distraction, but this relates to true lumbar flexion. In the healthy spine the distraction will be around 5 cm but in the patient with ankylosing spondylitis this is reduced.

FIBROMYALGIA

The assessment of fatigue and sleep disturbance is discussed in Chapter 9. However, in addition to these problems, patients with fibromyalgia present with several distinct hyperalgesic sites, which may be determined by digital palpation. These sites, which are illustrated in Figure 4.4 are normally uncomfortable to firm pressure, but the patient with fibromyalgia will experience marked tenderness and will wince or withdraw. In addition, negative control points are used where there should be no tenderness, for example the forehead or distal forearm. If tenderness is present wherever the patient is touched the diagnosis may be one of fabrication of symptoms or psychiatric disturbance (Doherty, 1993). For a diagnosis of fibromyalgia to be confirmed, the patient will experience pain at ten or more of the tender points illustrated, in a symmetrical pattern.

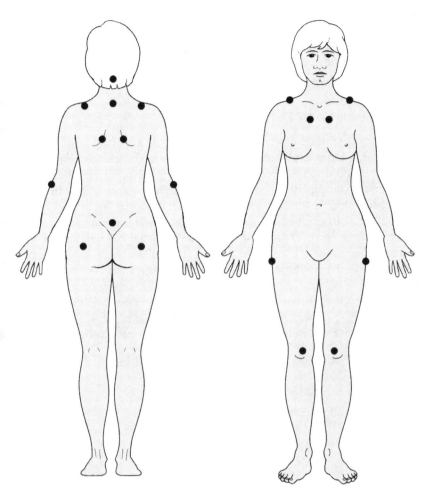

Figure 4.4 Tender points used to assess fibromyalgia.

OSTEOARTHRITIS

The Western Ontario McMaster Universities Arthritis Index (WOMAC) was devised by Bellamy *et al.* (1988). It was developed specifically to measure the clinically-significant, patient-relevant symptoms of osteoarthritis of the hip and knee. It comprises three subscales:

- pain – 5 items
- stiffness – 2 items
- function – 17 items

All the 24 questions relate to the patient's experience over the past 48 hours. There are different versions of this tool available and so scoring depends on which version is used. One uses five-point Likert scales when scoring consists of ticking none, mild, moderate, severe, extreme. Another version uses a visual analogue format.

SYSTEMIC LUPUS ERYTHEMATOSUS

There are several clinical assessment tools available for measuring disease status in systemic lupus erythematosus, but none are sufficiently sensitive or specific to be relied upon entirely (Hay et al., 1993). Because of the variety of clinical manifestations in this disease, the number of specialities involved in its management, and the fact that it is characterised by flares and remissions, it is difficult to evolve one instrument that is not too complicated and unwieldy to be practical. Those tools available are used in conjunction with the laboratory indicators.

The British Isles Lupus Assessment Group (BILAG) index was evolved by a group of British rheumatologists and scores disease activity separately in different organ groups. It has been tested for validity along with other tools (Liang et al., 1989) and was modified by Hay et al. (1991).

The tool comprises 86 items, related to eight organ based systems:

- mucocutaneous
- neurological
- musculoskeletal
- cardiovascular and respiratory
- vasculitic
- renal
- haematological
- other.

The scoring is based on a five-point ordinal scale and each system is scored separately and no total score is produced. If carried out manually, it is a lengthy and time-consuming assessment to complete, but there is now a computer programme available for this purpose (www.limathon.com/BLIPS).

SYSTEMIC SCLEROSIS

There are as yet no internationally agreed standards for assessing disease activity and severity in systemic sclerosis. However a skin score assessment is sometimes used. Work carried out in Denmark (Zachariae et al., 1994) demonstrated that increase in a simple skin score correlated with an increase in Type III procollagen, and thus Type III collagen. The degrees of skin thickening and pliability are judged over each of the following areas:

- face
- anterior chest
- abdomen
- upper arms
- forearms
- dorsum of hand
- fingers
- thighs
- lower legs
- dorsum of feet.

They are scored 0–3 as follows:

- normal skin – 0
- skin which is thickened – 1
- thickened, unable to pinch the skin – 2
- thickened, unable to move the skin (it is tethered) – 3.

OTHER INVESTIGATIONS

JOINT ASPIRATION

Aspiration is the removal of a sample of synovial fluid from a joint, by means of a needle and syringe using a strict aseptic technique. The fluid can be sent for laboratory tests such as microscopy and bacteriology and if required, biochemical analysis. Its appearance gives an indication of diagnosis; for example, in degenerative conditions it is more sticky or viscous. However, it is found to be more dilute in rheumatoid arthritis and other polyarthritides. A polarising microscope can be used to look for crystals such as uric acid or calcium pyrophosphate (Bird *et al.*, 1985; Maclean *et al.*, 1991).

SYNOVIAL FLUID EXAMINATION

This transparent and viscous fluid is found in:

- joint cavities
- bursae
- tendon sheaths.

The synovial membrane that lines joint cavities secretes synovial fluid and its composition is that of connective tissue. Examination of synovial fluid allows diagnosis through detection of crystals or infection (Wener, 2001).

ARTHROSCOPY

Arthroscopy is the examination of the interior of a joint using an optical device called an arthroscope. The most commonly examined joint using this method is the knee. A local or general anaesthetic can be used. A general anaesthetic can allow a more thorough examination and assessment of the:

- menisci
- cruciate ligaments
- loose bodies.

Arthroscopy also allows synovial biopsies to be taken. It is useful in the diagnosis of extrasynovial and synovial diseases and to monitor the progress of disease activity. Joint size can be indicative of the diagnosis. In rheumatoid arthritis and seronegative polyarthritis the joint capacity is often found to be large, whereas in osteoarthritis the joint capacity is often found to be small.

RADIOISOTOPE SCANNING

This technique involves using radioactive substances that are taken up by particular organs, when introduced into the body or a joint, usually intravenously. A scanner is then used to detect the emission of radiation. Radioisotope scans can assist in the early diagnosis of ankylosing spondylitis, the assessment of inflammation, detection of infection, secondary malignant deposits and Paget's disease (Bird *et al.*, 1985).

RADIOGRAPHS (X-RAYS)

Film, specially sensitised to x-rays or gamma rays, is used to make records of internal structures of the body. In rheumatology patients, radiological examination is an integral part of the assessment of clinically affected joints and for consideration of surgical intervention. In early rheumatoid arthritis, feet, hands and wrists are the most usual joints to be examined in this way. They often show early changes, such as soft tissue swelling around an affected joint and enlargement of the joint cavity. In contrast, in osteoarthritis, cartilage is lost and the two bones are found to have moved closer together. In rheumatoid arthritis, later changes can be seen, such as the development of bony erosions (osteopenia) and a decrease in the joint space, with the erosion and loss of cartilage (Bird *et al.*, 1985).

DUAL ENERGY X-RAY ABSORPTIOMETRY (DEXA)

Fracture rate is directly related to bone mineral density (BMD) and DEXA is a safe, noninvasive technique that provides a precise and rapid quantification of the density of bone. DEXA therefore plays an important role in the management of osteoporosis and can also be used to assess future fracture risk (Roy and O'Neill, 2001). Indeed, the Department of Health recommends that individuals who have a high risk of osteoporosis should have access to bone densitometry. The BMD is expressed as a T score or a Z score as follows:

- T score is the difference in standard deviation compared with peak bone mass in young adults of the same sex and race. A score less than −1 is considered to be low and the person osteopenic; a score of less than −2.5, osteoporotic (Wener, 2001).
- Z score is the difference in standard deviation compared with healthy age matched controls of the same sex and race.

Each of the diseases and conditions that affect patients cared for by a rheumatology team has its own set of assessment tools to monitor and record various aspects of disease severity and progress of treatment. In addition, there are many other assessments available for use in planning, monitoring, researching and auditing the care of patients with rheumatoid arthritis. Of necessity, this chapter is not comprehensive and other works describe many more of the outcome measures available (Katz, 2003). However, this chapter describes a range of assessments which will give an indication of disease progress, pain, ability and disability, psychological well-being and quality of life. These assessments will provide a basis for planning interventions and, by serial recording, a demonstration of benefit or otherwise of these interventions. They also have proven validity for use in research.

ACTION POINTS FOR PRACTICE

- A patient is newly diagnosed as having rheumatoid arthritis. Which assessments and measurements would you wish to record as a baseline?
- You are setting up a database of the patients with rheumatoid arthritis cared for by the multiprofessional team. Which assessment tools would you select to provide ongoing information about disease activity, efficacy of treatment, alterations in ability and quality of life? Consider not only those mentioned in this chapter, but also, using the reference and further reading lists, explore other possibilities. Discuss your reasons for making your selection.

ACKNOWLEDGEMENTS

The author would like to thank Jane Douglas and Catherine Sturdy who contributed to the first edition and whose work was combined and updated for this chapter.

REFERENCES

Arnett FC (1994) Histocompatability typing in the rheumatic diseases. *Rheumatic Disease Clinics of North America* 20:371–390.

Bellamy N, Buchanan WW, Goldsmith CH *et al.* (1988) Validation study of WOMAC: a health status instrument for measuring clinically important patient relevant outcomes to antirheumatic drug therapy in patients with osteoarthritis of the hip or knee. *Journal of Rheumatology* 15:1833–1840.

Bird H, Le Gallez P, Hill J (1985) Clinical assessments in rheumatology. In: *Combined Care of the Rheumatic Patient*. Berlin, Springer Verlag, p204.

Bondestam E, Hovgren K, Gaston Johannsen F *et al.* (1987) Pain assessment by patients and nurses in the early phase of myocardial infarction. *Journal of Advanced Nursing* 12:677–682.

British Society for Rheumatology (2000) *New treatments in arthritis: the use of TNFα blockers in adults with rheumatoid arthritis*. London, British Society for Rheumatology.

Carr A (2001) Defining the Extended Clinical Role for Allied Health Professionals in Rheumatology. *Conference Proceedings*, No 12. Chesterfield, Arthritis Research Campaign.

De Jong Z, Van Der Heijde D, McKenna SP *et al.* (1997) The reliability and construct validity of the RAQoL: a rheumatoid arthritis specific quality of life instrument. *British Journal of Rheumatology* 36:878–883.

DeVellis BM (1993) Depression in rheumatological diseases. In: Newman S, Shipley M (eds) *Psychological aspects in rheumatic disease. Bailliere's Clinical Rheumatology*, London, Bailliere Tindall, 7(2):241–258.

Doherty M (1993) Fibromyalgia syndrome. In: *Reports on rheumatic diseases*. Chesterfield, Arthritis and Rheumatism Council.

Doward LC, Spoorenburg A, Whalley D *et al.* (2003) Development of the ASQoL: a quality of life instrument specific to ankylosing spondylitis. *Annals of the Rheumatic Diseases* 62(1):20–26.

Evans DMD (1981) *Special Tests and their Meanings*, 12th edn. London, Faber.

Fries JF, Spitz P, Kraines RG *et al.* (1980) Measurement of patient outcomes in arthritis. *Arthritis and Rheumatism* 23:137–145.

Fuchs HA, Brooks RH, Callahan LF *et al.* (1989) A simplified twenty-eight joint quantitative articular index in rheumatoid arthritis. *Arthritis and Rheumatism* 32:351–357.

Griffiths I, Silman A, Symmonds D *et al.* (2004) BSR Biologics registry. *Rheumatology* 43:1463–1464.

Harth M, Pope J (2004) The measure of our measures. *Rheumatology* 1456–1457.

Hay E, Gordon C, Emery P (1993) Assessment of lupus, where are we now? *Annals of the Rheumatic Diseases* 52:169–172.

Hay EM, Bacon P, Gordon C *et al.* (1991) Development and testing of BILAG index (version 3). *British Journal of Rheumatology* 30:23.

Hewlett S (2004) Nurse clinics: using the right tools for the job. In: Oliver S (ed) *Chronic Disease Nursing – A Rheumatology Example*. London, Whurr Publishers.

Hewlett S, Cockshott ZC, Kirwan JR *et al.* (2001) Development and validation of a self-efficacy scale for use in British patients with rheumatoid arthritis (RASE). *Rheumatology* 40:1221–1230.

Hill J (1991) Assessing rheumatic disease. *Nursing Times* 87(4):33–35.

Hill J, Bird HA, Lawton CW *et al.* (1990) The arthritis impact measurement scales: an anglicised version to assess the outcome of British patients with rheumatoid arthritis. *British Journal of Rheumatology* 29:193–196.

Hill J, Hale C (2004) Clinical skills: evidence-based nursing care of people with rheumatoid arthritis. *British Journal of Nursing* 13(14):852–857.

Jamieson AH (1988) The McGill pain questionnaire thirteen years on. *Journal of Drug Development* 1:8–14.

Jordan K (2004) An update on gout. In: *Topical Reviews*, Chesterfield, 4.

Katz P (2003) Patient outcomes in rheumatology – a review of measures. *Arthritis Care and Research* 49(5-Suppl):S1–233.

Kee JL (1987) *Laboratory and Diagnostic Tests with Nursing Implications* (2nd ed) USA, Appleton and Lange.

Kirwan J, Reeback JS (1986) Stanford health assessment questionnaire modified to assess disability in British patients with rheumatoid arthritis. *British Journal of Rheumatology* 25:206–209.

Liang MH, Socher SA, Larson MG *et al.* (1989) Reliability and validity of six systems for the clinical assessment of disease activity in systemic lupus erythematosus. *Arthritis and Rheumatism* 32:1107–1118.

Lorig K, Chastain R, Ung E *et al.* (1989) Development and evaluation of a scale to measure perceived self-efficacy in people with arthritis. *Arthritis and Rheumatism* 32:37–44.

Mander M, Simpson JM, McLellan A *et al.* (1987) Studies with an enthesis index as a method of clinical assessment in ankylosing spondylitis. *Annals of the Rheumatic Diseases* 46:197–202.

Maclean D, Bateson M, Pennington C (1991) *Lecture notes on clinical investigation*. London, Blackwell Scientific Publications.

McRae IF, Wright V (1969) Measurement of back movement. *Annals of the Rheumatic Diseases* 28:584–593.

McGhee M (1993) *A Guide to Laboratory Investigations*, 2nd edn. Oxford, Radcliffe Medical Press.

McKenna SP, Doward LC, Whalley D *et al.* (2004) Development of the PsAQoL: quality of life instrument specific to psoriatic arthritis. *Annals of the Rheumatic Diseases* 63(2):162–169.

Meenan RF, Gertman P, Mason J (1980) Measuring health status in arthritis. *Arthritis and Rheumatism* 23(2):146–152.

Meenan RF, Mason JH, Anderson JJ *et al.* (1992) AIMS 2. The content and properties of the revised and expanded Arthritis Impact Measurement Scales health status questionnaire. *Arthritis and Rheumatism* 35:1–10.

Melzack R (1975) The McGill pain questionnaire: major properties and scoring systems. *Pain* 1:277–299.

National Institute of Clinical Excellence (2002) Guidance on the use of etanercept and infliximab for the treatment of rheumatoid arthritis. *Health Technology Guidance*. No 36. London, National Institute for Clinical Excellence.

Prevoo MLL, van't Hof MA, Kuper HH *et al.* (1995) Modified disease activity scores that include a 28 joint count. Development and validation in a prospective longitudinal study of patients with rheumatoid arthritis. *Arthritis and Rheumatism* 38(1):44–48.

Raiman J (1986) Towards understanding pain and planning for relief. In: *Nursing 11.* London, Bailliere Tindall, p411–422.

Ritchie D, Boyle J, McInnes J *et al.* (1968) Clinical studies with an articular index for the assessment of joint tenderness in patients with rheumatoid arthritis. *Quarterly Journal of Medicine* 147:393–406.

Rodin G, Craven J, Littlefield C (1991) *Depression in the medically ill an integrated approach.* New York, Brunner Mazel.

Roy D, O'Neill T (2001) Corticosteroid-induced osteoporosis – prevention and treatment. *Rheumatic Disease In Practice.* Chesterfield, Arthritis Research Campaign.

Ryan S (1999) The role of the rheumatology nurse. In: Ryan S (ed): *Drug Therapy in Rheumatology Nursing.* London, Whurr Publishers.

Seers K (1989) Assessing pain. *Nursing Standard* 3(15):33–35.

Steinberg AD (1978) On morning stiffness. *Journal of Rheumatology* 5:3–7.

Van Riel PL, Schumacher HR Jr (2001) How does one assess early rheumatoid arthritis in daily clinical practice? *Best Practice Research in Clinical Rheumatology* 15:67–76.

Whalley D, McKenna SP, De Jong Z *et al.* (1997) Quality of Life in rheumatoid arthritis. *British Journal of Rheumatology* 36:884–888.

Weller BF (1989) *Baillière's Encyclopaedic Dictionary of Nursing and Health Care,* 1st edn. London, Baillèire Tindall.

Wener MH (2001) Diagnostic Laboratory tests and imaging. In: Robbins L (ed): *Clinical Care in the Rheumatic Diseases.* 2nd edn. Atlanta: American College of Rheumatology.

Zachariae H, Bjerring P, Halkier-Sorensen L *et al.* (1994) Skin scoring in systemic sclerosis: a modification-relations to subtypes and the aminoterminal propeptide of type 111 procollagen (P111NP). *Acta Dermatological Venereolgica* 74:444–446.

Zigmond AS, Snaith RP (1983) The hospital anxiety and depression scale. *Acta Psychiatrica Scandinavica* 67:361–370.

II Addressing the Patient's Problems

5 The Psychological Aspects of Rheumatic Disease

S. RYAN
Haywood Hospital, Staffordshire, UK

The aim of this chapter is to promote an understanding and emphasise the importance of addressing the psychological aspects of rheumatological disorders. After reading this chapter the reader should be able to:

- describe the different models of control theory;
- discuss the features of chronic illness;
- discuss why control is important to well-being;
- understand the depression associated with rheumatological disorders;
- describe the role of the nurse in the assessment and management of psychological symptoms.

CHRONIC ILLNESS

Chronic conditions such as rheumatoid arthritis, ankylosing spondylitis and osteoarthritis have a global impact on an individual's life, affecting not only physical functioning but also their:

- selfe-esteem
- role
- relationships
- control perceptions
- level of mood.

Consequently, care management should not simply concentrate on disease suppression, but should enable patients to come to terms with the emotional and psychological impact of illness. In the case of rheumatoid arthritis, the course of the disease is difficult to predict and it has no known cure. A patient learns quickly that treatments are only palliative and that stressful flare-ups

Rheumatology Nursing: A Creative Approach, 2nd edn. Edited by Jackie Hill.
Copyright 2006 by John Wiley & Sons, Ltd.

can be encountered frequently (Parker and Wright, 1995). If the psychological consequences of chronic disability are neglected, negative control mechanisms can become established, increasing depression and social isolation (Parker and Wright, 1995). Sharpe *et al.* (2003) demonstrated that the use of cognitive behavioural interventions offered early in the course of RA resulted in improvements in psychological function.

THE FEATURES OF CHRONIC ILLNESS

Chronic illness has been defined as an altered health state that will not be cured by a single surgical procedure or a short course of medical therapy (Miller, 1992). It has been described as the 'fourth world' made up of millions of people alienated from everyday life and deprived of interaction because of the effects of the disease and its treatment (Copper, 1976).

Three main features of chronic illness have been identified by Reif (1975):

- Disease symptoms interfere with normal activities and routines.
- The medical regime is limited in its effectiveness.
- Treatment, although intended to mitigate the symptoms and long-term effects of the disease, contributes substantially to the disruption of the usual pattern of living.

These features could apply to a person with a rheumatic disease such as rheumatoid arthritis.

THE EFFECT OF CHRONIC ILLNESS ON THE INDIVIDUAL

Rheumatic disease, such as rheumatoid arthritis causes pain, stiffness, fatigue and in some cases deformity. The use of drug therapy including disease-modifying anti-rheumatic drugs such as methotrexate is variable in its effectiveness and does not always suppress the condition. Often the individual feels unwell due to the systemic nature of the condition, which in turn effects control perception (Ryan *et al.*, 2003). For example, the patient feels unable to influence events, which contributes to depression and poor coping.

The patient may also have to deal with the discontinuation of medication that is causing an adverse reaction or is ineffective, for instance the 30% of patients receiving biologic therapy who will not respond (Emery *et al.*, 1999). This can exert a heavy psychological toll. As symptoms increase, feelings of helplessness and hopelessness can occur which can cause the patient to lose faith in care management. In this situation, the role of the nurse is crucial. Support, explanation and reassurance will be needed to ensure that the patient remains an active participant in care and does not perceive further treatments as useless.

The uncertainty that patients face with rheumatological disorders is often derived from the inability to arrive at meaning in the illness-related event (Mishel, 1981). Sources of uncertainty are rife and include:

- inconsistency in symptom patterns;
- differences between expected and experienced illness related events;
- unfamiliarity with the situation.

A patient's perception of uncertainty will be influenced by their education, degree of social support from significant others and the relationship between the patient and the health-care professional.

Patients require information about their condition so that they can begin to exercise cognitive and behavioural control. A patient will feel less threatened by a flare if they have been taught what symptoms to expect if the disease moves into a more active phase and which self-help methods to implement, for example:

- application of an ice pack to an inflamed area;
- resting the affected joint;
- maximising analgesic intake.

Although this does not prevent the flare, it reduces the uncertainty by emphasising that although it is unpleasant, it is normal to experience certain symptoms in this situation. This information will enable the patient to take on an active role in care management, thus increasing the perception of control and removing feelings of helplessness that can occur in the face of such events.

Patients will require different psychological support at different stages of their illness, and they must know whom to contact for advice, should they enter an unfamiliar illness episode. Support will help to minimise the uncertainty of illness. Group work with family members can also be advantageous, as chronic illness can be bewildering for all concerned and sharing knowledge can help all parties to work together.

DISABILITY

Disability has been characterised as having four consecutive stages (Pope and Tarlov, 1991):

- pathology – the cellular abnormalities which accompany illness or injury;
- impairment – the dysfunction of organ systems which can accompany disease;
- functional limitations – the restriction of activities in everyday life due to illness or disease;
- disability/handicap – the limitations in performance of social roles due to environmental or societal constraints.

It is at this last stage that the patient perceives their illness through the affect it has on their role and their ability to carry out activities meaningful to them. From this perspective, disability is determined by more than the purely bio-medical aspects of disease. Disability can be minimised if psychological func-tional status can be preserved and if environmental and societal constraints can be minimised.

Krueger (1984) likens disability to loss and states that patients will go through several stages which include:

- shock
- retreat, denial or disbelief
- grief, mourning or depression
- hostility and anger
- adjustment.

Often, the initial lack of success of treatment leads to mourning that is analo-gous to normal grief such as at the death of a loved one. A feeling of hopeless-ness may also be experienced. For some patients it is the worsening of symptoms, despite taking the prescribed treatment that can adversely affect hope and lead to a negative perception of control. Here, the nurse has a vital role to play in educating patients about how they can live with the condition. Through enabling individuals and their families, the nurse will be endorsing a shared responsibility and enabling the patient to move towards the state of adjustment (Table 5.1).

THE ROAD TO MASTERY

Shaul (1995) conducted in-depth interviews with women with arthritis and concluded that they experienced three different stages before achieving an element of mastery over the condition.

Table 5.1 Characteristics of adjustment in arthritis

- Living with the illness
- Seeking information
- Employing self-management techniques such as pacing activities
- Remaining socially active
- Valuing one's self and one's contribution to society
- Sharing feelings with family and friends
- Working in partnership with health-care professionals
- Seeking help and advice when required

Becoming aware

The initial stage was one of becoming aware. The perception of the condition as a problem occurred when the symptoms did not go away, became worse or interfered with daily living. For many the first few years were the worst. As they struggled with the severe physical effects of their rheumatoid arthritis their emotional well-being suffered.

Learning to live with it

The second stage, learning to live with it, was characterised by a sense of disconnectedness and a feeling of alienation from the family. Some emerged from this stage knowing that certain strategies worked for particular problems, for instance pacing when fatigued, to conserve energy and reduce pain. These women incorporated the illness into themselves and although they could not predict its course, or when another flare would occur, they were better able to cope when an unfavourable situation did arise.

Mastery

The final stage was one of mastery. The women revealed a new identity, a different perspective on health. Knowledge was acquired about the disease and how to live with it. 'The women began as novices and emerged as experts in living with rheumatoid arthritis.' reported Shaul, 1995.

The achievement of mastery involves a learning process which includes:

* setting goals and expectations
* asking for help from others
* marshaling and managing energy
* maintaining connections with the family and community
* working with health-care professionals.

To achieve a sense of mastery, individuals must gain a sense of control over their situation and develop a repertoire of control strategies to enable them to cope with the changes in the process and context of the illness.

During the nursing assessment, it should be possible to determine which of the three stages the patient has reached by the use of open-ended questions as shown in Table 5.2.

ENABLING THE PATIENT TO ACHIEVE MASTERY

If the patient is at stage one (becoming aware) the nurse should give support through explanation of the condition, to minimise natural fear and anxiety. To be most effective, this should be given on an individualised basis, relevant to the patient's frame of reference.

Table 5.2 Nursing assessment, – the stages of mastery

Stage one	What symptoms does your arthritis cause?
	What does your arthritis prevent you doing?
	How do you cope on a daily basis?
Stage two	How do you try to minimise the pain?
	What would you do if a flare occurs?
	How often should you exercise?
Stage three	How do you feel about yourself in relation to your arthritis?

It must be remembered that a chronic illness is ever-changing. Mastery of one phase of the illness may be achieved, but if the individual finds themselves in an unfamiliar phase, they will revert to the position of novice.

To cope with any rheumatic illness the patient will need to learn how their illness affects their well-being. Treating patients as genuine participants, ought to be central to a profession that has human interpersonal relationships at its heart. Instead, participation has sometimes come to be thought of as merely an improbable by-product of involving patients in their own care plans (Ashworth *et al.*, 1992). The term participation can only be used correctly when the nurse is aware of the physical, psychological, social and emotional meaning of the illness. At the same time, the patient who is genuinely participating in the encounter has some awareness of the nurse as a person with a host of other demands and concerns. Participation involves mutual awareness of the stock of knowledge that constitutes each other's experiences. It would be a mistake for nurses to assume they intuitively know what the lived experience of any patient is like.

Any advice given to a patient will pass through a filter of lay beliefs, which are usually internally consistent and rational in their own terms. They are not static but change in the light of new experiences and the availability of believable information. Providing accurate information to the patient about their condition enhances predictability and a sense of cognitive control.

It is important to encourage patients to participate in as many treatment decisions as possible. When a patient chooses a course of action they are more likely to own it and persist with it, even if the benefits are not immediately apparent. Informing patients about treatment alternatives and allowing them a choice should heighten this sense of control and may play a key role in whether the treatment proves to be beneficial (Wallston, 1993). Nurses can help patients develop, secure and use resources that will promote a sense of control through a partnership based on mutual respect and trust. Knowledge is gained from the sharing of experience and through understanding the psychological and social influences surrounding their lives (Wallerstein and Bernstein, 1988).

THEORETICAL MODELS OF CONTROL

LOCUS OF CONTROL

The concept of locus of control stems from social learning theory which proposes that people relate their behaviour to outcomes and engage in a specific type of behaviour if they believe it will achieve the desired outcome (Rotter, 1966). For example, a patient will engage in relaxation if they believe it will influence their pain and they also desire to take an active part in pain management.

The construct of locus of control differs between individuals some of whom believe control is either:

- internal (dependent on the individual's own characteristics or behaviour) or
- external (dependent on the actions of other people or simply on chance).

Researchers have shown that an external locus of control is associated with less favourable clinical outcomes (Burckhardt, 1985). It is often characterised by passive coping mechanisms such as withdrawal, lack of goal setting, lack of self-involvement, denial and lack of information seeking.

Rotter's social learning theory predicts that when an individual finds themselves in a novel situation, for example faced with a chronic illness, it is their generalised expectations that determine behaviour. If so, a person having an internal locus of control would be best able to cope when faced with illness. Having a negative self-concept can limit what an individual can achieve; and a perception that they have no control over their life (*i.e.*, external locus of control) will make them more prone to feelings of helplessness and depression (Broome, 1989).

The onset of a chronic illness may challenge a person's belief that they can influence matters. As a result, a change from an internal to an external perception may occur until a level of mastery is achieved and an internal perception regained. As a person gains more experience of living with rheumatic disease, expectations in a specific situation will become more important predictors of behaviour than the individual's expectations in general. The belief that other people play a significant role in well-being does not necessarily imply a loss of control, especially if powerful others can be influenced to act in the patient's best interests.

Independence is not an issue unless it is threatened, patients require information, support and guidance to enable them to view themselves as normal (Pigg *et al.*, 1985).

LEARNED HELPLESSNESS

Learned helplessness is a theoretical construct which proposes that as a result of being subjected to uncontrollable adverse events, the individual acquires the beliefs that actions do not affect outcomes; for example, exercise does not influence pain. Someone in this situation comes to expect that further responding will be futile and stops trying to control symptoms through behavioural interventions (Bandura, 1977; Wallston, 1993).

Learned helplessness is related to psychological adjustment in patients with chronic rheumatoid arthritis (Nicassio et al., 1985; Callahan et al., 1988) and involves three types of deficit:

- cognitive deficit – a reluctance to develop new coping behaviours through a lack of information;
- motivational deficit – a reduced effort to engage in the activities of daily living;
- emotional deficit – a low self-esteem.

There appears to be a correlation between high levels of helplessness as recorded on the Rheumatology Attitude Index (Nicassio et al., 1985) and: low self-esteem, lower levels of formal education (Callahan et al., 1988), high anxiety and depression scores and impaired ability as assessed by the Stanford Health Assessment Questionnaire (Fries et al., 1980). Research on psychosocial adjustment in patients with systemic lupus erythematosus showed a correlation between engagement in activities of daily living and the development of new coping behaviour (Engle et al., 1990). There was also a correlation between lower levels of perceived helplessness and longer duration of disease, suggesting that coping behaviour develops over time.

SELF-EFFICACY

Self-efficacy is based on beliefs about control. It refers to personal judgement of performance capabilities, as distinct from actual accomplishments, in a given domain of activity (Lorig, 1989). According to the theory of self-efficacy (Figure 5.1), behavioural change and maintenance are a function of:

- expectations about the outcomes that will result from engaging in a particular behaviour;
- expectations about one's ability to engage in or execute the behaviour.

It should be emphasised that both outcome and efficacy expectations reflect a person's belief about their capabilities rather than their actual capabilities.

The theory postulates that a person's perceptions of their capabilities affect:

- how they behave, for example what activities will be accomplished;
- the acquisition of new behaviour;

- the level of motivation and effort expended on a task;
- emotional reactions such as anxiety, distress and thought patterns.

An individual with a low opinion of their ability to carry out a particular task may ponder their personal deficiencies rather than think about accomplishing the task in hand (O'Leary, 1985, Strecher *et al.*, 1986).

Self-efficacy is not a personality characteristic which operates independently of contextual factors. An individual's efficacy expectations will vary greatly, depending on the nature of the task which confronts them. Consequently, it is inappropriate to characterise a person as having a high or low self-efficacy, without reference to the specific behaviour and circumstances with which the judgement is associated (Strecher, 1986).

Skills that may be required to improve self-efficacy include:

- social skills – for example to explain to the family that rest is a necessary component of treatment;
- psychomotor skills – using joints in such a way as to prevent unnecessary pain and
- self-regulatory skills – to recognise frustration as a normal response in chronic illness and to adopt techniques such as pacing activities.

Self-efficacy has been found to correlate with daily pain and mood (Lefebvre *et al.*, 1999) and is one of the factors that determines patient demands for professional care (Riemsma *et al.*, 1998) and patient concordance with treatment programmes (Taal *et al.*, 1993). Although self-efficacy is based on self-judgement, the views of close associates will be an influencing factor. The

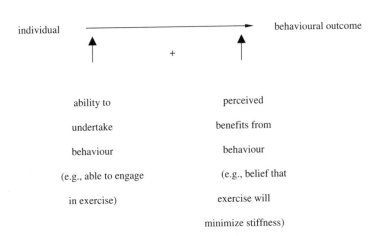

Figure 5.1 The theory of self-efficacy.

motivation to engage in exercise for example will be reduced by lack of family support or their non belief in its value. The time that an individual will persist with exercise may be affected by the fact that it does not always show an immediate result (O'Leary, 1985).

Self-efficacy theory has been applied to diverse domains of psychosocial functioning including anxiety disorders (Bandura et al., 1980; Bandura, 1982) and achievement behaviour (Schunk and Carbonaj, 1984). These studies have provided evidence that a person's perception of their efficacy significantly affects their level of motivation and psychosocial functioning.

Perceived self-efficacy for behaviours that affect health status will predict further health, given that subjects believe that the outcome of their behaviour will be improved health, and improved health is their objective. There may be secondary gains to not achieving health, such as increased social support. The patient's sense of self-efficacy in managing the symptoms and problems caused by rheumatoid arthritis is universally correlated with depression levels (Lorig et al., 1989). It has also been found that high self-efficacy scores are related to lower joint counts, fewer exhibitors of objectively assessed pain behaviours (Buescher et al., 1991) and improved patient perceptions of health status (Taal et al., 1993).

Further research by Lorig et al. (1993) has demonstrated that improved psychological function from attending a programme based on self-efficacy principles, can last as long as four years.

HEALTH BELIEFS

A person's beliefs about health are influenced by culture, social background, experience of health/illness and social network. These are complex factors and their origins difficult to discover; but they play a vital role in health behaviour (McAllister and Farquhar, 1992).

Four logic constraints contained in lay theories about causation of illness have been identified (Chrisman, 1977). These are:

• degeneration (ageing)
• balance (diet)
• invasion (germs)
• mechanical (blockage of blood vessels).

Their importance and dominance will vary from one culture to another but they must be taken into account when attempting to influence health behaviour and self-efficacy. The concept of illness causation amongst working class mothers was studied by Pitt and Stott (1983) who found that the majority believed germs to be the main causes of illness. These women, who regarded the causes of illnesses as external to the individual, were less likely to feel responsible for being ill. Those who felt some degree of responsibility for their illness were likely to be home owners and have more years of education. Their feelings of control in their lives may account for their greater sense of responsibility for health.

TYPOLOGY OF CONTROL

The complex influence of chronic illness on everyday life makes Lewis's typology of control (1986) valuable, in that it distinguishes between degrees of control and discriminates between beliefs and the possession of behavioural competencies. The typology provides the rheumatology nurse with a range of care options to enable the patient to have control.

PROCESSUAL CONTROL

This describes the situation in which a person is consulted but does not necessarily influence the decision. Lack of influence is of less importance to the individual than actually being consulted. Such tokenism can be beneficial even if the belief of control proves to be illusory, because the person believes they have been involved.

The belief that we have control and can influence events that relate to us as individuals, is central to self-concept and well-being. A correlation has been found between self concept and control, in that people with higher levels of self-esteem are better able to cope with the anxiety caused by illness and are less likely to adopt avoidance behaviour strategies such as denial (Tones, 1991).

The environment facilitates the exercise of control. Consequently it is necessary to move away from the classic characteristics of the hospital as a total institution, with its tendency to depersonalise and disempower individuals (Goffman, 1961). Control can be situationally determined and feelings of deference in communication with health-care professionals can create powerlessness in patients and the perception that their actions will not affect an outcome (Miller, 1992).

COGNITIVE CONTROL

Cognitive control occurs where a person cannot influence events but understands their reason and nature. This has clear psychological benefit. For example, a patient who understands what is involved in a painful investigative procedure may not be able to influence the level of discomfort but will be in a position to manage the event intellectually and thus reduce its threat. It has been shown that individuals with severe pain reported fewer days of pain-limited activity when they were able to derive benefit from the pain (Tennan et al., 1992). This phenomenon, where meaning is derived from an adverse stressor is described by Rothbaum *et al.* (1982) as secondary control. This cognitive adaptation addresses the heart of chronic illness and its significance for a patient's life.

BEHAVIOURAL CONTROL

Behavioural control is where a person is able to adopt behaviour that potentially or actually alters the objective qualities of an adverse event. Pain management techniques are examples of this.

CONTINGENCY CONTROL

This is similar to the concept of locus of control (Rotter, 1966). It concerns the extent to which individuals believe that events effecting them are controlled by either:

• their own effort (internal locus of control) or
• the influence of choice and powerful others (external locus of control).

EXISTENTIAL CONTROL

In existential control a person perceives they have no control over events but retains some degree of resilience through religious convictions. Newman (1993) views this as a negative coping strategy, as no attempt is made to influence the condition or learn to live with it.

Lewis (1986) makes clear that the essential ingredient in control is that the individual believes that they can influence events, even if their perception is incorrect.

Self-medication programmes have demonstrated that by involving patients in their own care and enabling them to have responsibility for drug administration within a supportive environment, a higher level of well-being is reported (Bird, 1990). Higher levels of psychological well-being have also been reported by patients with arthritis where they attempted to take control of their condition by engaging in physical activities and expressing their feelings (Newman, 1993).

Frequently society associates control with independence, power and strength, all positive attributes. Conversely, lack of control is often associated with dependency and viewed negatively. However, dependency is a relative term and can be part of re-normalisation (Wiener, 1975) where a person learns to accept new ways of carrying out activities. Patients require help and support to do this; it does not come automatically and patients must have information that will enable them to make informed decisions (Hill, 1995).

The rheumatology nurse should be well-equipped to support and teach, thus enabling patients to manage their own care by sharing responsibility.

This is an essential process for improving self-esteem and accepting the condition, so that effective coping strategies can be developed which will improve well being.

WALLSTON'S THEORETICAL MODEL OF CONTROL

Wallston (1995), influenced by the work of Lazarus and Folkman (1984) and Hobfoll (1989), has constructed a theoretical model on the stages influential in determining whether adaptation occurs or not. In this model, the presence of rheumatoid arthritis and its consequences such as pain and/or dysfunction, constitute a stressor for the patient and the patient's significant others. The threat value of the stressor relates to the amount of adaptation required to deal with the stressor. The individual appraises this and if the stressor is perceived as a threat then a secondary appraisal will occur. This will include a judgement of the adequacy of resources available. Resources can be either:

- internal – the patients belief about the controllability of the stressor, or
- external – the actual support available from the family.

If the secondary appraisal shows there to be sufficient resources to counter the threat, the person feels in control of the situation and this affects adaptation positively. Conversely, if the appraisal shows that resources are insufficient, for example if they are no longer able to attend to their hygiene needs and have no family to assist, one of two things may occur:

- Where the individual is predisposed to accept control, they may engage in a variety of coping behaviours in the hope that something can help the situation.
- Conversely, helplessness may set in and either no coping occurs or the coping is maladaptive.

The model states that both perceived control and coping influence the appraisal of whether the stressor is threatening or nonharmful. Both coping and the adaptation are also directly affected by the actual availability of resources, as well as by appraisal of their availability (Hobfoll, 1989). Adaptation is an ongoing process in which the outcome of one stage feeds back and influences appraisals made at the next stage.

THE HEALTH BELIEF MODEL

The health belief model evolved from an exploration of people's failure to take up screening and preventative programmes of health in the United States. It was later applied to the way in which people responded when they were ill, and whether they complied with treatment and advice. In the model, behaviour is dependent on two main variables:

* the value an individual places on a particular goal;
* the individual's estimation of the likelihood that a given action will achieve that goal.

The model is constructed from three dimensions.

Perceived susceptibility or vulnerability

This is often the strongest predicting factor of the model. However, people often neglect the true risk factors in relation to their situation, behaviour termed 'unrealistic optimism' (Weinstein, 1982). Thus whilst lack of mobility will increase the possibility of osteoporosis developing, patients remain reluctant to take responsibility for minimising the chances of this happening, by increasing exercise.

Perceived severity

The weakest predictor of behaviour is often cited as perceived severity because people are relatively unthreatened by long-term outcomes which are difficult to imagine and unlikely to happen. However this is not the case in rheumatoid arthritis where perceived severity has been shown to have a strong negative effect on behaviour (Hewlett, 1994).

Perceived benefits

Motivation plays a key role in the efforts required to influence behaviour and can be considered as the patient's perceptions of the rewards minus the costs. Exercise may be beneficial, but it is also painful and an exercise programme may reduce the time available to spend with the family. These factors, benefit and cost, will influence whether a person adopts the recommended exercise regime for their arthritis.

The model does not acknowledge the role of efficacy beliefs to the extent of incorporating them formally, nor does it acknowledge influences on past behaviour (Rutter, 1993).

THE THEORY OF REASONED ACTION

The theory of reasoned action differs from the health belief model in that it addresses beliefs and attitudes in general and is not specific to health (Rutter, 1993). The model is founded on the concepts of cognition and behaviour that are assumed to be products of reasoned information processing. Patients may fail to comply with medical advice because they do not understand or do not agree with the physician's stated rationale. This may be regarded as unreasoned behaviour, yet it is reasoned within the individual's lay belief system.

To predict behaviour from this model one must measure individual belief on two levels:

- personal belief – what is seen as a consequence of a particular behaviour, for example relaxation to ease pain;
- normative beliefs – the perception of important others on a particular behaviour, who may view relaxation as time-consuming and impinging on family activities.

The importance of normative beliefs is shown by the fact that social acceptance of behaviour relates positively to behavioural change and can influence healthier lifestyles (Jacobson, 1986).

However, research shows that personal beliefs more accurately predict behaviour than do normative beliefs. It was found that 20% of a sample of patients with rheumatoid arthritis ignored professional advice to rest, believing that this would be giving in and letting the arthritis win (Donovan, 1991). This research highlighted that patients do not always interpret the information given to them by doctors in the way it was intended. Patients wanted doctors to understand the severity of their problems as they perceived them, whereas doctors took a routine approach and tried to reassure all patients by stating that their condition was mild and in the early stages. For individual patients this did not make sense. From their perspective they were in considerable pain and feared the future. The idea that this was a mild form of the disease or at an early stage merely heightened anxieties, the opposite of what had been intended. The medical inattention to illness (the lack of appreciation by doctors of the difficulties of living with the results of sickness), is in part responsible for patient noncompliance, dissatisfaction with health care and inadequate clinical care (Lazare et al., 1975). This has led for a call for the development of a new framework for understanding and treating sickness. Patients weigh up the costs and benefits of various options open to them before choosing the most suitable treatment programme. Medical advice has to compete with a range of other suggestions and if it is not credible it may be dismissed. People's lay beliefs determine what advice is reasonable but actions also have to be possible within the constraints of everyday life. Some patients may reject advice to rest because it makes them stiff or interferes with family commitments. It is important to elicit lay beliefs to understand reasons for poor compliance.

The theory of reasoned action has important implications for nursing care, as it maintains that a person's personal belief will be the main influence on behavioural interventions. It is therefore necessary to discover the patient's beliefs, and explore their explanatory models, so that care, which is both meaningful and relevant to the individual, can be advocated.

A serious limitation of the model is that it applies only to behaviour perceived by the individual to be under their control. For example, a patient may have a positive attitude about attending the rheumatology clinic, but without a means of transport, they will not be able to carry out the behavioural intervention that will match their belief. What is missing is Bandura's element of self-efficacy, the conviction that one can execute the behaviour required to produce the outcome. There is also an assumption that all actions are reasoned and therefore rational. However, patients' explanatory models and to some extent those of medicine may be inconsistent and even self-contradictory, although they are usually relevant to the individual concerned (Klienman *et al.*, 1978).

It is of the utmost importance that the nursing assessment considers control orientation in the planning, implementation and evaluation of care. If patients do not believe that they can influence the symptoms of their arthritis, they will not adapt to their new situation. Advocating self-management principles to a patient with an external locus of control will not influence or alter their behaviour. The nurse must elicit individual lay beliefs and plan care accordingly in a shared partnership; if the proposed care does not appear relevant to the patient, it will be rejected. Enablement can only occur if time is spent understanding patients as individuals and their roles within their social context.

If the patient enters a new phase of their illness, it could alter their control orientation and return the experienced patient to the stage of novice. For this reason patients should be provided with a contact name so that they can be given relevant advice.

DEPRESSION

Depression is perhaps the most vexing and possibly the most widespread of the many types of psychological symptoms that can occur secondary to rheumatoid arthritis (Parker and Wright, 1995). Although the precise prevalence of major depression in rheumatoid arthritis is not known, it has been estimated to affect 21%–34% of patients (Creed *et al.*, 1990). Dickens and Creed (2001) suggest that RA patients are twice as likely to suffer from depression than the general population, yet it is often unrecognised and untreated.

Moldofsky and Chester (1970) describe two types of depression:

• depression that is more marked when joint tenderness is at its peak;
• depression that is more marked when joint tenderness is reduced.

The latter type has a less favourable outcome.

Major depression has been defined by Parker and Wright (1995) as that which is a 'profound, depressive syndrome of sufficient intensity to impair psychological, social and vocational functioning'. Features of depression are outlined in Table 5.3.

Depression can be measured by the Hospital Anxiety and Depression Scale (Zigmond and Snaith, 1983) or the appropriate scales from the Arthritis Impact Measurement Scales (AIMS) questionnaire (Meenan *et al.*, 1980). Both are described in detail in Chapter 4.

THE RELATIONSHIP BETWEEN DEPRESSION AND DISABILITY

In rheumatoid arthritis, psychological factors have been shown to be more accurate predictors of subsequent disability than conventional disease activity measures (McFarlane and Brooks, 1988). Depression in RA patients is associated with:

- social stress
- lack of social support
- increased levels of pain
- reduced ability to engage in activities.

The majority of studies in this area have been cross-sectional in design not allowing any causal inferences to be made (Dickens and Creed, 2001). Shaul (1995) undertook a qualitative study in which depression was mentioned as an outcome of physical limitations and as a companion to pain and fatigue. One participant stated, '*It is a vicious cycle with rheumatoid arthritis. You feel depressed so your arthritis acts up more, and the more it acts up the more depressed you get until you break it somehow*'.

Previous pain and the interaction of pain and sleep disturbances have been shown to be associated with subsequent depression (Nicassio and Wallston, 1992).

People with rheumatoid arthritis who had depressive symptoms performed 12% or fewer of their valued activities compared to patients with rheumatoid arthritis who were not depressed (Katz and Yelin, 1994). A later study found

Table 5.3 Features of depression

- Alteration in appetite
- Sleep disturbance
- Altered psychomotor activity
- Decreased energy
- Feelings of worthlessness
- Difficulty with concentration
- Recurrent thoughts of death
---

that a loss of 10% or more of individual valued activity was a significant predictor of late onset of depressive symptoms (Katz and Yelin, 1995). It is difficult to be certain of the cause and effect relationship, but it was concluded that the severity of the rheumatoid arthritis is the causative factor, and that the limitations it imposes on lifestyle heralds the onset of depressive symptoms. However, there were individuals in the study who experienced loss of valued activities who did not develop depressive symptoms, suggesting that other factors influence the relationship between activity loss and depressive symptoms. Control mechanisms may be one such factor. Learning different control mechanisms may enable the individual to undertake activities in other ways. For example, knowledge of joint protection techniques will enable behavioural control to develop and allow household activities to be carried out with minimal discomfort.

Depressed RA patients perceive their illness as being more serious, feel helpless about the lack of a cure (Murphy *et al.*, 1999) and have difficulty coping with a flare of their condition (Hurwicz and Berkanovic, 1993). Therefore patients require access to an expert clinician to discuss their cognitions and develop their coping strategies. As many as two-thirds of RA patients with depression would respond to a specific serotonin reuptake inhibitor (Anderson *et al.*, 2000).

The relationship between depression, pain and disability argues for a biopsychosocial approach to care management. Care should extend beyond the traditional approach, to embrace a genuine rehabilitation strategy where the maximisation of psychological and social functioning becomes a major treatment objective.

Chronic illness has a global impact on an individual and their significant others. Treatment of arthritis must not concentrate solely on the physical problems at the expense of the psychological manifestations. For an individual to have perceived control of their condition, all aspects of their arthritis must be considered from the patient's frame of reference. The role of the nurse must incorporate assessing the patient's perception of control from their lay beliefs, then planning or matching interventions to move the patient towards mastery and acceptance. A patient whose arthritis is suppressed by drug therapy, yet has little insight into how to live with the condition, will not adapt positively. A shared approach within an holistic framework is the way forward and nurses must not miss the opportunity to enter into a meaningful therapeutic relationship with patients.

ACTION POINTS FOR PRACTICE

- Next time you carry out a patient assessment, include questions to illicit the control orientation of the patient. This will influence how much involvement is required of the nurse in care interventions.

- List the characteristics you would expect a patient to exhibit if they had adjusted to living with their arthritis.
- Design an information sheet for patients on self-management techniques for pain control. This will influence behavioural control.
- Think about how depression is catered for in your clinical area. Provide a leaflet for colleagues informing them of how to recognise depression in their patients.

REFERENCES

Anderson IM, Nutt DJ, Deakin JFW (2000) Evidence based guidelines for treating depressive disorders with anti-depressants: a revision of the 1993 British Association for Psychopharmacology guidelines. *Journal of Psychopharmacology* 14: 2–30.

Ashworth PD, Longmate M, Morrison P (1992) Patient participation: its meaning and significance in the context of caring. *Journal of Advanced Nursing* 17:1430–1439.

Bandura A (1977) Self-efficacy-towards unifying theory of behavioural change. *Psychological Review* 84(2):191–215.

Bandura A (1982) Self efficacy mechanisms in human agency. *American Psychology* 37:122–147.

Bandura A, Adams NE, Hardy AB, Howells GH (1980) Tests of the generality of self efficacy theory. *Cognitive Therapy Research* 4:39–66.

Bird C (1990) A prescription of self help. *Nursing Times* 86:52–55.

Broome A (1989) *Health Psychological Processes and Applications*, 2nd edn. London, Chapman Hall.

Buescher KL, Johnston JA, Parker JC (1991) Relationship of self efficacy to pain behaviour. *Journal of Rheumatology* 18:968–972.

Burckhardt CS (1985) The impact of arthritis on quality of life. *Nursing Research* 34:11–16.

Callahan L, Brooks RH, Pincus T (1988) Further analysis of learned helplessness in rheumatoid arthritis. Using a rheumatology attitude index. *Journal of Rheumatology* 15(3):418–426.

Chrisman NJ (1977) The health seeking process; an approach to the natural history of illness. Culture, *Medicine and Psychiatry* 1:351–377.

Copper JS (1976) *Living with chronic neurological disease*. New York, WW Norton.

Creed F, Jayson MV, Murphy S (1990) Measurement of psychiatric disorder in rheumatoid arthritis. *Journal of Psychosomatic Research* 34(1):79–87.

Dickens C, Creed F (2001) The burden of depression in patients with rheumatoid arthritis. *Rheumatology* 40:1327–1330.

Donovan J (1991) Patient education and the consultation: the importance of lay beliefs. *Annals of the Diseases* 50:418–421.

Engle EW, Callahan L, Hochberg M, Pincus T (1990) Learned helplessness in systemic lupus erythematosus: using the rheumatology attitude index. *Arthritis and Rheumatism* 33:281–286.

Emery P, Panayi G, Sturock R, William B (1999) Targeted therapies in rheumatoid arthritis: the need for action. *Rheumatology* 38:911–916.

Fries JF, Holman HR, Kraines RG, Spitz P (1980) Measurement of patient outcome in arthritis. *Arthritis and Rheumatism* 23:137–145.

Goffman E (1961) *Asylums*. New York, Double Day.

Hewlett S (1994) Patients' views on changing disability. *Nursing Standard* 8(31):25–27.

Hill J (1995) Patient education in rheumatic disease. *Nursing Standard* 9(25): 25–28.

Hobfoll S (1989) Conservation of resources. A new attempt at conceptualising stress. *American Psychology* 44:513–524.

Hurwicz ML, Berkanovic E (1993) The stress process in rheumatoid arthritis. *Journal of Rheumatology* 20:1836–1844.

Jacobson D (1986) Types and timing of social support. *Journal of Health and Social Behaviour* 27:250–264.

Katz P, Yelin LH (1994) Life activities of persons with rheumatoid arthritis with and without depressive symptoms. *Arthritis Care Research* 7:69–77.

Katz P, Yelin LH (1995) The development of depressive symptoms among women with rheumatoid arthritis, the role of function. *Arthritis and Rheumatism* 38:49–56.

Klienman A, Eisenberg L, Good B (1978) Culture care and illness. *Annals of Internal Medicine* 88:251–258.

Krueger DW (1984) *Rehabilitation Psychology*. Maryland, Aspin.

Lazare A, Eisenthal S, Wasserman L (1975) The customer approach to patienthood. *Archives of General Psychiatry* 32:553–558.

Lazarus RS, Folkman S (1984) *Stress Appraisal and Coping*. New York, Springer.

Lefebvre JC, Keefe FJ, Affleck G, Raezer LB, Starr K et al. (1999) The relationship of arthritis self-efficacy to daily pain, daily mood and daily pain coping in rheumatoid arthritis patients. *Pain* 80:425–435.

Lewis FM (1986) The concept of control a typology and health related variable. In: Tones K (ed) Health Promotion Empowerment and the Psychology of Control. *Journal of the Institute of Health Education* 29(11):17–25.

Lorig K, Mazonson PD, Holman HR (1993) Evidence suggesting that health education for self management in patients with chronic arthritis has sustained health benefits whilst reducing health costs. *Arthritis and Rheumatism* 36:439–446.

Lorig K, Chastain R, Holman H, Shoors, Ung E (1989) The beneficial outcome of the arthritis self management course are not adequately explained by behavioural change. *Arthritis and Rheumatism* 32:91–95.

McAllister G, Farquhar M (1992) Health beliefs a cultural division. *Journal of Advanced Nursing* 17:1447–1454.

McFarlane AC, Brookes PM (1988) Determinants of disability in arthritis. *British Journal of Rheumatology* 27:7–14.

Meenan R, Gertman P, Mason J (1980) Measuring health status in arthritis. *Arthritis and Rheumatism* 23(2):146–152.

Miller JF (1992) *Coping with Chronic Illness Overcoming Powerlessness*, 2nd ed. FA London, Davies.

Mishel M (1981) The meaning of uncertainty in illness. *Nursing Research* 30:258–268.

Moldofsky HP, Chester WJ (1970) Pain and mood pattern in patients with rheumatoid arthritis. A prospective study. *Psychosomatic Medicine* 32:309–318.

Murphy H, Dickens CM, Creed FH, Bernstein R (1999) Depression, illness perception and coping in rheumatoid arthritis. *Journal of Psychosomatic Research* 46:155–164.

Newman SP (1993) Coping with rheumatoid arthritis. *Annals of the Rheumatic Diseases* 52:553–554.

Nicassio PM, Callahan LF, Herbert M, Pincus T, Wallston KA (1985) The measurement of helplessness in rheumatoid arthritis. The development of the arthritis helplessness index. *Journal of Rheumatology* 12:462–467.

Nicassio PM, Wallston KA (1992) Longitudinal relationships among pain, sleep problems and depression in rheumatoid arthritis. *Journal of Abnormal Psychology* 101(3):514–520.

O'Leary A (1985) Self efficacy and health. *Behavioural Research and Therapy* 23(4):437–451.

Parker JC, Wright GE (1995) The implications of depression for pain and disability in rheumatoid arthritis. *Arthritis Care and Research* 8(4):279–283.

Pigg JS, Caniff R, Driscoll PW (1985) *Rheumatology Nursing. A Problem Orientated Approach.* New York, John Wiley.

Pitt R, Stott NCH (1983) *A Study of Health Beliefs, Attitudes and Behaviour among Working Class Mothers.* Department of General Practice. Cardiff, Welsh National School of Medicine.

Pope AM, Tarlov AR (1991) *Disability in America. Towards a National Agenda for Prevention.* Washington DC, National Academy Press.

Reif L (1975) Beyond medical intervention strategies for managing life in the face of chronic illness. In: Davies M, Kramer M, Straiss A (eds) *Nurses in Practice. A Perspective on Work Environments.* St Louis, Mosby pp. 261–273.

Riemsma RP, Klein G, Taal E, Rasker JJ, Weigman O (1999) The supply and demand of informal and professional care for patients with rheumatoid arthritis. Scandavian *Journal of Rheumatology* 27:7–15.

Rotter JB (1966) Generalised expectancies for internal versus external control of reinforcements. *Psychological Monographs* 80(1):1–28.

Rothbaum F, Snyder S, Weisz J (1982) Changing the world and changing the self. A two process model of perceived control. *Journal of Personality and Social Psychology* 42:5–37.

Rutter D (1993) *Social Psychological Approaches to Health.* London, Harvest Wheatsley.

Ryan S, Hassell A, Dawes P, Kendall S (2003) Control perceptions in patients with rheumatoid arthritis; the impact of the medical consultation. *Rheumatology* 42:135–140.

Schunk D, Carbonaj J (1984) Self efficacy models In: Matarazzo J (ed) *Behavioural Health: A Hand Book of Health Enhancement and Disease Prevention.* New York, John Wiley.

Sharpe L, Sensky T, Timberlake N, Ryan B, Allard S (2003) Long-term efficacy of a cognitive behavioural treatment from a randomised controlled trial for patients recently diagnosed with rheumatoid arthritis. *Rheumatology* 42:435–441.

Shaul MP (1995) From early twinges to mastery: The process of adjustment in living with rheumatoid arthritis. *Arthritis Care and Research* 8(4):290–297.

Strecher VJ, Becker M, Devills B, Rosenstock I (1986) The role of self efficacy in achieving health behaviour change. *Health Education Quarterly* 13(1):73–91.

Taal E, Riemsma RP, Brus HL, Seydel ER, Rasker JJ, *et al.* (1993) Group education for patients with rheumatoid arthritis. *Patient Education and Counselling* 20:177–187.

Tennen H, Affleck G, Higgins PM, Mondola R, Urrows S (1992) Perceiving control, constructing benefits and daily processes in rheumatoid arthritis. *Canadian Journal of Behavioural Science* 24(2):86–203.

Tones K (1991) Health promotion empowerment and the psychology of control. *Journal of the Institute of Health Education* 29(1):17–25.

Wallston K (1993) Psychological control and its impact on the management of rheumatological disorders. *Baillière's Clinical Rheumatology* 7(2):281–296.

Wallston K (1995) Adaptation, coping and perceived control in persons with rheumatoid arthritis. *Rheumatology in Europe* 2:291–304 (suppl), Eular Publications.

Wallerstein N, Bernstein E (1988) Empowerment education. Friere's ideas adapted to health education. *Health Education Quarterly* 15(4):379–394.

Wiener CL (1975) The burden of rheumatoid arthritis - tolerating the uncertainty. *Social Science and Medicine* 9:97–104.

Weinstein ND (1982) Unrealistic optimism about future life events. *Journal of Personality and Social Psychology* 39:806–20.

Zigmond A, Snaith RP (1983) The hospital anxiety and depression scale. *Psychiatry Scandinavian* 67:361–370.

6 The Effects of Rheumatic Disease on Body Image and Sexuality

J. HILL
University of Leeds, West Yorkshire, UK

The aim of this chapter is to provide an insight into the effects that rheumatic disease has on body image, sexuality and issues such as comfortable sexual intercourse. Parenting and contraception are also discussed. After reading this chapter the reader should be able to:

• understand how rheumatic disease impacts on body image;
• define the term 'sexuality';
• discuss practical aspects of sexual intercourse with patients;
• determine why sexuality is an aspect of patient care that is often neglected by nurses;
• outline the problems of pregnancy and parenting;
• summarise the methods of contraception available to the rheumatic patient and their partner.

Changes to body image and impingement on sexuality can be consequences of some forms of rheumatic disease. Unfortunately, although nurses aim to provide holistic care for their patients, sexuality remains an area that many feel unable to discuss (Irwin, 1997; Law, 2001). This is somewhat regrettable, as sexuality appears to be an important aspect of the lives of the majority of people and is a suitable topic for nurses to address. This is highlighted in a discussion and guidance document produced by the RCN (2000) which states categorically that it is.

BODY IMAGE

Society largely determines what is normal and this picture of normality will be the only one that is accepted by many (Drench, 1994). Our society is pre-occupied with physical attractiveness. Emphasis placed on physical beauty

Rheumatology Nursing: A Creative Approach, 2nd edn. Edited by Jackie Hill.
Copyright 2006 by John Wiley & Sons, Ltd.

and perfection predisposes the disabled or disfigured person to stigmatisation (Chandani *et al.*, 1989). This may affect the way an individual:

* is viewed by society
* views themselves
* perceives the way in which others view them.

Jones (1994) suggests that body image has three aspects as follows:

* the body ideal – what we aspire to (This is strongly influenced by the society in which we live, the cultures within that society, all forms of media, and within that context, what we personally want to reflect to others.);
* the body reality – what nature actually gave us;
* body presentation – how we choose to present our body to the rest of society, that is, the way that we express our individuality.

Body image is a very vulnerable part of our make-up (Price, 1990) and a damaged body image can significantly harm a person's whole identity. Illness or injury that distorts the body structure may alter the individual's image of the body. It may also interfere with the entire self-image including interrupting social and vocational roles that may ultimately affect the individual's self-esteem (Webb, 1985; Drench, 1994).

SELF-CONCEPT

Self-concept develops as part of our personality and results from how we think that others view us. It involves notions about femininity, masculinity, physical prowess, endurance and capabilities (Drench, 1994). Body image is closely linked to self-concept as it is the part that involves attitudes and experiences pertaining to the body.

SELF-ESTEEM

Self-esteem is how a person values himself or herself. The loss of a job that afforded status can alter a person's perception of the way that others value them and how they value themselves. Self-esteem combined with self-worth is the basis from which man functions. If people feel well, they feel positive about themselves. They have the energy to invest in life and in relationships, and give the impression of health and vigour to other people, who may see them as attractive and worthwhile. However, the impression given may be radically altered for a person experiencing the effects of a progressive degenerative disease such as one of the forms of rheumatic disease (Webb, 1985; Webb, 1987).

WHAT DO WE MEAN BY THE TERM 'SEXUALITY'?

Sexuality is defined in the Collins English Dictionary (1986) as:

- the state or quality of being sexual;
- preoccupation with or involvement in sexual matters;
- the possession of sexual potency.

This definition provides a very limited view of sexuality and the health-related literature expands on this. In essence, sexuality is more than the act of sexual intercourse. Freud (1936) made a fundamental distinction between sex and sexuality. He stated, *'Sex is something we do, sexuality is something we are.'*

Sexuality appears to be an integral part of the whole person. In his book on motivation and personality, Maslow (1970) maintains that sexual behaviour is multidetermined: *'Sexual behaviour is multidetermined, that is to say, determined not only by sexual but also by other needs, chief among which are love and affection needs.'*

An individual's expression of sexuality is influenced by a number of factors (Jones, 1994) including their:

- background;
- accumulated life experiences;
- values of the society in which they have been brought up;
- attitudes, personality and views;
- and the attitude of others.

To a large extent, our sexuality determines who we are and is an integral factor in the uniqueness of every person (Savage, 1990; Stuart and Sundeen, 1979).

SEX AND DISABILITY

Disabled people tend to be perceived by the general public to be asexual, and their need for sexual fulfilment regarded as inappropriate, or even unthinkable (Hahn, 1981). Work carried out in the 1980's suggested that this belief was also held by many caring professionals who were excessively puritanical in their outlook. The majority tended to give no consideration to the sexual needs of their clients. However, it was noted that during the preceding decade, there had been some improvement, the sexual needs and difficulties of the disabled were being given some attention but there were still many exceptions (Carolan, 1984).

Dawson-Shepherd (1984), a disabled person herself, acknowledged the beginning of an increased awareness that sexuality did exist despite disability.

This must have been encouraging, as disabled people need to be given choices, opportunities and support in this most fundamentally important aspect of their lives.

THE EFFECTS OF RHEUMATIC DISEASE

DOES ILLNESS IMPACT ON SEXUAL ACTIVITY?

When people become ill, sexuality is unlikely to be a priority! When the illness is acute, such as influenza or perhaps an acute appendicitis, once the illness resolves then people resume their normal routines, including their sexual activity. When the illness is a chronic rheumatic disease with no prospect of cure, what happens then? There has been some research undertaken in the rheumatic diseases, but this is not rife. However, common sense tells us that a painful chronic disease has the potential to lead to loss of libido.

EXPRESSING SEXUALITY

Chronic disabling conditions, such as rheumatoid arthritis and more severe osteoarthritis, may result in the patient experiencing a decrease in sexual desire and ability to express sexual love through bodily movement (Cochrane, 1984; Smith, 1994). Research has demonstrated that this can be due to a number of problems (Hill *et al.*, 2003; Hill and Reay, 2004). They include:

- reduced mobility
- lack of manual dexterity
- pain and discomfort
- reduced general well-being.

Additionally, many people suffer from anxiety, depression and damaged body image, and any or all of these problems can contribute to a lack of desire for sexual activity. Loss of independence may result in a change in role for both the patient and their partner, which may affect how they view one another sexually. For example, a wife who takes on the role of caregiver may no longer view herself as a wife and lover (Webb, 1987).

Although some patients may not wish to have sexual intercourse, there is often an increase in the need for love, reassurance and physical closeness for both the patient and their partner. The patient may worry that they will not be able to demonstrate this because of the symptoms of their disease (Chesson, 1984). The patient's partner may be inhibited from showing any physical love by the anxiety of causing their loved one pain. For the patient, even a hug may be too painful to give or to receive. The action of hugging may be impossible to perform because of joint stiffness or disorganisation of the shoulder or elbow joints reducing movement. Kissing may be a painful experience if the temporomandibular joints are affected (Cochrane, 1984). Potentially, anticipation of pain may colour entirely pain-free periods for both the patient and their partner. This can result in the weakening of even the strongest emotional bonds (Lee and Moll, 1987).

PERSONAL APPEARANCE

The patient's self-esteem can be affected if deformities or skin problems such as psoriasis or a lupus rash affect their body causing worries that others will no longer find them attractive. Rheumatoid arthritis commonly affects the small joints of the hand. If the patient's condition deteriorates, the hands can become deformed and holding small objects such as a make-up brush becomes impossible. For those wishing to wear make-up this can be a devastating blow and the help of the occupational therapist should be sought to find ways of overcoming the difficulty. If patients are unable to present themselves to society in the way that they feel most comfortable it affects their confidence and self-worth leading to feelings of low self-esteem (Smith, 1994).

The psychological impact of rheumatic disease on the young can be devastating (Chapter 17). This may be more severe for those who are first afflicted in their teens than those whose disease starts at an earlier age, as very young children tend to accept disability. However, adolescents and older teenagers may experience particular difficulties in establishing a satisfactory self-image, believing themselves to be unattractive, unlikely to find a sexual partner and likely to be unable to express physical love as they would wish.

TOUCH

The hands are an important, if not the ultimate tool of touch. Patients with hand involvement will be less inclined to touch their partner and can be less willing to be touched themselves. When the small joints are swollen and painful, even holding hands can be traumatic. Therapeutic touch can be used to the benefit of many patients, especially if they are disfigured, alone and lacking human contact. Massage can help to overcome problems of body image (Chapter 13). Touching is a natural and literal reaching out of one human being to another, but some cultures find it difficult to show their warmth through touch. The problem with touch is circular. When there is little physical touching in a culture it begins to take on a mysterious connotation and hence it is mistrusted and little used. Yet when touching occurs it is usually experienced as perfectly natural and not at all discontinuous with the flow of communication between those involved (Mearns and Thorne, 1988).

EFFECTS ON RELATIONSHIPS

Cohen (1991) suggests that patients with chronic illness or disability tend to withdraw from life, breaking off contact with friends and showing less interest in going out or entertaining. This can lead to increasing isolation, which makes it difficult for the patient to develop new relationships. However, the majority of problems tend to occur if the arthritis develops after the relationship has started (Smith, 1994; LeGallez, 1993). This indicates that when the arthritis is there from the start, both partners may know what they potentially have to cope with. Even so, because of the unpredictability of rheumatoid arthritis, some problems may not have been anticipated and once rheumatoid arthritis has taken a significant hold on the patient, the impact is intense (Le Gallez, 1993). Le Gallez's study highlighted a number of indicators that influence the outcome of relationships, including:

- the patient's ability to adjust to the disease;
- acceptance of the physical limitations that it imposed;
- the amount of support that the partner was prepared to give;
- the partner's acknowledgement of the existence of the patient's disease.

Le Gallez believes that many marriages break down under the strain of one partner becoming totally dependent on the other, most commonly when the wife has become disabled. There is evidence that for men it is not the care, but the housekeeping and caring for the children that causes the majority of problems as these are not considered part of the natural role of the male (Greengross, 1976; Le Gallez, 1993). Whatever their gender, the patient's self-esteem is likely to be affected when they realise that they are unable to contribute to the running of the home or to achieve even the simplest of goals due to their disabilities (Chesson, 1984, Smith, 1994).

A study by Hill et al. (2003) found that a large minority of patients thought that their rheumatoid arthritis had put a strain on their relationship with their partner and that a number of patients blamed themselves for any problems that arose. The strained relationship arose because of:

- curtailment of activities;
- changes in the balance of the relationship;
- emotional impact;
- reduced finances.

Patients also thought that their partners had become short-tempered and lacked patience since the onset of their disease. However, on the positive side patients do tend to communicate with their partners (Hill, 2004). For instance 88% of patients surveyed in a study by Ryan et al. (1996) discussed their relationship with their partners and only five patients thought that their partners did not understand their problems.

SEXUAL INTERCOURSE

For some patients the act of sexual intercourse can be painful and physically difficult and this is often due to the symptoms and ensuing physical problems that arise from rheumatic diseases (Hill *et al.*, 2003; Hill and Reay, 2004; Kraaimaat *et al.*, 1996). These include:

- joint or muscle pain
- joint stiffness
- joint swelling
- fatigue
- reduced range of movement
- joint deformity
- anaemia
- loss of tactile sensation
- dry vagina due to Sjögren's syndrome
- drug therapy
- reduction in libido.

Psychological problems such as anxiety, depression and loss of self-esteem have been shown to contribute to the intrusiveness of rheumatoid arthritis on sexual activity (Kraaimaat *et al.*, 1996). One note of caution, it should not be assumed that people with rheumatic disease are unable to have pleasurable sexual intercourse. Many couples coping with a rheumatic disease are able to maintain a satisfying sexual relationship (Majerovits and Revenson, 1994) and have no problems at all. Even those with the most severe disability can overcome difficulties. As is the ethos of nursing, each patient should be treated as an individual.

Providing practical verbal and written advice can help patients and their partners to enjoy sexual intercourse and it also gives them the permission to try different techniques that many seek.

PLANNING SEXUAL INTERCOURSE

Although spontaneous unplanned intercourse is often pleasurable, the limitations caused by the disease symptoms may mean that the time that intercourse takes place needs to be planned. At first sight this seems cold and calculating, but it should be viewed in a positive light. Patients and their partners should be reminded that the anticipation of planning ahead could heighten rather than diminish their pleasure!

Although many people have intercourse either last thing at night or on waking in the morning, these are not always the best times for someone with a disease such as rheumatoid arthritis. The joints are often less mobile and stiff in the morning, and by the end of the day patients can be very fatigued. The middle of the day tends to be favoured by many.

If pain is a problem, planning intercourse when nonsteroidal anti-inflammatory drugs are at their most effective can be helpful. Alternatively, an analgesic taken about half an hour before intercourse reduces pain.

Some limbering-up exercises followed by a warm shower or bath that will also help the patient to relax can relieve joint stiffness. Gentle massage can act as a form of pain relief and this can be incorporated into foreplay and be pleasurable for both patient and partner.

POSITIONING

There are many positions in which intercourse is possible and no matter which joints are affected there is usually at least one that couples find pleasurable. The conventional position in which the man lays on top and the woman is underneath with her legs spread may not be suitable for someone with arthritis. For instance if the woman is the patient and has hip involvement which prohibits abduction a side-lying or standing position may be more suitable. If the male has shoulder or elbow involvement he may be better lying on his back with his partner sitting or lying over him.

Painful joints or those with reduced or fixed range of movement may need to be supported by pillows or cushions.

A number of patients undergo prosthetic surgery of the hip (Chapter 14) and need advice regarding when and how sexual intercourse can be resumed. Genital intercourse is not usually recommended during the first six weeks postoperatively. Cochrane (1984) recommends that the side-lying position is adopted for the following six weeks as this will avoid the adduction and internal rotation of the prosthesis and so avoid dislocation.

SEX AIDS

Not everyone feels comfortable with the idea of using sex aids, but for those who do they can be a valuable asset to foreplay. Vibrators can give pleasure to both the disabled and able-bodied partner. They are particularly helpful for those with impaired, painful hands.

Vibrators are available in a wide variety of shapes, sizes and powers and can be useful for increasing stimulation of the:

- penis
- vagina
- clitoris.

Catalogues of sex aids are available and simply offering this to a patient may make them feel that using mechanical sexual stimulation is both permissible and acceptable.

Sexual satisfaction does not necessarily rely on penetration. Other ways of giving and receiving sexual pleasure include:

- kissing and cuddling
- oral sex
- masturbation.

Even these methods can cause discomfort. Oral sex may be painful if the patient has temporomandibular involvement, or unpleasant with the reduced salivary production of Sjögren's syndrome. Masturbation may prove difficult if they have reduced manual dexterity. Although masturbation can provide a satisfying alternative or addition to sexual intercourse, it attracts more than its fair share of taboos, myths and smutty jokes. Patients need to be made aware that it is an acceptable and harmless form of sexual pleasure.

VAGINAL DRYNESS

Vaginal dryness can cause painful intercourse for both the woman and her male partner. A secondary condition that often occurs in rheumatoid arthritis is Sjögren's syndrome. Venables (1985) describes this syndrome as a group of diseases characterised by a common pathological feature, namely:

- inflammation
- destruction of exocrine glands.

The salivary and lachrymal glands are principally involved giving rise to dry eyes and a dry mouth, though other exocrine glands including those of the pancreas, sweat glands and mucus-secreting glands of the bowel, bronchial tree and vagina may be affected. Although many patients are given artificial tear eye drops and artificial saliva sprays, very few women with rheumatoid arthritis are given any advice regarding their vaginal dryness. Lubricants such as water-soluble jelly are available from pharmacies and their use can ensure painless sexual intercourse. The use of oils and other lotions are not recommended as they may give rise to infection.

It is generally assumed that people know how to get help or can actually work things out for themselves. This is not always the case and nurses should not shy away from their responsibilities in the area of providing practical sexual advice, or if they are not confident in their abilities, make sure that patients are referred to another professional.

DRUGS AND SEXUAL INTERCOURSE

Some drugs are known to have an effect on sexual function (Table 6.1) but this varies from person to person and is also dose-dependent. Those listed do

Table 6.1 Drugs that affect sexual function

Drug	Effect on desire	Effect on arousal	Effect on orgasm
Alcohol	Initially increased, later reduced	Reduced	Much reduced
Analgesics			
Opiates	Reduced	Reduced	Reduced
Nonopiates	Reduced	Reduced	Retarded ejaculation
Antihypertensives			Failure or retrograde ejaculation
Anticholinergics	Often reduced	Erectile impotence	Reduced
Antidepressants	Often reduced	Reduced	Reduced monoamine oxidase inhibitors (MAOIs) give retarded ejaculation
Antihistamines	Often reduced	Reduced lubrication	
Beta blockers	Reduced	Erectile impotence	
Cimetidine		Some erectile dysfunction	
Diuretics		Erectile impotence common, some reduction of lubrication	
Hormones			
Contraceptive pill	Variable	Variable	Variable
Androgen	Raised (rare in androgen-deficient male)	Raised (rare in androgen-deficient male)	Raised
Oestrogen		Increased vaginal lubrication in oestrogen-deficient female	
Antiandrogens	Reduced	Reduced	Reduced
Minor tranquilizers (benzodiazepines)	Reduced	Reduced	Reduced
Major (phenothiazides)	Reduced	Delayed ejaculation in male	Reduced

not always induce sexual dysfunction, sometimes they can cure it. For example, lack of arousal in the clinically depressed patient is sometimes resolved by the introduction of tricyclic antidepressants, on the other hand these drugs can also induce problems.

If particular drugs are necessary to the patient, it may not be possible to eliminate the side effects. In these cases the nurse should discuss the side effects with the patient and suggest alternative ways of giving and receiving sexual pleasure.

SEXUALITY AND THE NURSING ROLE

Some nurses do not believe that broaching the topic of sexuality is a legitimate area for nurses to address. However, the discussion and guidance document produced by the Royal College of Nursing (2000) states, '*Nurses need to recognise that sexuality and sexual health is an appropriate and legitimate area of nursing activity, and that they have a professional and clinical responsibility to address it.*' However, before nurses undertake this responsibility they must be competent. This means that further training and support needs to be available to ensure that nurses are able to develop their professional competence.

Nursing patients with a rheumatic disease requires a holistic approach that encompasses the whole individual. This being the case, any aspect that is perceived to impact on the lives of those with a rheumatic disease should be addressed. The recent literature has demonstrated that rheumatoid arthritis (Hill *et al.*, 2003; Ryan *et al.*, 1996) and osteoarthritis (Hill and Reay, 2004) have a detrimental effect on the sexual lives and relationships of patients and their partners. Unfortunately research undertaken by Waterhouse (1996) has indicated that nurses are not proactive in discussing sexuality and wait for patients to raise the issue. Patients also find this topic a difficult issue to bring up and consequentially it remains largely unaddressed even when they have been diagnosed for many years and have consulted many members of the multidisciplinary team. There are many possible reasons for this void in care and some of these are set out in a Royal College of Nursing discussion and guidance document (2000). They include:

- poor training or education in sexuality and sexual health;
- lack of relevant experience;
- religious or personal views;
- the belief that the topic is not important or appropriate;
- embarrassment.

Interestingly, nurses working in rheumatology do appear to be aware of issues surrounding sexuality in their practice. A small survey of qualified nurses working in the speciality showed that they believed addressing the subject of sexuality was an important nursing function, but they felt they needed additional training (Wylie, 2001).

Many nurses feel uneasy when dealing with the most intimate aspects of patient care and this may even lead them to avoid the patient altogether. In general, nurses are not taught how to help patients with their sexuality and as a result may experience discomfort and embarrassment when confronted with a patient expressing their problems (Andrew and Andrew, 1991).

It should always be remembered that sexuality is complex and multidimensional and must be addressed by the nurse in a holistic fashion. To achieve this it is crucial to make the distinction between the patient's physical sexual needs and their need to enjoy love and nonsexual relationships.

ASSESSING SEXUAL EXPRESSION

When a nurse writes up her patient assessment, the sections relating to patients' expression of sexuality are often left blank, or read 'likes to wear make-up' or 'shaves on alternate days'. However, Roper *et al.* (1980) have urged the assessor to seek the answers to the following questions:

- How does he/she express sexuality?
- What factors influence his/her expression of sexuality?
- What does he/she know about expressing sexuality?
- What does he/she feel about expressing sexuality?
- What difficulties does he/she have in expressing sexuality?

When asked about expressing sexuality, most people think directly of the sexual act or acts, and this may be an entirely inappropriate concern for a person who is ill. As the expression of human sexuality and body image are virtually inseparable, in health and illness, it may also be appropriate to include questions regarding:

- how the patient sees their own body image;
- how their disease has affected their image of themselves;
- how their disease has affected their quality of life.

THE TIMING OF ASSESSMENTS

The timing of undertaking the assessment of sexual expression can be crucial. Smith (1994) suggests that sexuality should be treated like any other problem and should be addressed as part of a routine assessment on ward admission. However, this may not be the most appropriate time. The patient may not have had enough time to develop a relationship with the nurse to the point where they feel that they can put their trust in him/her. Annon (1976) who has devised a model for helping people with sexual difficulties acknowledge this. People often feel embarrassed about their sexual problems and may need permission to ventilate their feelings and worries. He suggests that the patient will need time and evidence that the nurse is willing to listen, and suggests that the subject should be raised when it is felt appropriate, which may be later on in the admission. If the nurse raises the subject of the patient's sexuality too early, the patient may feel under pressure to answer questions that cause him/her a great deal of embarrassment.

Unfortunately, many patients will only express their problem when it has reached crisis point (Smith, 1994). This is particularly so of those with rheumatic disease, who tend to be exceptionally stoical and uncomplaining. Many patients come into hospital with a flare in their arthritis and are in a state of crisis. They are at their lowest ebb and their sexual problems and body image are generally low on their agenda, their primary concern being the pain of the flare. This is illustrated by Maslow's hierarchy of need (Maslow, 1970). In this theory Maslow asserts that basic needs must be met before the person can consider satisfying their less essential wants. Only when the symptoms of the flare subside and they are able to mobilise and carry out basic activities of daily living do other problems take precedence. They begin to think about their experience and worry about issues such as:

- What caused the flare?
- Will I be able to cope with relationships?
- Will I manage financially?
- How will my family cope?
- Will I manage on a day-to-day basis with my disabilities?
- Will my joints become disfigured?
- What will I look like?
- Will other people find me attractive?

Patients often feel depressed even if they are not actually clinically depressed, they are often low in mood, tearful and in need of support and help. It is therefore important that the nurse is sensitive to the patient's difficulties in expressing their feelings and to the delicacy of the subject. Patients who are met by a judgmental attitude or embarrassment on the part of the nurse, are unlikely to raise the subject again.

PATIENT EDUCATION

Sexual education is a delicate subject and needs to be dealt with sensitively and with discretion. Information should be given to the patient when they ask for it as most people find it difficult to discuss the intimate details of their sexual lives. If the request is ignored they may not feel able to broach the subject again. From the professional viewpoint, information on sexuality should be an accepted part of the care package. Patients who do not seek information should be offered it when the nurse feels that the time is right for the patient and themselves. This can be done as part of routine activities, for instance when carrying out an articular index (Hill, 1991). If the hips, hands or knees are painful on movement or to pressure it is natural to ask, 'Does this cause you a problem when you make love?' During an explanation of Sjögren's syndrome it is easy to mention that it can cause the vagina to become dry which can naturally lead to the question: 'Have you found this at all?' If the answer is yes then it should be followed up by asking if it causes a problem with love-making. These types of question tell the patient that the nurse is happy to discuss the topic without placing any undue pressure on the patient.

Another important aspect is to assess whether to involve the patient's partner and if so, whether the nurse has the knowledge to cope with counselling or teaching two people. Nurses should recognise that if they do not feel knowledgeable, comfortable or capable of offering advice they can suggest to the patient that they could be referred to somebody more qualified to deal with their problem (Glover, 1982). It is very important that nurses are aware of:

- the boundaries of their knowledge
- the scope of their abilities
- how and where to get backup for themselves and their patients.

The Arthritis Research Campaign (ARC) and Arthritis Care also produce leaflets that cover many aspects of arthritis, including problems related to body image, sexuality and parenting. This material should be readily available on wards and in outpatient clinics. Information in this form may be all that the patient requires and further intervention by the nurse may not be necessary. However, the nurse needs to be familiar with the effect that illness and disability may have on the patient's sexuality and watch for verbal and non-verbal signals that indicate the patient may require additional help.

PARENTING

There are multitudes of factors that may influence a patient's decision to have children. For example, it is commonly believed that rheumatoid arthritis is hereditary and patients fear that the disease will be passed to their offspring. In fact, the risks are just as great for children of healthy parents as for those with parents who have rheumatoid arthritis (Cochrane, 1984; Smith, 1994).

When contemplating parenthood, a person with a systemic rheumatic disease has to take into account his or her ability to care of a child (Cochrane, 1984). Problems that may be encountered include the progressive nature of a disease such as rheumatoid arthritis. The mother may encounter difficulties caring for her child and may have to give up her role as carer if her disabilities increase. This may lead to a great deal of emotional distress for both the mother and the child, especially if the child is too young to understand. It is not only the mother who experiences problems in parenting; for men with rheumatic disease fulfilling a parental role can also problematic. They may be unable to share in activities with their children and have to hand over their parental role to someone else, possibly leading them to experience loss of self-esteem and self-worth (Locker, 1983). Family dynamics are changed and illness may result in the patient being unable to fulfill their usual role. Other family members may have to take on additional responsibilities and the patient's need for rest imposes limitations on other family members (Blau and Blau, 1991).

As well as being able physically to care for their children, the patient also has to consider whether they will be able to support their family financially, especially in view of the possibility that both partners may be unable to work in the future. The patient might worry that their children may suffer as a result of them having a disabled parent. However, there is little researched evidence to support this view. Le Gallez (1993) found that for seventy-five percent of the children in her study, the effect had been far from detrimental and that living with a sick parent had brought them closer together as a family. Even so, twenty-five percent of the children in the study expressed resentment, anger and guilt, all of which was directed at the sick parent.

PREGNANCY AND ARTHRITIS

For those who decide they want a child and who take medications for their arthritis, it is essential for the safety of the foetus that they plan their pregnancy. Some drugs are teratogenic (Le Gallez, 1988) and others such as methotrexate, which is given for rheumatoid arthritis, psoriatic arthritis and myositis needs to be stopped a number of months prior to conception. The problems associated with drugs and pregnancy are discussed in Chapter 12.

Pregnant women with arthritis may undergo additional difficulties compared to healthy women. They may experience more backache if they have ankylosing spondylitis or exacerbated pain in the knees and ankles as they gain weight. However for those with rheumatoid arthritis, pregnancy can bring welcome but temporary relief from their symptoms, even though they often return within eight months of giving birth.

ANTENATAL ASPECTS

Fatigue is quite normal during pregnancy, but for women with rheumatic disease who already suffer from fatigue, the effect is additive. Extra rest is important and teaching the principles of energy conservation should be a priority. Tiredness may also be brought about by the anaemia that often accompanies rheumatoid arthritis and iron and vitamin supplements will need to be taken.

A healthy diet is important to rheumatic patients (Chapter 10) but this is particularly so during pregnancy. About 300 extra calories a day are needed during pregnancy and 500 extra calories are required during lactation (Richardson, 1992). It is important to advise the patient that excess weight postpartum will cause extra stress on already damaged lower limbs and so this needs to be avoided.

THE BIRTH

Rheumatic diseases do not usually pose significant problems during labour or at delivery. Sometimes involvement of the hips means that the woman has difficulty or is unable to abduct her hips to give birth vaginally. The anaesthetist may encounter difficulty administering spinal anaesthetics to those patients with spinal problems. If a general anaesthetic is required, patients with rheumatoid arthritis who have cervical spine involvement should wear a cervical collar to prevent hyperextension causing injury to the spinal cord.

CARING FOR THE CHILD

Caring for babies and children is difficult and tiring even for a healthy person. For those with an energy depleting, painful disease it is doubly so. Patients will need a lot of support and advice during this time. It may be necessary to provide extra help in the form of a home helper to ease the situation. If the patient has shoulder or elbow involvement, cuddling and feeding the baby may be difficult. If the elbow joint is weak, a hinged elbow brace may provide additional support. If the upper limbs are painful, a transcutaneous electrical nerve stimulation (TENS) unit worn whilst feeding or nursing can sometimes bring relief. Some women find physical contact is easier to achieve in comfort if they lie on a bed supported by pillows with the baby at their side.

BREAST OR BOTTLE

One of the earliest decisions the mother must make is whether to breastfeed or to bottle-feed. There are pros and cons for both methods. Breastfeeding is not contraindicated in the rheumatic diseases, but mothers need to be aware that any drugs they take will pass into the breast milk. Most health professionals advocate breastfeeding, even if it is for a short period of time as the baby receives some immunity from the mother. Breastfeeding also has the advantage of being less work in terms of bottle washing and sterilisation and it is also cheaper.

However bottle feeding is advantageous in that partner, family or friends can do the feeds! For patients with painful hands or reduced dexterity, teats can be rather fiddly to clean and of course it is essential that they are scrupulously clean.

The best method of feeding is that with which the mother is most comfortable and on which the baby thrives.

CONTRACEPTION

Family planning is an important decision whether the couple are healthy or not. If one or both partners have a rheumatic disease the timing and spacing of pregnancies is crucial. The opportunity to discuss pregnancy and family planning often arises when patients begin disease-modifying drug therapy. Drugs such as sulphasalazine reduce the sperm count and patients need to be informed about this. It is then natural to follow this up with questions about family planning. Fertile women who are considering cytotoxic drugs should be counselled about the reliability of their preferred method of contraception and the consequences to the foetus if they become pregnant.

Those patients who wish to avoid pregnancy may experience a great deal of anxiety at the prospect of an unwanted pregnancy and potential problems with contraception may add to this anxiety. There are a growing number of methods of birth control and some are more reliable than others. An in-depth discussion of contraception is outside the scope of this chapter but there are some problems specific to rheumatic diseases.

Apart from sterilisation, hormonal contraception is the most effective method of fertility control but the effectiveness might be slightly reduced if the patient is taking nonsteroidal anti-inflammatory drugs (Smith, 1994).

Intrauterine devices (IUDs or 'coils') are highly effective but they sometimes cause menorrhagia, which can pose particular problems for those women with rheumatoid arthritis who are prone to anaemia.

Condoms and diaphragms are barrier methods of birth control that should be used in conjunction with spermicidal creams. Condoms or sheaths are available for both males and females and can be bought from pharmacies and supermarkets. They are effective if used properly, but for patients with painful hands or decreased manual dexterity, the male condom in particular can be difficult to put on. If this is the case then the able-bodied partner may need to assist. Diaphragms pose a similar problem.

ACTION POINTS FOR PRACTICE

- Describe how illness and disease may influence self-image.
- Write a case history of a patient with severe rheumatoid arthritis and outline what effect it has had on their sexuality.

- A patient has expressed problems with his/her sexuality. Describe how you would respond to this patient and how you think you would feel. Discuss the available resources and describe the help that the patient should receive.
- Mrs Smith is a 34-year-old woman who has had rheumatoid arthritis for three years. She has one five-year-old child. Her rheumatoid arthritis is very aggressive and has caused deformities of her hands and feet. She has synovitis at the metacarpophalangeal joints which means she is unable to wear her wedding ring, a very important symbol of her love. She finds playing with her child difficult and very tiring. She used to like socialising and would wear smart clothes and beautiful high-heeled shoes, which is now no longer possible. She has a loving husband who is 36 years old but she fears he may in her words 'stray'. She no longer feels attractive. Pain and hip involvement make sexual intercourse painful and she feels that her relationship is, along with her health, deteriorating. Detail how you can help this patient.

ACKNOWLEDGEMENTS

This chapter is an updated version of that in the first edition. I would like to thank Juliet Prady and Angela Vale who contributed to the original chapter on which this chapter is based.

REFERENCES

Andrew C, Andrew H (1991) Sexuality and the dying patient. *Journal of District Nursing* 8–10.

Annon JS (1976) The PLISSIT model: a proposed conceptual scheme for behavioural treatment of sexual problems. *Journal of Sex Education Therapy* 2(2):1–15.

Blau SP, Blau B (1991) Sexuality and family life. In: Spiera H, Oreskes I (eds) *Rheumatology for the Health Care Professional*. USA, Warren H Green.

Carolan C (1984) Sex and disability. *Nursing Times* 80:28–30.

Chandani AT, Mass F, McKenna KT (1989) Attitudes of university students towards the sexuality of physically disabled people. *British Journal of Occupational Therapy* 52(6):233–236.

Chesson S (1984) Social and emotional aspects of rheumatoid arthritis. *Nursing* 31:914–915.

Cochrane M (1984) Immaculate infection. *Nursing Times* 80:31–32.

Cohen M (1991) Sexuality and family life. In: Spiera H, Oreskes I (eds) *Rheumatology for the Health Care Professional*. USA, Warren H Green.

Collins Dictionary of the English Language 2nd Edn. Ed: Hanks P. Glasgow, William Collins Sons & Co Ltd.

Dawson-Shepherd R (1984) Why the carpet is no longer big enough. *Nursing Times* 80:33–34.

Drench ME (1994) Changes in body image secondary to disease and injury. *Rehabilitation Nursing* 19(1):31–35.

Freud A (1936) *The Ego and Mechanisms of Defence*. London, Hogarth Press.

Glover J (1982) Psychosexual counselling. *Nursing* 35:1509–1512.

Greengross W (1976) *Entitled to love*. London, Malby Press.

Hahn H (1981) The social component of sexuality and disability: some problems and proposals. *Sexuality and Disability* 4(4):220–233.

Hill J (1991) Assessing rheumatic disease. *Nursing Times* 87(4):33–35.

Hill J (2004) The impact of rheumatoid arthritis on the patients' sex lives. *Nursing Times* 100(20):34–35.

Hill J, Bird H, Thorpe R (2003) Effects of RA on sexual activity and relationships. *Rheumatology* 42:280–286.

Hill J, Reay N (2004) Patients perceptions of the effects of osteoarthritis on their sexual relationships. *Annals Rheumatic Diseases* 63(1):suppl. 543.

Irwin R (1997) Sexual health promotion in nursing. *Journal of Advanced Nursing* 25:170–177.

Jones H (1994) Mores and morals. Sexuality, older people. *Nursing Times* 90(47): 55–58.

Kraaimaat FW, Bakker AH, Janssen E *et al.* (1996) Intrusiveness of rheumatoid arthritis on sexuality in male and female patients living with a spouse. *Arthritis Care and Research* 9(2):120–125.

Law C (2001) Sexual health and the respiratory patient. *Nursing Times* 97: X11–X12.

Lee MV, Moll JMH (1987) *Nursing care of the rheumatic patient – principles and practice*. London, Croom Helm.

Le Gallez P (1993) Rheumatoid arthritis: effects on the family. *Nursing Standard* 7(39):30–34.

Le Gallez (1988) Teratogenesis and drugs for rheumatic disease. *Nursing Times* 84(27):41–44.

Locker D (1983) *Disability and Disadvantage – The Consequences of Chronic Illness*. London, Tavistock Publications.

Majerovitz SD, Revenson TA (1994) Sexuality and rheumatic disease: the significance of gender. *Arthritis Care and Research* 7(1):29–34.

Maslow A (1970) *Motivation and Personality*. New York, Harper & Row.

Mearns D, Thorne B (1988) *Person-centred counselling in action*. London, Sage Publications, p69–70.

Price B (1990) *Body Image – Nursing Concepts and Care*. New York, Prentice Hall.

Richardson A (1992) Rheumatoid arthritis in pregnancy. *Nursing Standard* 6(45):25–28.

Roper N, Logan WW, Tierney AJ (1980) *The Elements of Nursing*. Edinburgh, Churchill Livingstone.

Royal College of Nursing (2000) *Sexuality and Sexual Health in Nursing Practice*. London, Royal College Nursing.

Ryan SJ, Dawes PT, Mayer B (1996) Does inflammatory arthritis affect sexuality? *British Journal Rheumatology* 35(suppl.2):19.

Savage J (1990) Sexuality and nursing care – setting the scene. *Nursing Standard* 4(37):24–25.

Stuart GW, Sundeen SJ (1979) *Principles and Practice of Psychiatric Nursing.* St. Louis, Mosby.

Smith PJ (1994) Rheumatoid arthritis and sexual relationships. *Rheumatology in Practice*, Winter:12–13.

Royal College of Nursing (2000) *Sexuality and Sexual Health in Nursing Practice.* London, Royal College Nursing.

Venables P (1985) Sjögren's syndrome. In: *Collected reports on the rheumatic diseases.* Arthritis and Rheumatism Council for Research, UK, p93.

Waterhouse J (1996) Nursing practice related to sexuality: a review and recommendations. *Nursing Times Research* 1(6):412–418.

Webb C (1985) Gynaecological nursing – a compromising situation. *Journal of Advanced Nursing* 18:47–54.

Webb C (1987) *Sexuality, Nursing and Health.* Chichester, John Wiley.

Wylie E (2001) Let's talk about sexuality. *Rheumatology* 40(suppl.1):141.

7 The Social Implications of Rheumatic Disease

S. RYAN

Haywood Hospital, Staffordshire, UK

This chapter explores the effect that living with a rheumatological disease has on social relationships, the family unit, changes in role at home and in the workplace. The chapter concludes with a section on pregnancy. After reading this chapter the reader should be able to:

- describe the implications for the family unit of living with a rheumatological condition;
- discuss the function of social support;
- understand both the advantages and disadvantages of social support;
- describe the advantages of a telephone helpline service;
- describe the role of the nurse in supporting and educating both the patient and family members;
- understand how rheumatological conditions can affect a person's ability to work;
- discuss the implications of rheumatic disease for pregnancy.

Rheumatological conditions have a global impact on the well-being of the patient and their family, Maycock (1988) has described it as 'the tightrope between freedom and a life sentence'. Although many of the symptoms of chronic disease are physical, such as pain, stiffness and synovitis, the patient also faces restraints on valued aspects of everyday life. These include the ability and option of remaining active and contributing socially and remaining in employment. A person with a rheumatic disease may find it impossible to continue with activities that bring meaning to their life, such as engaging in sports, and this will require a major adjustment in lifestyle. Not surprisingly these changes exact a heavy psychological toll on some patients. Yelin *et al.* (1987) suggest that one-half to two-thirds of persons with rheumatoid arthritis experience:

Rheumatology Nursing: A Creative Approach, 2nd edn. Edited by Jackie Hill.
Copyright 2006 by John Wiley & Sons, Ltd.

- losses in social relationships
- disrupted leisure activities
- limitation in work activities
- transportation problems.

THE FAMILY

The family is a dynamic social unit that undergoes many changes in the course of life and fulfils many functions that are essential for physical, psychological and social well-being (Table 7.1). It is within the family that an individual is able to share thoughts and be themselves, benefiting from an environment of mutual trust and respect. The family unit can be an area of retreat which acts as a protective framework from the strains of everyday life. It is often in the family where ties or relationships are cemented, and the individual has concerns and cares for their partner and children.

The family has a paramount role when one of its members is faced with chronic illness such as arthritis (Bury and Anderson, 1988). The social support offered from within the family unit influences the individual's response to illness and also has a major bearing on subsequent outcomes such as adherence to treatment and rehabilitation. This is especially true as the repercussions for family members are considerable. They have to cope with the social, emotional and financial impact of the disease not only on the affected family member, but on the family unit as a whole.

THE EFFECT ON THE FAMILY

The family can be affected in one of three ways:

- The arthritis brings the family unit closer together.
- The family experiences minimal alteration in role responsibility or division of labour.
- There is a negative effect on relationships with family members as a consequence of the illness.

(Affleck *et al.*, 1988)

Table 7.1 Function of the family

- Emotional support such as love and affection
- Sexual well-being
- Physical assistance with everyday tasks such as personal hygiene
- Recreational activities and social commitments

Prior to the illness, different family members will have adopted certain responsibilities for the various functions outlined in Table 7.1. Members will be comfortable with their present roles as they will have been negotiated within the unit, and accepted largely from choice and desirability. Roles will also have been influenced by cultural norms, women often undertaking responsibility for the domestic management of the unit. The onset of a rheumatological condition such as rheumatoid arthritis in one of its members will cause the family to look at itself and alter role responsibility within it. This can cause great disruption especially as the patient's emotional reaction to the illness may lead to feelings of helplessness. This can place great stress on the whole unit as other family members may find it difficult to adapt to new roles such as carrying out domestic tasks. It will be a time of great adjustment. Family members must learn when to give and when to withhold help, as being oversupportive or providing support at the wrong time may produce negative outcomes (Revenson, 1990).

THE EFFECT ON SOCIAL CONTACT

The affects of arthritis can place significant restrictions on social contact (Table 7.2). In an attempt to minimise this, the patient may become expert at disguising the pain, fatigue and other symptoms of the condition to the outside world. This will be more difficult within the family unit, where members will recognise alterations in habits and mood. Unless the family has received information, education and guidance from the nurse about the nature of the condition and its manifestations, this can prove very bewildering and relationships can be placed under great strain. For example, if the family is unaware of the importance of pacing activities in conditions such as rheumatoid arthritis and systemic lupus erythematosus, a patient's resting time may be perceived by family members as lazy and wasteful. Similarly, a patient with rheumatoid arthritis can experience a vast daily variation in the severity of symptoms, such as stiffness. Unless the implications of the condition have been discussed with a health professional, family members may find this difficult to comprehend.

Table 7.2 Factors affecting social contact

- Impairment of mobility
- Pain, stiffness and fatigue
- Symptom control
- Time required for treatment interventions such as exercise
- Emotional status
- Self-esteem

LIMITATION IN FAMILY ROLE FUNCTIONING

Research demonstrates that a reduction in the extent to which the family functions as a unit is associated with diminished well-being as measured by life satisfaction and depressive symptoms (Reisine *et al.*, 1987). Activities within the family unit can be divided into two main areas:

- instrumental activities – cooking, cleaning, financial management and shopping;
- nurturing activities – making family arrangements, maintaining family ties, looking after family members and listening to others.

(Gove, 1984)

It is the latter category that is often highly valued by both the individual and the family (Reisine, 1995).

A rheumatological condition such as rheumatoid arthritis or osteoarthritis can impact negatively on both instrumental and nurturing function. Yelin *et al.* (1987) describe the most affected areas being:

- shopping
- cleaning
- maintaining family ties.

The severity of the illness can also be influential. Women with severe rheumatoid arthritis are able to undertake a significantly smaller proportion of household tasks compared to those with mild arthritis, or those unaffected by the disease (Allaire *et al.*, 1991; Allaire, 1992).

In women with rheumatoid arthritis the level of involvement in each role is dependent on both the women's situation and age. Younger women generally carry out more roles than those who are retired or who have raised children. Women with children tend to have significant levels of involvement with their families that decrease during active phases of their condition. Eventually, temporary changes in role responsibility evolve into a redistribution of duties, some shared, others delegated and some former activities foregone. Women who work outside the house tend to push themselves at work and then retire early to bed (Shaul, 1995).

Family and friends are the sources of physical and emotional support most often cited by patients. Frequently, patients with rheumatoid arthritis are able to discuss their situation more openly with a friend, because friends can offer empathy without having to take full responsibility for the consequences (Bury and Anderson, 1988).

Due to the complexity of chronic illness many patients will have difficulty understanding what is happening and may experience feelings of denial, hostility and fear. However they may not voice concerns to their partner for fear of burdening them with emotional pressures when they may already feel they are burdening the family with physical limitations. This is part of the problem of discovering meaning, both in terms of practical consequences and in terms of the wider significance of the disease as a crippling condition (Bury and Anderson, 1988). The depth of impact depends not on the degree of disability but on how well each patient is able to adjust to the disease and accept the physical limitations it imposes (Le Gallez, 1993).

ISOLATION

Arthritis does not only affect household activities, it can also limit social activity leading to social isolation. This can be very destructive and often causes depression. Families frequently become isolated but do not seek outside help, possibly because our culture encourages family emotions to be kept within the family (Broome, 1989). From childhood, social attitudes emphasise the containment rather than the expression of emotion. Discussion outside the family can be interpreted as betrayal. Equally, there can be a lack of awareness as to which agency to approach for help.

EFFECTS ON THE SPOUSE AND MARRIAGE

Living with a rheumatological condition can cause considerable stress on the healthy partner, as the partner with the illness faces a complex set of illness-related demands including:

- pain
- in some cases disability
- uncertainty about disease progression
- frequent medical care.

Family cohesion has been found to be a significant factor in influencing pain perception, disability and psychological functioning in patients with rheumatoid arthritis and fibromyalgia (Nicassio and Radojenic, 1993). The importance of the family role in patient outcome was illustrated in a study of the benefits of behavioural intervention to minimise pain in patients with rheumatoid arthritis. The intervention incorporating family support was more effective in reducing pain than the intervention with the patient alone (Radojenic *et al.*, 1992).

The extent to which partners are prepared to acknowledge the existence of illness and provide support is more important than the level of disability in influencing patient well-being. Families with a severely disabled member often cope better than families with fewer disabilities (Le Gallez, 1993). Spouses of patients with rheumatoid arthritis can have poor perception of the disability, pain and stiffness their partners live with (Phelan *et al.*, 1994).

These negative perceptions have been shown to lessen by attendance at an education programme aimed at improving knowledge about the condition. The spouse may report greater and longer lasting distress than the patient, causing anxiety and depression, which can have a negative effect both within the home and the workplace (Flor *et al.*, 1987). However, work by Revenson and Majerovitz (1991) found that the level of depressive symptoms in the healthy spouse was no greater than that found in community samples.

ROLE ALTERATION

The disabling effect of arthritis can herald a change in the role of both the patient and the partner. This change of role is recognised by the majority of female patients but by only a minority of male patients. Men largely accept the role of caring for their female partner. However, whilst the female partner is as willing as the male to accept the responsibility of caring, some male patients are unable to accept this offer, viewing it as a threat to their perceived role as head of the house and family provider (Le Gallez, 1993).

Communication within the family unit is essential. It is not unusual for there to be conflict, especially between feelings of overprotectiveness on one hand, and anger and resentment at the disruption of their lives on the other. In a study into the lived experience of rheumatoid arthritis, one female patient stated *'he was bewildered he did not know whether to answer back or try and console me'* (Ryan, 1996a). It will take time for all members to adjust to the new situation in which the family finds itself. When carrying out an assessment on the patient it is of vital importance that the rheumatology nurse assesses the patient's social circumstances. The family may have certain limitations in insight which adversely affect communication links. If so, the nurse can include this in the care management plan and provide the intervention required to improve communication and understanding.

THE EFFECT OF MARRIAGE

Many studies have demonstrated that married people have fewer health problems and a lower mortality rate than those who are single, divorced, separated or widowed (Reisine, 1993). It has been suggested that the benefits of marriage are due to having a more supportive social network. One study of patients with rheumatoid arthritis supports this theory. Married women perceived better access to help with instrumental tasks, experienced more physical affection and had greater feelings of being needed by others compared to those who were not married (Manne and Zautra, 1989).

Although there is data to support the notion that marriage constitutes a special social tie that confers health protection to those who are married, negative aspects of the marital relationship can affect coping and psychological adjustment. High levels of spouse criticism are directly related to maladaptive coping behaviour (Reisine, 1995) and in one survey, 17% of patients believed that their RA had been the cause of their divorce (NRAS, 2003).

SEXUAL RELATIONSHIPS

Patients with RA report a reduction in the frequency of sexual intercourse due to:

- joint pain and stiffness
- joint function
- fatigue (Hill *et al.*, 2003; Gutweigner *et al.*, 1999; Ryan, 1996b).

The nurse was cited as the most appropriate person to provide support in this area. However, if nurses are to take on this role, they must be given adequate training and preparation. Only then will the nurse feel able to include it in the assessment stage and plan interventions that match identified need. This area is discussed further in Chapter 6.

THE FUTURE

Central to the experience of illness is the uncertainty and worries about prognosis of variable and fluctuating disorders such as rheumatoid arthritis (Weiner, 1975). Patients with rheumatoid arthritis are often unduly pessimistic about their future and are frequently inaccurate in their perceptions of their illness (Hewlett, 1994). Negative beliefs whether well-founded or not, may affect a person's ability to cope and to learn positive methods of living with their illness. If they are convinced of a negative future, they may lose faith in prescribed treatments and inadvertently cause more pain and other manifestations by ignoring advice relating to analgesia taking, exercise, pacing activities.

The nurse must find time to ascertain what most concerns the patient about their condition and perception of the future. Being admitted to hospital can be a bewildering and frightening experience. As one participant stated *'being on the ward and seeing all these people with twisted joints or using wheelchairs, you do wonder if that is going to happen to me'* (Ryan, 1996a). Talking through fears may help the patient to see them as more manageable. If the fear is of something specific, for example a reduction in mobility, the nurse can discuss remedies such as:

- exercise regimes
- suitable footwear
- the possibility of surgical intervention.

Active involvement in care can be used as a coping strategy and the nurse must endeavour to inform fully on all aspects, so choices can be made and alternatives offered. The patient needs to feel in control of the situation through knowledge and through full participation. Consistency is important; being given conflicting information by members of the health care team will only heighten feelings of anxiety. Fear is a natural expression of concern, but intervention is required if it prevents the patient from taking action that is in their best interest (Pigg *et al.*, 1985). Knowledge and involvement will foster hope. If hope is threatened, a spiral of decline can occur involving depression and isolation.

THE EFFECT ON CHILDREN

Nearly three-quarters of children living with a parent who had rheumatoid arthritis have been found to be afraid of developing the disease but did not communicate this fear to their parents (Le Gallez, 1993). Silences such as this within the family unit makes the support and education of all family members an essential role of the nurse (Chapter 15).

It has also been found that the self-esteem of adolescent children living with a parent who has arthritis, was lower than that of children living with healthy parents, but comparable to that of children living with a parent suffering depression. Greater family and peer support did not effect their self-esteem in any positive way (Hirsch and Reishch, 1985). For adolescents whose parents had arthritis, involvement of friends with their family presents more opportunities for friends to see the disability, and so to view the whole family in a negative light. In this way the parent's physical disability might adversely affect the adolescents' ability to draw on friendship for support (Revenson, 1993). However this was not substantiated in work by Le Gallez (1993) who found that 75% of children living with a parent with rheumatoid arthritis experienced either a minimal impact on their lives or that it brought them closer together as a family. These children expressed deep concern and displayed a nurturing attitude towards the ill parent. The 25% of children who felt living with a parent with arthritis was detrimental, could be divided in to two groups:

- those whose parents were unable to accept the pain and physical limitations;
- those children who resented the fact that a parent was ill and as a result showed little consideration or compassion for them.

SOCIAL SUPPORT

Social support refers to the process by which interpersonal relationships promote:

- physical
- psychological
- social well-being
- emotional well-being.

The functions of social support are shown in Table 7.3. The need for this support is especially heightened at the time of chronic illness, where the effects on an individual invade all domains of life. The person will often experience anger, resentment and grief at their new situation. The degree and type of support offered is probably one of the most important factors in determining how both the individual and the family unit accept the disease.

Coping with arthritis patients is helped by three factors:

- being given the opportunity to express feelings and concerns;
- receiving encouragement, hope and optimism;
- receiving advice and information.

(Affleck *et al.*, 1988)

MECHANISMS OF SUPPORT

There are two common models for support:

- The stress-buffering model which states that support acts as a protector at a time of crisis (Cohen and Wills, 1985).
- The direct-effect model which states that support is beneficial regardless of the stress experienced; that support can enhance well-being at all times and not just in the face of chronic illness (Revenson, 1993).

The validity of these models has been tested in patients with rheumatoid arthritis, using pain as the stressor. It was found that irrespective of the level of pain experienced, greater support was related to reduced levels of depression and that this correlation prevailed after six months (Brown *et al.*, 1989). This work supports the direct effect model.

Table 7.3 Functions of social support

- Expressing positive affect
- Encouraging communication of feelings
- Providing information and advice
- Validating beliefs, emotions and actions
- Enhancing psychological well being
- Providing material aid

Regardless of disability, greater levels of social support are also associated with an increased level of self-esteem and lower reported depression levels (Fitzpatrick et al., 1988). This is not surprising as patients living with a rheumatological condition experience a fluctuating pattern of symptoms and progression. The knowledge that support is available constantly and not just at times of acute activity must contribute to general well-being.

The stress-buffering model might be more appropriately applied to individuals experiencing acute illness, such as appendicitis, where support will be required for a limited time.

THE BENEFITS OF SOCIAL SUPPORT

Social support has numerous benefits:

- Patients with arthritis who received support from family and friends exhibit greater self-esteem (Fitzpatrick et al., 1988), psychological adjustment (Affleck et al., 1988), life satisfaction (Burckhardt, 1985), and report less depression (Revenson and Majerovitz, 1991).
- Involvement of the family in patient care increases sensitivity to the perception of functional disability, pain and stiffness experienced by the patient. Maycock (1988) refers to a young person, newly diagnosed with rheumatoid arthritis, who complained that because the arthritis was not visible, that family could not comprehend the severity of the illness.
- Social support increases the motivation to partake in instrumental action and reduces the emotional stress that may impede other coping efforts, so increasing patients' adherence to treatment (Cohen, 1988). For example, if the family accepts the need for exercise it can be incorporated in the family routine.
- Support may encourage the performance of positive health behaviour, thus preventing or minimising illness and the reporting of symptoms (Cohen, 1988).
- Patients with arthritis who have a greater number of close friends and relations report fewer activity losses and make activity modifications (Katz, 1995).
- Social support may be important in predicting health outcomes in patients with rheumatoid arthritis. Both unmarried men and married women with a poor social support network, predict greater impairment and depression (Revenson, 1993).

NEGATIVE ASPECTS OF SOCIAL SUPPORT

Social support is not beneficial in all circumstances and negative effects can occur.

Patients may resent their need for support and reject it when it is offered, viewing its acceptance as reducing self-autonomy and reinforcing the concept of powerlessness

The family may become overprotective, encouraging the patient to constantly rest rather than partake in exercise. This will have negative consequences causing increased pain, stiffness and muscle wasting.

Patients can become overly dependent on the family, adopting disability as a way of life, and ceasing to be an active participant in care management. In effect the patient withdraws into a childlike condition, allowing everything to be done for them in a paternalistic environment.

Patients may be less likely to seek help if they feel they are not able to return the support, causing a reduction in self esteem.

Support from some family members can become a form of social control in the relationship that limits patient participant in self management (Rook, 1990).

EFFECTIVENESS OF SUPPORT

Social support can positively influence a patient's perception of control over the daily symptoms of their condition (Ryan *et al.*, 2003). The aspects of social support that influence control perception include:

- remaining involved in family activities;
- receiving ongoing support from family members;
- achieving a balance between support needs and support provision.

The balance between the recipient's support needs and the amount of support offered influence the effectiveness of support. For example, a newly diagnosed patient with inflammatory arthritis will require information about how to self-manage the condition in a supportive educational partnership with the nurse. It would certainly be inappropriate at this stage in a person's condition to discuss surgical intervention as this would not be addressing the patient's perceived needs. If the nurse is underpinning her practice with the therapeutic care philosophy described in Chapter 1, and providing care that has both meaning and relevance for the patient, the nurse will engage in a partnership with the patient and their significant others to draw up a plan of care that is appropriate to the individual's situation (Figure 7.1).

THE TELEPHONE HELPLINE

Although many rheumatology nurses are involved in operating a telephone helpline service for patients there is little published about the types of services offered (McCabe *et al.*, 2000). The Royal College of Nursing provides guid-

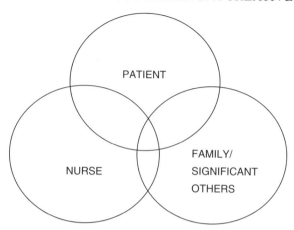

Figure 7.1 The care partnership.

ance on providing a telephone consultancy service (RCN, 1999). The objective of a telephone helpline service is to provide a designated point of contact for the patients should they need advice regarding any aspect of their condition. This is reassuring for the patient and their family as they know they can easily access and communicate with a professional involved in their care. A twelve-month audit of a helpline demonstrated that patients' most frequent needs include advice on:

* drug therapy
* pain control
* how to cope with a flare
* benefit entitlements.

The nurse is able to provide advice directly to the individual concerned and coordinate further action if it is required. A patient with a swollen joint may require aspiration and injection to relieve the inflammation, and this can be arranged quickly by liaison with the appropriate member of the rheumatology team. It may be the nurse herself that will conduct this procedure, so providing comprehensive care for the patient, and reinforcing the relationship of trust that will have developed during the communication period. Patients with osteoarthritis who received biweekly telephone contact for six months reported increased levels of perceived support and less pain (Weinberger *et al.*, 1989).

The telephone helpline can also provide direct access for other members of the team involved in the patient's medical and nursing care. A general practitioner for example may ring for advice regarding whether gold injections should be discontinued due to the presence of haematuria. The advice may be to continue and this will prevent treatment being stopped unnecessarily. It will also enable a consistency of care management to develop between members of the primary and secondary health care team. This will reinforce communication links and promote a greater appreciation of the different roles of these two groups, who are both key providers in the patients care.

SUPPORT GROUPS

Some patients become members of support groups to obtain an additional source of support and as a means of obtaining more information about living with the condition. This can empower the patient and the family on many different aspects of their condition, for instance the purpose of drug therapy. Support groups can also be active in raising public awareness of the problems faced by people living with arthritis. For some patients it prevents isolation and provides a regular point of contact with a group of people living with similar difficulties and limitations in lifestyle. Those attending the group and who are coping well may serve as role models and motivators for those members who are coping less well. It is important that the facilitator of the group maintains a positive attitude, with the emphasis on education and support. If this is not done, the group could be used unconstructively as a forum for complaints and no longer serve its members in a positive way.

THE ROLE OF THE NURSE

Revenson (1993) states that practitioners can work towards a number of goals including:

- teaching patients how to develop and maintain family ties;
- teaching patients how to recognise and accept the help and emotional encouragement provided by family members;
- improving family member skills for determining the patient support needs and offering help;
- facilitating positive appraisals of support.

WHEN IS SUPPORT MOST BENEFICIAL?

Different types and levels of support will be needed at different stages of the illness. After diagnosis and commencement of therapy, a patient with inflammatory arthritis will expect that the condition will be controlled and that they can return to the pattern of life they enjoyed prior to the illness. However, if the treatment is not effective and the disease remains active, the patient will experience increased pain and stiffness, and their ability to carry out activities of daily living independently will be reduced. It is at this stage that a patient may experience feelings of anxiety, despondency and depression. Whereas, in the initial phase of illness the role of the nurse may have centred around the provision of information, a negative response to treatment will necessitate a change in care provision to emotional support, guidance and motivation. Conditions such as rheumatoid arthritis, with its fluctuating pattern of symptoms, will require the nurse to be receptive to the patient's needs at various stages of the illness and match the support required with the patient's identified needs. The types of support the nurse can provide are described in Table 7.4.

THE THERAPEUTIC RELATIONSHIP

The nurse will need to enter into a therapeutic relationship with the patient as described in Chapter 1, and spend time relating and communicating with them on a personal level. This will allow care to be planned that has meaning and relevance for the patient. The patient will be able to identify with the care programme and to become an active participant in it, promoting a worthy relationship between patient and nurse, seeking common goals and objectives. Once a problem such as unrelenting pain has been identified, the nurse and the patient will need to agree on the necessary interventions to minimise the problem. This will involve ascertaining the patient's lay beliefs. Exercise may be recommended but a patient who doubts its efficacy is unlikely to persist if there are no immediate benefits.

The care management plan will require regular evaluation. This may be a weekly occurrence whilst the patient learns to implement self management techniques such as pacing activities. As the patient and the family begin to develop effective coping skills, the evaluation will be needed less frequently.

Experiencing frequent flares will be stressful to both the patient and their family. As social support needs change, carers must learn when to give and

Table 7.4 Types of support the nurse can provide

* Emotional – providing the opportunity for discussing feelings about the condition
* Instrumental – arranging for the occupational therapist to carry out an assessment of the home environment
* Informational – providing self-management information on how to cope with a flare of the condition

when to withhold help, as providing too much support or providing it at the wrong time, may produce negative outcomes such as reducing autonomy and self-worth. Attempts at achieving the necessary balance of support can be difficult because individuals do not automatically know how to provide support that does not demean the recipient (Coyne *et al.*, 1988). This is why it is so important to involve family members and significant others in all aspects of care planning so that information and subsequent understanding can be shared. This will enable the family to function as a unit rather than in isolated parts.

THE EFFECT ON ROLE

The most difficult task the nurse faces is to help the patient and their family recognise that roles and relationships have changed (Pigg *et al.*, 1985). The nurse needs to assist patients to communicate their feelings about the change in lifestyle that the condition has caused. The individual can often feel afraid and lost if they see their traditional role being eroded. If a person is unable to return to paid employment, the despondency this causes the individual will have repercussions within the family, especially if the healthy partner has to increase their working activity for financial reasons. The nurse needs to encourage and support the patient and assist them to explore ways in which their skills can be used positively and constructively. This may include:

- referral to the disability employment officer for advice on retraining;
- active involvement on a committee of a support group;
- participating in a personal development programme through voluntary agencies such as arthritis care;
- assisting with teaching of junior staff or general practitioners through an expert patient partners programme.

(Dinsdale, 1999)

The nurse will need to assess family reactions to the illness at the time of patient assessment. This should be done by the use of open-ended questions such as:

'How did your family react to your illness?'

or

'How do the family support you?'

The response may reveal limitations in insight that can be addressed by providing information or family counselling. It may be useful for the family members to meet others in a similar situation and the nurse can facilitate this.

SHARING FEELINGS

The nurse needs to encourage the patient to share their feelings. Sometimes the patient feels unable to do this within the home situation due to the emotional pressure it places on family members. The nurse can act as an emotional support and work through the patient's feelings with them. If the patient reveals signs of clinical depression a referral to the psychiatrist for appropriate management might be necessary. However, for the vast majority of patients coming to terms with living with a chronic illness, the nurse will be able to provide adequate support. By knowing the patient through a therapeutic relationship, the patient will feel able to trust the nurse and share their feelings openly.

FAMILY INSIGHT

If they are to support the patient, the family needs a similar knowledge base and understanding. Family members who do not believe that a person's disease is a major or serious problem may be unable to support measures such as rest or pacing activities that will change the family's lifestyle. Unless it is explained to them and they are included in the family discussions, children may not understand the reason that their father can no longer play sport with them. A family with unrealistic expectations places an unnecessary burden on the patient, especially if they believe that all will be well if only the patient works hard enough.

WORK

The experience of chronic illness operates simultaneously at two levels:

- biological functioning
- cultural competence.

Society often defines a person by their occupation, and the status associated with particular work effects self-esteem.

The impact of musculoskeletal condition on employment is of concern to:

- the individual, who faces the loss of income as well as role alteration;
- family members, who may alter their own employment, sometimes by leaving the workforce to provide care or by entering the workforce to compensate for the lost income;
- society, that must meet the cost of benefit payments.

Several studies have evaluated work disability, the relationship between the type of work undertaken and the extent to which the disease impairs the ability to carry out that work (Yelin et al., 1987). In the work characteristic model it is the interaction between the impairment caused by the disease and the job requirement that affects the work disability rate. If an individual, employed in a job that requires manual dexterity, develops hand and wrist synovitis, they may no longer be able to carry on in that particular job. Equally if an individual has rheumatoid arthritis and needs to leave work for regular monitoring of treatment, the probability of ceasing employment is increased if the job offers no flexibility.

Persons with a musculoskeletal condition are more likely to stop working if they:

- are older
- are female
- have fewer years in education
- have pain and comorbidity
- have experienced limitation in function (Yelin, 1995).

In Great Britain work loss due to back disorders has doubled in five years, accounting for 52.6 million days lost from work in 1988–1989 and for one-seventh of all sickness invalidity benefit payments. Back disability is growing faster than any other form of disability (Frymoyer and Cats-Baril, 1991).

In the United States 57% of people with a musculoskeletal condition were not working and 64%–72% of people with rheumatoid arthritis were unemployed (Pincus et al., 1989; Yelin and Callahan, 1995). In the National Rheumatoid Arthritis Survey 54% of participants attributed not being in paid employment to their RA and 30% of employed participants worked part-time due to their RA (NRAS, 2003).

The intrusiveness of rheumatoid arthritis is greatest in the areas of active recreation, work and health. The degree of interference with active recreation and work is equivalent to that found in individuals with multiple sclerosis (Devins et al., 1993). Furthermore, the intrusiveness of rheumatoid arthritis increases as physical function worsened (Devins et al., 1992).

Most patients with rheumatoid arthritis stop work within ten years of developing the disease (Meenan et al., 1981; Le Gallez, 1993) with 40% of patients stopping work within five years of diagnosis (NICE, 2002). As the condition most commonly affects individuals in their third and fourth decade of life, patients may face many years without being able to work. It is of particular importance that the individual concerned and their family are given time to adjust to this radical change in their lifestyle. It is also important that the person believes their limitations to be real, rather than accepting the judgement of someone else, such as the doctor. This will prevent them aimlessly wondering whether they could have returned to work and prevent wishful thinking which can be viewed as a negative coping strategy (Newman, 1993).

During this difficult stage, substantial counselling and support should be made available to both the patient and their family to help them adjust. Boredom and a sense of uselessness needs to be faced, and alternative interests found. This is particularly important for men, who often have a poor support network (Le Gallez, 1993). Unemployment will affect self-perception, lead to an alteration of role and have financial implications. The nurse must be proactive in this area, referring patients to the appropriate agencies, for example to social work for advice on benefits, whilst at the same time providing the family with guidance and support.

PREGNANCY

An individual's decision about whether or not to have children is likely to be influenced by:

• how the woman is coping with the condition
• disease activity
• drug therapy
• practical support
• family finances.

Preconception counselling and education are vital to ensure that prospective parents are given the necessary information regarding their disease to enable them to make a fully informed decision.

PRECONCEPTION ADVICE

Patients planning a family should be encouraged to seek advice from the rheumatology team. Women with rheumatoid arthritis often need to achieve disease suppression to increase their chance of conceiving. Decisions regarding the withdrawal of potentially toxic drug therapy, need to be made in good time, since many drugs can affect the vulnerable stage of embryogenesis. Women should discontinue teratogenic agents such as methotrexate, azathioprine and cyclophosphamide at least six months before attempting conception or two years if taking leflunomide. Ideally all drug therapy should be avoided during pregnancy and lactation. The implications of taking the most frequently prescribed medication in arthritis are described in Chapter 12.

ANTENATAL CARE

In rheumatoid arthritis 75% of women experience some remission of their condition during pregnancy but often return to a disease status comparable with their prepregnant state within eight months of giving birth.

The effect of pregnancy is less predictable in systemic lupus erythematosus. If the patient has renal involvement close monitoring will be required, as deteriorating renal function is also associated with toxaemia.

In ankylosing spondylitis 80% of patients may experience a worsening of symptoms or no alteration in their condition during pregnancy (Le Gallez, 1988).

During the antenatal phase the nurse will need to provide:

- advice on pacing activities (Fatigue is quite normal in pregnancy but may be compounded by disease activity so there must be a balance between rest and activity. Good quality sleep, gentle exercises such as swimming and early maternity leave are all important (Richardson, 1992).);
- advice on coping with pain (This should include relaxation techniques, the application of hot and cold therapy and the use of diversion techniques. The occupational therapist may also be involved at this stage to offer advice on joint protection and the suitability of proposed baby equipment.);
- advice on diet (An additional 300 calories a day will be needed during pregnancy and extra 500 calories a day during lactation.).

MANAGEMENT OF LABOUR AND DELIVERY

Hip involvement in musculoskeletal disorders may limit thigh abduction or pelvic measurements. If a caesarean section is indicated and the patient has cervical spine disease a cervical collar will be required to prevent hyperextension.

POST-NATAL CARE

The support of the community rheumatology sister and the health visitor will be essential in providing both physical and psychological support. If the mother has physical limitations and is unable to lift the baby, their advice will be required and alternative methods found such as supporting the baby on a pillow across the knees, or lying on the bed to provide physical contact.

Breastfeeding is not contraindicated but all drugs taken by a nursing mother will pass in to the breast milk. The actual amount of drug passing to the baby will depend on the maternal rates of:

- absorption
- metabolism

* distribution
* elimination.

Women who develop an exacerbation of rheumatoid arthritis postpartum will need to recommence their suppressive drug therapy and individual advice from the rheumatology nurse will be required if the mother is breastfeeding. Due to the demands placed on lifestyle by a new baby, it may be necessary to plan a specific time for sexual activity (Chapter 6).

Patients living with a rheumatological condition will find it has a vast impact on their social life and the family unit and the social support offered needs to match their needs. In this area the rheumatology nurse can be proactive; supporting, guiding, motivating, informing and involving the patient and their significant others in all areas of care management. This will ensure that the family unit works in unison, sharing the same knowledge base and treatment objectives.

ACTION POINTS FOR PRACTICE

* List the functions of the family unit.
* Plan a teaching session for colleagues to illustrate the effects on the family, when one of its members has arthritis.
* Look at ways of involving the family more fully in care planning.
* Design a poster informing patients where they can receive advice regarding employment and benefit entitlements.
* Provide a handout for family members explaining the ways in which the family can provide positive support.
* Provide information for patients on the local support groups in the area.

REFERENCES

Affleck G, Fifield J, Pfeiffer C, Tennen H (1988) Social support and psychological adjustment to rheumatoid arthritis. *Arthritis Care and Research* 1:71–77.
Allaire SH (1992) Employment and work disability in women with rheumatoid arthritis. *The Journal of Applied Rehabilitation and Counselling* 23:44–50.
Allaire SH, Anderson JJ, Meenan RF (1991) The impact of rheumatoid arthritis on the household performance of women. *Arthritis and Rheumatism* 34:669–678.
Broome A (1989) *Health Psychology Processes and Applications.* London, Chapman and Hall.
Brown EK, Nicassio PM, Wallston KA (1989) Social support and depression in rheumatoid arthritis; a one year prospective study. *Journal of Applied Social Psychology* 19:1164–1181.
Burckhardt CS (1985) The impact of arthritis on quality of life. *Nursing Research* 34:11–16.

Bury M, Anderson R (1988) *Living with Chronic Illness. The Experience of Patients and their Families.* London, Unwin Hyman.

Cohen S, Wills TA (1985) Stress social support and the buffering hypothesis. *Psychological Bulletin* 98:310–357.

Cohen S (1988) Psychological models of the role of social support in the aetiology of physical disease. *Health Psychology* 7:269–297.

Coyne JC, Lehman D, Wartman CB (1988) The other side of support, emotional over-involvement and miscarried helping. In: Gottlieb BH (ed) *Social Support, Formats Processes and Effects* 305–330. Newbury Park CA, Sage Publications.

Devins GM, Edworthy SM, Guthrie NG, Martin L (1992) Illness intrusiveness in rheumatoid arthritis, differential impact on depressive symptoms over the adult lifespan. *Journal of Rheumatology* 19:709–715.

Devins GM, Eworthy SM, Klein GM, Mandin H, Paul LC, *et al.* (1993) Differences in illness intrusiveness across rheumatoid arthritis, end stage renal disease and multiple sclerosis. *Journal of Neurology and Mental Disorders* 181:377–381.

Dinsdale P (1999) Gain from pain. *Nursing Times* 95(41): 34–35.

Fitzpatrick R, Lamb R, Newman S, Shipley M (1988) Social relationships and psychological well-being in rheumatoid arthritis. *Social Science and Medicine* 27: 399–403.

Flor H, Scholz OB, Turk DC (1987) Impact of chronic pain on the spouse; marital, emotional and physical consequences. *Journal of Psychosomatic Research* 31: 63–71.

Frymoyer JW, Cats-Baril WL (1991) An overview of the incidence and costs of low back pain. *Orthopaedic Clinical North America* 22:261–271.

Gove WR (1984) Gender differences in mental and physical illness. The effect of fixed roles and nurturant roles. *Social Science Medicine* 19:77–84.

Gutweigner S, Kopp M, Mur E, Gunter V (1999) Body image of women with rheumatoid arthritis. *Clinical and Experimental Rheumatology* 17(94):413–417.

Hewlett S (1994) Patients views of changing disability. *Nursing Standard* 8(31): 25–29.

Hill J, Bird H, Thorpe R (2003) Effects of rheumatoid arthritis on sexual activity and relationships. *Rheumatology* 42:280–286.

Hirsch BJ, Reishch T (1985) Social networks and developmental psychopathology, a comparison of adolescent children, of a depressed, arthritic or normal parent. *Journal of Abnormal Psychology* 94:272–281.

Katz P (1995) The impact of rheumatoid arthritis on life activities. *Arthritis Care and Research* 8(4):272–278.

Le Gallez P (1988) Teratogenesis and drugs for rheumatic disease. *Nursing Times* 84(27):41–44.

Le Gallez P (1993). Rheumatoid arthritis effects on the family. *Nursing Standard* 7(39):30–34.

McCabe C, McDowell J, Cushnaghan J, Butts S, Hewlett S, *et al.* (2000) Rheumatology telephone helplines; an activity analysis. *Rheumatology* 39:1390–1395.

Manne SL, Zautra AJ (1989) Spouse criticism and support: their association with coping and psychological adjustment among people with rheumatoid arthritis. *Journal Personal Social Psychology* 56:608–617.

Maycock J (1988) The image of rheumatic disease. In: Salter M (ed). *Altered Body Image. The Nurse's Role.* New York, J Wiley.

Meenan RF, Espstein VW, Newitt M, Yelin EH (1981) The impact of chronic diseases, a socio-medical profile of rheumatoid arthritis. *Arthritis and Rheumatism* 24(3):544–548.

Newman SP (1993) Coping with rheumatoid arthritis. *Annals of the Rheumatic Diseases* 52:553–554.

Nicassio PM, Radojenic V (1993) Models of family functioning and their contribution to patient outcome in chronic pain. *Motivation Emotion* 17:295–316.

National Institute for Clinical Excellence (2002) Guidance on the use of etanercept and infliximab for the treatment of RA. *Technology appraisal guidance NO 36.* London, NICE.

National Rheumatoid Arthritis Society (2003) *The National Rheumatoid Arthritis Society Survey,* April 2003. Berkshire, NRAS.

Phelan M, Campbell A, Byrne J, Hough Y, Hunt J, et al. (1994) The effect of an education programme on the perception of arthritis by spouses of patients with rheumatoid arthritis. *Scandinavian Journal of Rheumatology,* Suppl 74.

Pigg JS, Caniff R, Driscoll PW (1985) *Rheumatology Nursing. A Problem Orientated Approach.* New York, John Wiley.

Pincus T, Burkhausen R, Mitchell J (1989) Substantial work disability and earning losses in individuals less than 65 years with osteoarthritis: comparisons with rheumatoid arthritis. *Journal of Clinical Epidemiology* 42(5):449–457.

Radojenic V, Nicassio PM, Weisman MH (1992) Behavioural interventions, with and without family support for rheumatoid arthritis. *Behavioural Therapy* 23:13–30.

Reisine S (1993) Marital status and social support in rheumatoid arthritis. *Arthritis and Rheumatism* 36:589–592.

Reisine S (1995) Arthritis and the family. *Arthritis Care and Research* 8(4): 265–271.

Reisine S, Goodenow C, Grady KE (1987) The impact of rheumatoid arthritis on the homemaker. *Social Science Medicine* 25:89–95.

Revenson TA (1990) Social support processes among chronically ill elders; patient and provider perspective. In: Giles H, Coupland N, Wiemann J (eds). *Communication, Health and the Elderly* 92–113. Manchester, University of Manchester Press.

Revenson TA (1993) The role of social support. In: Newman S, Shipley M (eds) *Pychological Apects of Teumatic Dseases. Bailliere's Clinical Reumatology* 7(2):377–396.

Revenson TA, Majerovitz DM (1991) The effects of illness on the spouse: social resources as stress buffers. *Arthritis Care and Research* 4:63–72.

Richardson A (1992) Rheumatoid arthritis in pregnancy. *Nursing Standard* 6(45): 25–29.

Rook K (1990) Social networks as a source of social control in older adults lives. In: Giles H, Coupland N, Weimann JM (eds). *Communication, Health and the Elderly* 45–63. Manchester, University of Manchester Press.

Royal College of Nursing (1999) *Nurse Telephone Consultation Services-Information and Good Practice.* London, RCN.

Ryan S (1996a) Living with rheumatoid arthritis: a phenomenological exploration. *Nursing Standard* 10(41):34–37.

Ryan S (1996b) Does inflammatory arthritis affect sexuality. *British Journal of Rheumatology* (Suppl 2) 35:19.

Ryan S, Hassell A, Dawes P, Kendall S (2003) Control perceptions in patients with rheumatoid arthritis: the impact of the medical consultation. *Rheumatology* 42:135–140.

Shaul M (1995) From early twinges to mastery. The process of adjustment in living with rheumatoid arthritis. *Arthritis Care and Research* 8(4):290–297.

Yelin E, Henke C, Esptein W (1987) Work dynamics of the person with rheumatoid arthritis. *Arthritis and Rheumatism* 30:507–512.

Yelin E (1995) Musculoskeletal conditions and employment. *Arthritis Care and Research* 8(4):311–317.

Yelin E, Callahan L (1995) The economic cost and social and psychological impact of musculoskeletal conditions. *Arthritis and Rheumatism* 38:1351–1362.

Weiner CE (1975) The burden of rheumatoid arthritis: tolerating the uncertainty. *Social Science and Medicine* 9:97–104.

Weinberger M, Bootier P, Katz BP, Tierney WM (1989) Can the provision of information to patients with osteoarthritis improve functional status? A randomised controlled trial. *Arthritis and Rheumatism* 32:1577–1583.

8 Pain and Stiffness

J. HILL
University of Leeds, West Yorkshire, UK

Pain and stiffness are two of the most disabling symptoms of rheumatic disease. The aim of this chapter is to help the nurse to understand these symptoms, the effect they have on their patients and the various treatments available to minimise these effects. After reading this chapter the reader will be able to:

- understand the meaning to the patient of pain and stiffness;
- determine some of the causes of pain and stiffness;
- demonstrate knowledge of the nociceptor sensory system;
- describe influences that effect the perception of pain;
- discuss the use of assessment tools;
- select appropriate treatments for each individual.

PAIN

Pain is one of the most discomforting symptoms of rheumatic disease and is the primary reason that many seek medical advice (Symmons and Bankhead, 1994). Patients with rheumatoid arthritis (RA) cited pain as their most important symptom (Parker *et al.*, 1988; Minnock *et al.*, 2003) and it has been linked with impaired quality of life, depression and disability in both osteoarthritis (OA) and RA (Covic *et al.*, 2000; Sprangers *et al.*, 2000). It has been found that the patients' current experience of pain is likely to predict their subsequent pain and disability, and it makes a major contribution to both physician and patient assessment of general health status (Kazis *et al.*, 1983).

Pain is usually perceived as being unpleasant, and the relief of pain and the provision of comfort are considered as two of the main functions of the nurse (Maycock, 1984). This makes it incumbent on nurses to increase their knowledge of pain and its management.

Rheumatology Nursing: A Creative Approach, 2nd edn. Edited by Jackie Hill.
Copyright 2006 by John Wiley & Sons, Ltd.

DEFINITIONS OF PAIN

Although pain is a common symptom it is a difficult sensation to elucidate. Pigg *et al.* (1985) has likened it to love, a feeling most people understand but have difficulty explaining! Pain is a complex phenomenon, which does not occur in isolation. It is an emotional, sensory and physiological event, which no two people experience in the same way. This makes it impossible to quantify in absolute terms.

The International Association for the Study of Pain (1994) has stated that 'Pain is an unpleasant sensory and emotional experience associated with actual or potential tissue damage, or described in terms of such damage'. Pain is always subjective and individuals learn the application of the word through experience related to injury in early life. It is unquestionably a sensation in a part of the body but is also always unpleasant and therefore always an emotional experience. Many people report pain in the absence of tissue damage or any likely pathophysiological cause. There is no way to distinguish their experience from that due to tissue damage (Merskey, 1979).

Within the realms of nursing, the most accepted definition is that suggested by McCaffery (1983): 'Pain is whatever the experiencing person says it is, existing whenever he says it does'. This accepts that pain is an individual, emotional and subjective experience which makes the patient the authority on their pain, and their impressions on frequency and intensity must be believed.

THE PURPOSE OF PAIN

The primary purpose of the pain is protection (Harvey, 1987). Pain tells us that there is something wrong with our body. For instance someone with appendicitis will feel pain due to the inflammation of their appendix. Once the appendix has been removed, the system will return to normal and become pain-free. Pain also protects us from harming ourselves. Notice how quickly a very hot item is dropped, usually before the pain from the burn is perceived.

Although pain can arise because of a noxious stimuli, chronic pain can occur in the absence of any organic pathology, these are termed somatoform pain disorders.

THE NOCICEPTOR SENSORY SYSTEM

PAIN RECEPTORS

The sensation that we know as pain is brought about by the excitation of receptors in the nociceptive sensory system known as nociceptors. However, pain should not be equated with nociception alone as it can arise in its absence. Conversely, nociception may be present without the sensation of pain (Jones, 1997).

Two types of pain receptors have been identified:

• mechano nociceptors
• polymodal nociceptors.

Mechano nociceptors are activated by pinching or heavy pressure and polymodal nociceptors by heat, cold and pain-producing chemicals. The intensity of the stimulus determines the frequency of nerve impulses (frequency coding), and this is an important element in the severity of pain perception (Campbell, 1995).

Nociceptors are attached to fibres projecting to the dorsal horn of the spinal cord. Two different types of sensory fibres are responsible for signalling different qualities of pain. These are:

• A delta – small myelinated fibre
• C fibre – smaller unmyelinated fibres.

A delta-mediated pain is pricking or sharp and well-localised. This is also called first pain. By comparison, C fibre pain, known as 'second pain', feels dull, burning or throbbing and is poorly localised. Although some pain is easy to determine in these terms, many people with rheumatic disease have difficulty discriminating between the two types.

TRANSMISSION OF PAIN TO THE BRAIN

Nociceptors are sensory neurones that carry impulses to the central nervous system. All sensory nerves enter the spinal cord via the dorsal (posterior) horn (Figure 8.1). From here, they cross over the spinal cord to the opposite anterior horn where they ascend the spinothalamic tract to the medulla, thalamus and on to the cerebral cortex for interpretation and action (Figure 8.1). Simultaneously, impulses are carried from the thalamus to the limbic system, which is associated with basic emotions such as pleasure, fear, anxiety and anger. Impulses arising in the cerebral cortex are also carried to the thalamus and limbic system, modifying their responses (Gallop, 1983).

PAIN GENERATION

Pain in the rheumatic diseases is caused by inflammation, pressure or mechanical disorganisation. Inflammation is particularly prevalent and causes pain through hyperalgesia which occurs as a result of nociceptor sensitisation. Inflammation damages cells and releases chemical mediators that cause

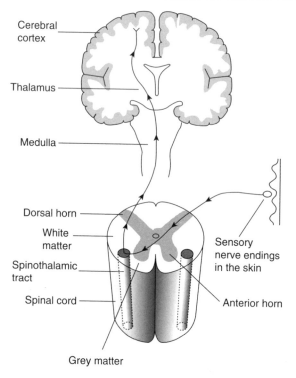

Figure 8.1 Sensory nerve pathway to the cerebral cortex.

chemical sensitisation. These include bradykinin, histamine and prostaglandins.

Pigg *et al.* (1985) has suggested that the causes of pain in the rheumatic diseases can be placed into several discreet categories which include:

- physical changes
- biological
- chemical irritation.

PHYSICAL CHANGES

Disease activity

Many rheumatic diseases cause physical changes within and around joints. The joint capsule, periosteum, blood vessels and deep subcutaneous fascia are well-supplied with nerves capable of carrying pain signals, and these structures are the most sensitive to pain. Muscle, fat and synovial membranes are less receptive and compact bone and articular cartilage are insensitive.

However, the pain from rheumatic diseases is often deeply located and widely dispersed around the joints and often bears little relationship to the tissue affected, be it periosteum, ligament or fascia (Pigg *et al.*, 1985).

Pressure

In the rheumatic diseases, inflammatory effusion and synovial hypertrophy exert increased pressure on the joint capsule and on any exposed bone within it. Pressure at the site of attachment of capsule to sensitive bone can also cause pain. Increased venous pressure, caused by hyperaemia induced by inflammation is an additional stressor. Obesity can be an additional problem, as the excess weight puts further pressure on the diseased joints.

MECHANICAL DAMAGE

Mechanical damage within the joint usually occurs as a result of long-term aggressive disease from RA and OA. The loss of cartilage and erosion of bone leaves the joint disorganised and misaligned. Although the cartilage itself is insensitive to pain, its loss leaves the bone surfaces exposed and unprotected, allowing them to come into contact. In this situation, pain tends to occur on movement and when the patient is bearing weight. Small overgrowths of bone can cause pain both within the joint capsule, and at the heel or spine. They sometimes press on nerve roots, causing excruciating, severe pain. A further source of pain are fractures. These can sometimes develop in subchondral bone in RA and are common in osteoporosis.

BIOLOGICAL CAUSES

Biological causes of pain are those which involve microbial agents. These acute infections are known collectively as 'septic arthritis'. The most common septic arthritis is gonococcal arthritis, but this is less destructive and less serious than that caused by the staphylococcus (Mahowald, 1993). The inflammation and pressure within the joint cause pain whatever the bacterium involved. Once the causative agent has been eliminated the pain will cease. If appropriate treatment is started early in acute gonococcal or streptococcal infections, pain will subside in about two weeks, but it may take longer in staphylococcal and gram-negative infections. In joints with previous disease, or when joint damage has occurred due to the infection, pain can become chronic.

CHEMICAL ORIGINS

Gout, calcium pyrophosphate dihydrate deposition disease and apatite crystal disease are examples of chemically induced pain.

The pain during acute attacks of these crystal deposition diseases can be excruciating, even light pressure, such as that from a bed sheet can be unbearable.

TYPES OF PAIN

The International Association for the Study of Pain (IASP) classifies pain according to its duration (IASP, 1994), namely:

* acute – of recent onset and probably of limited duration;
* chronic – lasting for long periods of time.

Whilst acute pain may serve as an indicator of the presence of disease, chronic pain rarely serves any biological function but causes a great deal of human suffering and is financially costly to the individual, society and the state.

ACUTE PAIN

There are five main features of acute pain:

* It happens suddenly.
* There is an identifiable cause.
* Healing takes place.
* Its duration is short.
* It has a predictable end.

Infections, injury, or surgery usually cause acute pain. Common everyday examples are tonsillitis, fractured limbs or hernia repair. Although most patients with rheumatic disease experience chronic pain, there are instances where arthritis causes acute pain. An instance would be the concurrent development of septic arthritis, bursitis, tenosynovitis or a flare. In these circumstances, the patient is able to differentiate between the different types of pain and often state that the pain they are feeling is different from their usual arthritis pain. Nurses should always take care to listen to their patients and investigate their symptoms; after all, they are the experts.

Some patients with rheumatic diseases undergo surgery for the relief of pain and improvement of function. Postoperative pain is classed as acute pain. Anecdotally, some patients who have endured severe, disabling, chronic pain do not perceive their postoperative pain to be as severe as those who have not had this experience.

CHRONIC PAIN

Chronic pain is usually defined as that which lasts for three months or longer. McCaffery (1983) makes three further classifications.

Limited pain

This is when there is a known and existing pathology, which is time-limited, although the pain may go on for months or years. Examples are carcinoma, which is limited by death, or slow healing injuries such as burns or repetitive strain injury.

Intermittent pain

Here the patient has pain-free periods. The pathology may by understood, but this is not always the case. Examples are migraine or back pain.

Chronic non-malignant pain

This is pain due to non-life-threatening causes, which is not responsive to currently available methods of pain relief and may continue for the remainder of the patient's life (McCaffery and Beebe, 1989). This category applies to many patients with RA and OA.

Chronic nonmalignant pain is seen as a downward spiral that leads some patients to experience feelings of hopelessness when they can see no end to it. Nurses are apt to be less pessimistic preferring to view the pain as a vicious circle as this can be intercepted at some point, and the pain therefore moderated or alleviated (Figure 8.2). Unfortunately, the longer patients have their

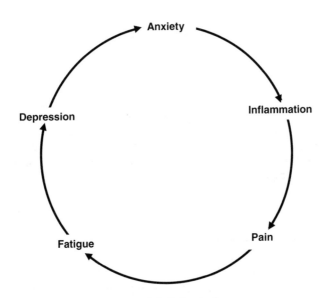

Figure 8.2 Pain circle.

pain, the less able some tolerate it. They sometimes become desperate for relief, using inappropriate drugs and techniques. Increasing passivity and dependency can occur, and worried spouses, family and friends can unwittingly support this. Health professionals can become frustrated at their inability to diminish pain, and tend to accuse patients of exaggerating its severity.

FACTORS THAT INFLUENCE PAIN

The intensity of the pain experience cannot simply be equated with tissue damage or the severity of disease (Bellamy and Bradley, 1996) and so other factors must be implicated. In his extensive review of pain and pain control, Weisenberger (1977) considered the following factors to be influential in the pain experience:

- the circumstances in which pain occurs;
- socialisation;
- past experience;
- personality and mood of the person in pain;
- the meaning or significance of the pain to that person.

There is also widespread agreement that anxiety exacerbates pain (Skevington, 1993). Donovan (1989) has identified a number of beliefs about pain:

- Pain is a punishment.
- Pain is a warning that something is wrong.
- Pain is an emotion (therefore separating psychogenic from somatic aspects of pain).
- Pain is a neurotransmission.
- Pain is a challenge to science.
- Pain is a complex interaction between mind and body.

We all have our own ideology of pain and so if optimum alleviation is to occur, it is important for nurses to examine their own beliefs as well as those of the patient and their caregivers. For instance, a nurse who does not believe there is merit in aromatherapy for the treatment of pain is unlikely to practise its use, thereby reducing the chances of a successful outcome for some patients.

The attitude of nurses is crucial to pain control, and a number of studies into postoperative pain serve to underline this (Davis, 1988; Lloyd, 1994). Nurses frequently underestimate the patient's pain (Seers, 1989), the level of pain experienced by the patient cannot be read by the nurse (Jacques, 1992).

THE GATE CONTROL THEORY

The basic elements of the traditional pain pathways (Figure 8.1) fail to account for a variety of clinical phenomena such as phantom limb pain and the absence of pain from major sporting and wartime injuries. Patients and health professionals alike owe much to Melzack and Wall (1965) for their pioneering work on the 'Gate Control Theory'. This was the first attempt to incorporate physiological and psychological mechanisms into a feasible theory that underpins many of the pain-relieving techniques used by nurses.

THE SITE OF CONTROL

The grey matter of the dorsal horn in the spinal cord is capped by the substantia gelatinosa, which is thought to be the site of control. The theory postulates a gate between the peripheral and higher centres of the central nervous system. When the gate is closed, impulses cannot gain access to the brain. When the gate is open, impulses have free access to the spinal cord and ascend to the brain where the feeling of pain is perceived.

OPENING AND CLOSING THE GATE

Gate closure can be achieved by a number of methods including:

- increasing large diameter fibre activity, for example by skin stimulation;
- increasing brainstem activity, for instance by distraction from the painful sensation;
- altering thalamic activity by reducing anxiety;
- altering cortical function by changing the significance of painful sensations.

Two important features of gate control are:

- Substance P – an excitatory neurone transmitter, which is released by nociceptor afferent (sensory) neurones at the substantia gelatinosa;
- A beta fibres – thick, heavily myelinated fibres which release inhibitory neurotransmitters at the substantia gelatinosa.

The gate is closed when the input of A beta fibres is greater than the input of the A delta and C fibres (nociceptive input), and open when nociceptive input exceeds A beta input. It is thought that A beta stimulation can be achieved by gentle massage or rubbing, or by the application of heat or cold. It has been suggested that the reason why many patients with rheumatic disease find rocking chairs comfortable, is that the rhythmic rocking of the chair stimulates a barrage of impulses which inhibit nociceptive transmission (Wyke, 1981).

A number of other factors at other sites are also though to be implicated in gate control. For instance, McCaffery and Beebe (1989) suggest that feelings of confidence and control cause inhibitory signals from the cerebral cortex, which help to close the gate.

ENDOGENOUS OPIOIDS

The first evidence to support the presence of endogenous analgesia pathways was published in the late 1960's. Reynolds (1969), and Hughes *et al.* (1975) isolated the first endogenous opiate substances shortly thereafter. Endogenous opiates are naturally produced by the body and have properties similar to morphine. They are thought to be neuromodulators, which close the gate by inhibiting the release of substance P. Acupuncture and low-frequency transcutaneous electrical nerve stimulation (TENS) increase the production of endogenous opiates.

ASSESSMENT OF PAIN

Pain is a complex phenomenon and so there is no single method of assessment that encapsulates the experience. The most comprehensive assessment will include both:

• measurement of the pain
• observation of the expression of pain.

PAIN MEASUREMENT

When measuring pain, a number of factors need to be recorded. These include its:

• onset
• intensity
• location
• frequency.

Pain is a subjective phenomenon that can only be assessed by the person experiencing it. Patients who are able to do this will need to be taught pain measurement techniques and their recording systems. However, if patients are incapable of recording their own pain, for instance immediately following surgery, the nurse should undertake this task.

ASSESSMENT TOOLS

There are a number of commonly used pain assessment tools and these are discussed in Chapter 4. Consideration should be given as to the most appropriate tool for use at a given time. For instance, those patients who are seen in the outpatient clinic at monthly or two-monthly intervals could use a simple daily diary card. This usually consists of a five-point numerical scale with space to record optional analgesic intake (Figure 4.3). Patients should be encouraged to record any activity that exacerbates their pain, and any therapy or activity that relieves it.

FREQUENCY OF MEASUREMENT

The appropriate timing and frequency of assessment depends on the circumstances, and should be assessed individually for each patient. Assessment should be made whenever the patient and the nurse feel it is appropriate, and this can vary within a 24 hour period, depending on the efficacy of intervention.

A patient who has been admitted to a ward with septic arthritis may need to assess their pain every four hours in the first instance. As they begin to improve and their pain decreases, frequency of assessment will gradually diminish until discharge.

Pain assessment should not be regarded as a single encounter between the patient and nurse; it has far wider implications. Firstly, the collaborative, two-way communication that is essence of pain assessment can help to build a strong nurse/patient relationship. Secondly, discussions can also be used as an educational opportunity. By recording their pain and their ability to control it, patients become more confident in their self-management and coping skills, which can in itself help to reduce their pain.

EXPRESSING PAIN

When someone is in pain they communicate it:

- verbally
- bodily.

People with chronic rheumatic disease often experience some degree of pain for many years. As they adapt to their disease, many patients learn to control both their verbal communications in the belief that other people get tired of hearing complaints. Lack of verbal expression can be misleading, and maybe one of the reasons that the literature records that nurses constantly underestimate their patients' pain (Seers, 1989).

Patients should be encouraged to discuss their pain as this will help to assess its presence and severity accurately. A study by Jacox (1979) demonstrated that patients being interviewed about their pain began by denying pain or discomfort. However, after ten or fifteen minutes encouragement, they admitted to a minimum or mild discomfort.

Additional visual observation of the patient is essential, and video recorded assessments have shown that observing pain behaviour is a reliable method of assessing pain (Bradley, 1993). Research has been undertaken on pain behaviours associated with both OA (Keefe *et al.*, 1987) and RA (McDaniel *et al.*, 1986).

Behaviours adopted by patients with OA are:

- guarding
- active rubbing
- unloading joints
- rigidity
- joint flexing.

Those with RA shared some of these characteristics, and used these methods:

- guarding
- bracing
- grimacing
- sighing
- rigidity
- passive rubbing
- active rubbing.

These behaviours and facial expressions should be watched for and noted as they can signal the presence of unvocalised pain.

MANAGEMENT OF PAIN

It is a misconception that those who have intractable pain get used to it. It is more likely that they will become more fearful of it, as their anxiety about their inability to control it and cope with it increases. However, it is important that patients realise that the responsibility for pain control lies partly with them. Nurses and other health professionals should help them to set realistic goals, in the realisation that complete relief may not be possible. Care should incorporate coping techniques as well as pharmacological and complementary therapies.

There are a number of factors to consider when caring for patients in pain. These include:

- environment
- equipment
- handling and positioning.

These are discussed in Chapter 11.

PAIN RELIEF MEASURES

Relieving or palliating physical and psychological pain is one of the primary functions of the rheumatology nurse. As the causes of pain are so diverse, it is incumbent on nurses to equip themselves with a battery of interventions and skills. The most commonly used treatments are:

- drug therapy
- physiotherapy
- transcutaneous electrical nerve stimulation
- heat/cold
- patient education
- patients' own remedies.

DRUG THERAPY

Pharmacology plays an important role in pain control and the drugs used are discussed in more depth in Chapter 12. The most common medications are:

- simple and compound analgesics
- nonsteroidal anti-inflammatory drugs (NSAIDs)
- steroids
- antidepressants.

ANALGESICS

Analgesics are usually classified as nonopioid or opioid drugs. Both act on the central nervous system (Magliano and Morris, 2000).

Nonopioids

Simple analgesics such as paracetamol work by blocking the synthesis and secretion of prostaglandins, thereby preventing nociceptor sensitisation (Speight, 1987). These drugs are quite mild and usually prescribed at a maximum dose of eight 500 mg tablets a day. Perhaps the most commonly prescribed analgesic for rheumatic diseases is a compound analgesic, coproxamol. This is a combination of paracetamol and the opioid dextropropoxyphene. Again the maximum dose is two tablets, four times a day.

Opioids

Opioid analgesics are potent drugs that work by fitting into the opioid receptors of the brain and the spinal cord. Controversy surrounds their use in nonmalignant pain (Hill and Ryan, 2000), as side effects and dependence is said to occur in most patients (Justins, 1996). They are used following surgery, and occasionally and with great caution, when rheumatic pain is very severe.

Different analgesics suit different patients at different times. The way in which drugs are used is probably more important than which drug is prescribed (McCaffery and Beebe, 1989).

When treating the rheumatic patient, analgesics are rarely prescribed alone. In RA they are usually prescribed in addition to a nonsteroidal anti-inflammatory drug (NSAID) and a disease-modifying antirheumatic drug (DMARD). In OA they are the first drugs of choice, but as the disease progresses and the pain increases, they are often combined with an NSAID.

Analgesics are usually taken at the discretion of the patient. They should be informed of the maximum dose and advised to take them before the pain gets severe. This means that if they are in a flare, it may be necessary to take the maximum dose on a regular basis, but if pain is mild, an occasional ingestion will suffice.

Analgesics can also be taken prophylactically, to prevent predictable pain in chronic disease. A good example is taking analgesics half an hour before sexual activity. Many analgesics are quickly absorbed and have a short half-life. For the quickest effect, they can be taken on an empty stomach, but this is contraindicated if the patient is using aspirin-based analgesics as these are gastric irritants. Particular care is needed when elderly patients are taking aspirin products as they are at increased risk of gastric bleeding (Jordan and White, 2001). Baum (2003) advocates that patients taking aspirin for mild OA should be prescribed the enteric coated form.

If patients habitually need the maximum dose, or are overdosing on their analgesics, this is an indicator that they are not working as they are intended. In these cases, pain should be reassessed and new therapies initiated.

NON STEROIDAL ANTI-INFLAMMATORY DRUGS (NSAIDS)

The NSAIDs are one of the mainstays of drug therapy in the rheumatic diseases (Chapter 12). They come in the form of tablets, suppositories, gels and creams. Tablets and suppositories are taken as a regular regimen, gels and creams are used as necessary. They can take effect extremely quickly, reducing pain and joint stiffness. They also have an antipyretic effect. Efficacy usually increases as the levels of drug in the plasma rise and steady state is reached.

Tablets should always be taken with or after food, as this reduces the chance of gastric irritation. Many patients take their first NSAID of the day as soon as they wake up. If they are in hospital, this means that they will need an early morning snack with which to take them.

STEROIDS

Steroids are commonly administered via these routes:

- oral
- intramuscular
- intra-articular
- intravenous.

When used at the right time, via the correct route and in the correct dose, steroids can be very effective at reducing pain and stiffness (Chapter 12). One of the most common applications is intra-articular treatment to a single or small number of inflamed joints. This treatment can have a dramatic effect on pain. In a recent study, triamcinolone hexacetonide was shown to bring about greater sustained pain relief in rheumatoid knees, than hydrocortisone succinate or triamcinolone acetonide (Blyth et al., 1994). Nurses administering intra-articular injections should refer to the guidelines produced by the Royal College of Nursing.

ANTIDEPRESSANTS

There is a clear relationship between pain and depression even if the causal relationship remains unclear (Oliver and Ryan, 2004). Depression is known to affect the perception of pain (Gray, 2001) and if the patient is depressed, antidepressants can help. Amitriptyline is an antidepressant that is used in the rheumatic diseases as a pain modulator. It is usually taken at night, which helps the patient to sleep. Having slept, they feel less tired and more able to cope with their pain.

SELF-ADMINISTRATION OF DRUGS

Some rheumatology wards have incorporated self-administration schemes into their ward practice. Following her research, Bird (1990) concluded 'Self-administration of drugs would appear to be a more appropriate method than the conventional system for selected hospital patients'. Rheumatic patients are certainly in this category. They need to be able to take their drugs both prn and prophylactically, and if indicated, with or directly following food. This becomes very difficult if patients have to wait to be given their drugs by nurses.

PHYSIOTHERAPY

Pain relief is a multidisciplinary process and liaison with the physiotherapist is imperative. Physiotherapy can help to control pain in a number of arthritic conditions, including RA, OA and back pain (Minor and Sanford, 1993). The

Clinical Standards Advisory Group (1994) has published an epidemiological review of low back pain. It highlights the necessity for active rehabilitation within the first six weeks of onset, which helps to prevent long-term pain and disability.

OA of the patelofemoral compartment of the knee has been shown to be an important cause of knee pain (McAlindon et al., 1992). The medial application of tape to this area has been shown to reduce pain in this condition (Cushnaghan, 1993).

Referring patients to the physiotherapist at an early stage in their disease may help to prevent malalignment and so prevent pain from occurring.

TRANSCUTANEOUS ELECTRICAL NERVE STIMULATION (TENS)

This is a noninvasive therapy in which electrical current is applied via electrodes placed on the skin. There are two types of TENS, which work in distinctly different ways (Davis, 1994):

- high-frequency
- low-frequency.

High-frequency TENS (15–150 Hz) works by stimulating A fibre activity which closes the gate, inhibiting the transmission of pain sensations to the brain via the C fibres.

Low-frequency TENS (2 Hz) works by increasing the production of endogenous opiates. TENS is felt by the patient as a buzzing, tingling or vibrating sensation, but it does not appear to cause many side effects. Skin irritation has been reported by some patients, usually associated with the electrode, gel or tape application (Richardson, 1985). TENS helps some patients with arthritis (Lewis et al., 1984), but by no means all. It is worth trying on particularly painful joints and it has the advantage to the patient of being self-administered. The application, contraindications and effectiveness are discussed in more depth elsewhere (Hayes, 1996).

HEAT AND COLD

Patients often feel that warming a joint reduces their pain, and many patients report global improvement following heat treatments. Heat is thought to contribute to pain relief in several ways. They include:

- increasing blood flow
- washing out pain producing metabolites
- decreasing muscle guarding.

Two types of heat are used to reduce pain:

- superficial heat
- deep heat.

As the name implies, superficial heat only penetrates the skin to a depth of a few millimetres. Its effects are thought to occur through reflex vascular and neural responses. Common ways of applying superficial heat are:

- hot packs
- heat lamps
- warm baths/showers
- wax baths.

Heat is usually applied for about twenty minutes. It is an easy treatment for the nurse to apply, and convenient, cheap and safe for the patient to use at home.

Deep heat is usually administered by a physiotherapist using:

- ultrasound
- short-wave diathermy.

It works in the same way as superficial heat, but penetrates deeper, reaching muscles and connective tissue.

Contraindications to the application of heat are discussed by Hayes (1996).

Some patients feel quicker and longer lasting pain relief by the local application of cold to their joints.

This can be provided by:

- ice packs
- cold packs
- iced water
- vapocoolant sprays.

Applications of cold decreases three of the symptoms of arthritic disease, namely:

- pain
- swelling
- inflammation.

Pain relief is brought about by slowing or blocking nerve conduction or releasing endorphins. Reduction of swelling is through vasoconstriction, and the reduction of inflammation is aided by blocking the release of histamine. Cold is particularly effective for acutely inflamed joints, close to the skin surface. It is also an effective therapy for tendonitis and bursitis.

Side effects include:

• ice burns
• hypersensitivity
• joint stiffness.

Cold should not be used on patients with impaired peripheral circulation.

PATIENT EDUCATION

Patient education is the keystone of successful treatment and this is discussed in Chapter 15. The foundation of many patient education programmes is grounded in self-efficacy theory. The term self-efficacy refers to the belief that one can manage a specific challenging situation (Bandura, 1977). Teaching patients about their disease and treatments has been shown to bring beneficial effects (Hill, 1995; Reimsma et al., 2002; Hill, 2003), and a number of studies have shown that patient education can help to bring pain relief to those with rheumatic disease (Lorig et al., 1987).

Pain behaviour is related to belief in self-efficacy, rather than being solely accounted for by disease activity (Buescher et al., 1991). Depression has been shown to effect pain perception (Wolfe and Hawley, 1993), but anxiety and depression occur as a result of pain rather than being the cause of it (Smedstad et al., 1995).

Teaching patients about their disease helps to relieve anxiety and lift depression, which helps to relieve their pain (Hill, 1991a). It has also been shown to enhance adherence (Hill et al., 2001). Verbal education should always be backed up by written information.

PATIENT'S OWN REMEDIES

Expectations regarding outcome are also important. The patient's beliefs must be taken into account. If someone believes that a treatment will help, then it has more chance of being successful. If patients expect to feel pain, or do not expect a treatment to work, their expectations tend to be fulfilled. Once expectations are formed, it is hard to change them. Providing they are not harmful, incorporate the patient's own remedies into the treatment plan.

COMPLEMENTARY THERAPIES

As well as conventional treatments for pain relief, nurses have access to an array of techniques to complement these therapies. They include:

- massage
- relaxation
- therapeutic touch
- aromatherapy
- reiki
- reflexology
- visualisation
- guided imagery.

Many of these therapies are discussed in Chapter 13. All treatments must be with the agreement of the patient, and many of these therapies can be undertaken safely by the patient or carer at home. For instance, someone who is close to the patient can undertake simple massage, or essential oils can be used in the bath.

JOINT STIFFNESS

Stiffness is a major problem for those with rheumatic disease. It can alter the quality of their lives and ability to function normally (Brown *et al.*, 1987). Although it is often worse first thing in the morning when it is known as morning stiffness, it can occur at other times of day, usually following rest when it is termed inactivity stiffness (Hill, 1991b). When patients with rheumatic diseases are admitted to a ward, consideration will need to be given to the effect that their stiffness has on their mobility. An unhurried atmosphere is essential and they will need extra time to limber up and mobilise in the mornings. Washing and dressing will take longer and they may require an early hydrotherapy treatment or a warm bath or shower before other patients.

DEFINITIONS OF STIFFNESS

Stiffness is a very complex sensation and so has proved a remarkably difficult symptom to define. The Dictionary of the Rheumatic Diseases (1982) defines early morning stiffness as 'the subjective complaint of localised or generalised lack of easy mobility of the joints upon arising'.

For those experiencing stiffness it is often defined by its effects. These terms include:

- immobility
- limitation of movement
- resistance to movement
- tightness.

CAUSES OF STIFFNESS

In the rheumatic diseases, joint stiffness is usually caused by:

• inflammation
• soft tissue thickening
• changes to the articular surfaces of the bones
• loss of mechanical integrity
• environmental factors.

Inflammation causes tissue swelling or oedema that leads to an increase in the amount of synovial fluid within the joint. This causes the feeling of tightness of which many patients complain. Baker's or popliteal cysts in the knee are a common cause of stiffness and tightness. Roughening of the articular surface can increase friction within the joint, which limits movement. This is often described by the patient as the sensation of stiffness.

MUSCLE STIFFNESS

Most people are affected by muscular stiffness at some time, perhaps as a result of unaccustomed exercise or following an extra vigorous exercise routine. Most muscle stiffness resolves spontaneously after a few days. Patients with rheumatic disease are not exempt from this type of stiffness and unfortunately when it happens, it may be more pronounced and of longer duration (Pigg et al., 1985).

THE RELATIONSHIP BETWEEN PAIN AND STIFFNESS

Stiffness can be perceived in the absence of pain, but for patients with rheumatic disease, it often coexists. A study that investigated morning stiffness qualitatively and quantitatively showed that 40% of patients with RA and noninflammatory conditions mentioned pain as often as stiffness as descriptors (Hazes et al., 1993). This finding concurred with that of Rhind et al. (1987), who found that 68/100 patients interviewed indicated that limited movement was accompanied by pain.

Stiffness can also be a symptom of pain. If this is the case, then treating the pain will help the stiffness.

ASSOCIATION OF STIFFNESS AND DISEASE ACTIVITY

Although stiffness is unpleasant at any time, morning stiffness is of particular significance in inflammatory arthritis, and a significant indicator of disease activity in RA. For many years the duration rather than the severity of morning stiffness has been used as a measure of disease activity. Although the duration of morning stiffness is placed at the head of the most recent criteria for the classification of RA (Arnett *et al.* 1988), this rational has recently been questioned by Hazes *et al.* (1993). In their study, the severity of morning stiffness was found to be a better discriminator between active and inactive rheumatoid arthritis.

From the patient's viewpoint, it is usually the duration of morning stiffness, rather than its severity that has the most profound effect. Prolonged morning stiffness creates many practical problems that stem from limited and slow movement and reduction in grip strength. These include:

- getting out of bed
- washing/bathing
- dressing
- preparing food
- eating food
- driving.

These difficulties are compounded if the patient is a young mother who has to care for a baby or is trying to get the children off to school.

MEASURING STIFFNESS

A measurement of the duration and severity of stiffness will help the nurse to assess the patient's problems and formulate a meaningful care plan. Sequential readings will help to evaluate the effects of any treatments.

Objective measurement of stiffness has been attempted, but for practical purposes, stiffness measurement relies upon the patient's subjective assessment. Unfortunately, some patients have great difficulty dissociating their stiffness from their pain and the nurse needs to take the time to explain the difference. Another area that causes confusion is that patients often have morning stiffness, which is followed by inactivity stiffness if they rest or sit for prolonged periods. This may then be proceeded by evening stiffness. The type of stiffness the patient is required to note will depend on why it is being recorded. A thorough explanation to the patient of what is required and why it is needed will help accurate measurement.

The most sensible way to record morning stiffness is on a daily diary card similar to that used to record pain. If the patient completes it each day, they will get into the habit of noting:

- duration of stiffness
- severity
- location
- what, if anything causes stiffness
- treatments that are helpful.

The stiffness diary card can then be used as a teaching aid as well as an assessment tool.

RELIEVING STIFFNESS

Many of the treatments that relieve pain also relieve stiffness. They include:

* drug therapy
* exercise
* hydrotherapy
* splinting
* heat
* massage
* patient education.

DRUG THERAPY

NSAIDs reduce stiffness by decreasing inflammation. Indomethacin, which can be given as a suppository in the evening, is particularly effective for morning stiffness. If the cause of joint stiffness is an excess of synovial fluid, this can be aspirated and when inflammation is also present, an intra-articular injection of steroid may be efficacious. When patients are in pain they often tense their muscles, which exacerbates stiffness and increases pain. Analgesics will help the stiffness by reducing the pain that is causing the stiffness.

If the morning stiffness is caused by disease activity, the introduction of a DMARD will help to alleviate it over time.

EXERCISE

Morning stiffness can be prolonged for those with active rheumatoid arthritis. There are a number of activities that patients can undertake that will ease their morning stiffness:

* gentle limbering-up movements before getting out of bed;
* a daily exercise regime;
* gentle range of motion exercises before going to bed.

In addition to these methods, inactivity stiffness can be relieved by:

* frequent changes of position
* frequent gentle stretching movements
* range of movement exercises.

Patients need to get into a routine of exercising, but they often find this difficult as in addition to their stiffness, they may be in pain, feel debilitated and fatigued. The best way to ensure that patients undertake exercise is to make sure that they believe that it will make a difference. The exercise regime should not be too long, and when possible it should be incorporated into their daily routine. The nurse's role is to encourage, guide and enable the patient. Once they begin to notice the benefits, they will become more confident in their own self-efficacy ability, which will foster their willingness to carry out their exercise programme.

SPLINTING

Splinting tends to bring greater relief from pain than from morning stiffness. However, splints do help to reduce inflammation and consequently this can help to alleviate stiffness. For instance, a resting or night splint may help to relive pain and morning stiffness.

The elastic or stretch glove is a type of soft splint that is worn specifically to reduce morning stiffness. It works by gently compressing the hand and providing neutral warmth, and there is some research to show that it is effective (Erlich and DiPiero 1971). However, for those patients with carpal tunnel syndrome, it should be provided with caution as they can exacerbate paraesthesia.

HEAT

Heat can be very comforting and relaxing and this may well help to alleviate stiffness. For patients who are hospitalised, prolonged morning stiffness can be lessened by hydrotherapy. This should be scheduled as early as possible and prior to their exercise regime. If hydrotherapy is not available, or the when the patient is at home, a warm bath or shower taken first thing in the morning helps to alleviate or moderate their morning stiffness. Local applications of superficial heat are cheap and easy to apply both in hospital and at home. Stiff hands and feet can be placed into warm water, and the addition of flexing and stretching movements will make them feel more flexible. Contrast baths consist of dipping the hands or feet alternately into warm and cool water. This technique works for some people, but should be avoided if the patient suffers from circulatory problems or Raynaud's phenomenon.

MASSAGE

Massage can help to reduce stiffness and its application is discussed in Chapter 13. Gentle stroking massage has been advocated to reduce oedema and stiffness (Pigg et al., 1985). Patients can carry this out for themselves if the area is accessible, but it is more relaxing when undertaken by a carer or friend.

PATIENT EDUCATION

The patient's knowledge of the causes of their stiffness and the treatments available to relieve it should be assessed and whenever possible relatives and carers should also be included. Patients may be unaware of the association between lengthening morning stiffness and increasing disease activity. It is important that they and their significant others are taught to discriminate between the differing causes of stiffness so that they can choose the most effective treatments to manage it.

The effective management of pain and stiffness are major challenges to both nurses and patients alike. Patients place the alleviation of pain and stiffness high on their list of priorities, and it is incumbent on nurses to try to meet their aspirations as far as it is possible. To be successful, nurses require a high degree of knowledge and skill to enable their patients to cope with these debilitating symptoms. Uncontrolled, chronic pain leads to loss of grace and dignity in any human being. It can be destructive to both the person who feels it and to those who witness it, this includes family, friends and health professionals alike. Elimination of pain is rarely achievable in the rheumatic diseases, but moderation to a level which is acceptable to the patient must be.

ACTION POINTS FOR PRACTICE

- Describe the nociceptor receptor system, and discuss its effects on the perception of pain.
- Keep a reflective diary whilst working in a situation when you are nursing a patient in pain. Note the critical incidents that occur and demonstrate how your knowledge of pain affects your ability to care for the patient.
- Write a case history of a patient with severe rheumatoid arthritis. Discuss the tools used to assess their pain and stiffness and the treatments used to alleviate their symptoms.
- Write a list of the causes of pain and stiffness. In the opposite column, write a list of all the possible treatments. Include complementary therapies and the patient's own remedies.

REFERENCES

Arnett FC, Edworthy SM, Bloch DA et al. (1988) The American rheumatism association 1987 revised criteria for the classification of rheumatoid arthritis. Arthritis and Rheumatism 31:315–324.
Bandura A (1977) Self-efficacy: toward a unifying theory of behavioural change. Psychological Review 84:191–215.

Bellamy N, Bradley LA (1996) Workshop on chronic pain, pain control and patient outcomes in rheumatoid arthritis and osteoarthritis. *Arthritis and Rheumatism* 39(3):357–362.

Bird C (1990) A prescription for self help. *Nursing Times* 86(43):52–55.

Blyth T, Hunter JA, Stirling A (1994) Pain relief in the rheumatoid knee after steroid injection a single-blind comparison of hydrocortisone succinate, and triamcinolone acetonide or hexacetonide. *British Journal of Rheumatology* 33:461–463.

Bradley LA (1993) Pain measurement in arthritis. *Arthritis Care and Research* 6:178–186.

Brown GMM, Dare CM, Smith PR, Meyers OL (1987) Important problems identified by patients with chronic arthritis. *South African Medical Journal* 72:126–128.

Buescher KL, Johnston JA, Parker JC et al. (1991) Relationship of self-efficacy to pain behavior. *Journal of Rheumatology* 18(7):968–972.

Campbell J (1995) Making sense of pain management. *Nursing Times* 91(27): 34–35.

Clinical Standards Advisory Group (1994) *Epidemiology review: the epidemiology and cost of back pain.* HMSO, London.

Covic T, Adamson B, Hough M (2000) The impact of passive coping on rheumatoid arthritis pain. *Rheumatology* 39(9):1027–1030.

Cushnaghan J (1993) Tackling pain. *Nursing Times* 89(22):32–34.

Davis PS (1994) Reducing pain. In: Davis PS (ed) *Nursing the Orthopaedic Patient.* Edinburgh, Churchill Livingstone, ch7, p133.

Davis PA (1988) Changing nursing practice for more effective control of post operative pain through a staff initiated education programme. *Nurse Education Today* 8:325–331.

Dictionary of the Rheumatic Diseases (1982) Signs and symptoms. Atlanta, American Rheumatism Association.

Donovan MI (1989) An historical view of pain management. *Cancer Nursing* 12(4):257–261.

Erlich GE, DiPiero AM (1971) Stretch gloves: nocturnal use to ameliorate morning stiffness in the arthritic hand. *Archives of Physical Medicine and Rehabilitation* 51:479–480.

Gallop SM (1983) Patient teaching: pain and pain control. In: Wilson-Barnett J (ed) *Patient teaching.* Edinburgh, Churchill Livingstone, ch10, p178.

Gray E (2001) Linking chronic pain and depression. *Nursing Standard* 15(25): 33–36.

Harvey A (1987) Neurophysiology of rheumatic pain. *Bailliere's Clinical Rheumatology,* 1(1):1–26.

Hayes KW (1996) Physical modalities. In: Wegener ST (ed) *Clinical Care in the Rheumatic Diseases.* Atlanta, American College of Rheumatology, ch13, p79–82.

Hazes JMW, Hayton R, Silman AJ (1993) A re-evaluation of the symptom of morning stiffness. *Journal of Rheumatology* 20(7):1138–1142.

Hill J (2003) An overview of education for patients with rheumatic diseases. *Nursing Times* 99(19):26–27.

Hill J (1995) Patient education in rheumatic diseases. *Nursing Standard* 9(25): 25–28.

Hill J (1991a) Caring and curing. *Nursing Times* 87(45):29–31.

Hill J (1991b) Assessing rheumatic disease. *Nursing Times* 87(4):33–35.

Hill J, Ryan S (2000) Rheumatology: *A Handbook for Community Nurses*. London, Whurr Publishers.

Hill J, Bird H, Johnson S (2001) Effect of patient education on adherence to drug treatment for rheumatoid arthritis: a randomised controlled trial. *Annals of the Rheumatic diseases* 60:869–875.

Hughes J, Smith TW, Kosterlitz HW *et al.* (1975) Identification of two related pena peptides from the brain with potent opiate antagonist activity. *Nature* 258: 577–579.

International Association for the Study of Pain (1994) *Classification of Chronic Pain: Descriptions of Chronic Pain Syndromes and Definitions of Pain Terms* (2nd ed) Seattle, IASP.

Jacox A (1979) Assessing pain. *American Journal of Nursing* 79:895–900.

Jacques A (1992) Do you believe I'm in pain? *Professional Nurse* 249–251.

Jones AKP (1997) *Pain and its perception*. Topical Reviews, Chesterfield, Arthritis and Rheumatism Council.

Jordan S, White J (2001) Non-steroidal anti-inflammatory drugs, the clinical issues. *Nursing Standard* 15(23):45–52.

Justins DM (1996) Management strategies for chronic pain. *Annals of the Rheumatic Diseases* 55:588–596.

Kazis LE, Meenan RF, Anderson JJ (1983) *Pain in the rheumatic diseases*: investigation of a key health status component. *Arthritis and Rheumatism* 26(8): 1017–1022.

Keefe FJ, Caldwell DS, Queen K *et al.* (1987) Osteoarthritic knee pain: a behavioral analysis. *Pain* 28:309–321.

Lewis D, Lewis L, Sturrock R (1984) Transcutaneous electrical nerve stimulation in osteoarthritis: a therapeutic alternative? *Annals of the Rheumatic Diseases* 43:47–49.

Lloyd G (1994) Nurses' attitudes towards management of pain. *Nursing Times* 90(43):40–43.

Lorig K, Konkol L, Gonzalez V (1987) Arthritis patient education: a review of the literature. *Patient Education and Counselling* 10:207–252.

McAlindon TE, Snow S, Cooper C, *et al.* (1992) Radiographic patterns of osteoarthritis of the knee joint in the community: the importance of the patellofemoral joint. *Annals of the Rheumatic Diseases* 51:844–849.

McCaffery M (1983) *Nursing the Patient in Pain*, 2nd edn. London, Harper & Row.

McCaffery M, Beebe A (1989) Pain. *Clinical Manual for Nursing Practice*. St Louis, CV Mosby.

McDaniel LK, Anderson KO, Bradley LA *et al.* (1986) Development of an observation method for assessing pain behavior in rheumatoid arthritis patients. *Pain* 24:165–184.

Mahowald M (1993) Infectious arthritis: bacterial agents. In: Schumacher HR, Klippel JH, Koopman WJ (eds.) (1997) *Primer on the Rheumatic Diseases*, 10th edn. Arthritis Atlanta, Foundation, p192–197.

Magliano M, Morris V (2000) Use of Analgesics in Rheumatology. *Rheumatic Disease Topical Reviews: 7*. Chesterfield, Arthritis Research Campaign.

Maycock J (1984) Pain – a different approach. *Nursing* 31:924–925.

Melzack R, Wall PD (1965) Pain mechanisms: a new theory. *Science* 150:971–978.

Merskey H (1979) Pain terms: a list with definitions and notes on usage recommended by the IASP subcommittee on taxonomy. *Pain* 6:249–252.

Minnock P, Fitzgerald O, Bresnihan B (2003) Women with established rheumatoid arthritis perceive pain as the predominant impairment in health status. *Rheumatology* 42:995–1000.

Minor MA, Sanford MK (1993) Physical interventions in the management of pain in arthritis: an overview for research and practice. *Arthritis Care and Research* 6:197–206.

Oliver S, Ryan S (2004) Effective pain management for patients with arthritis. *Nursing Standard* 18(50):43–52.

Parker J, Frank R, Beck N *et al.* (1988) Pain in rheumatoid arthritis: relationship to demographic, medical and psychological factors. *Journal of Rheumatology* 15(3):433

Pigg JS, Driscoll PW, Caniff R (1985) *Pain.* In: Rheumatology Nursing a Problem-Oriented Approach. New York, John Wiley, ch5, p107.

Reimsma R, Kirwan J, Taal E (2002) *Patient education for adults with rheumatoid arthritis.* The Cochrane database of Systematic Reviews (3):CD003688.

Reynolds DV (1969) Surgery in the rat during electrical analgesia induced by focal brain stimulation. *Science* 164:444–445.

Rhind VM, Unsworth A, Haslock I (1987) Assessment of stiffness in rheumatology: the use of rating scales. *British Journal of Rheumatology* 26:126–130.

Richardson C (1985) Plugged in to pain control. *Nursing Mirror* 160(5):6–8.

Seers K (1989) Assessing pain. *Nursing Standard* 15(3):32–34.

Skevington SM (1993) The experience and management of pain in rheumatological disorders. *Baillier's Clinical Rheumatology* 7(2):319–335.

Smedstad LM, Vaglum P, Kvien TKm, *et al.* (1995) The relationship between self reported pain and sociodemographic variables, anxiety and depressive symptoms in rheumatoid arthritis. *Journal of Rheumatology* 22(3):514–520.

Speight TM (1987) *Avery's drug treatment.* Edinburgh, Churchill Livingstone.

Sprangers MA, de Regt EB, Andries F, *et al.* (2000) Which chronic conditions are associated with better or poorer quality of life? *Journal of Clinical Epidemiology* 53(9):895–907.

Symmons D, Bankhead C (1994) *Health care needs assessment for musculoskeletal diseases: the first step – estimating the number of incidents and prevalent cases.* Chesterfield, Arthritis and Rheumatism Council.

Weisenberger M (1977) Pain and pain control. *Psychological Bulletin* 84(5): 1008–1044.

Wolfe F, Hawley DJ (1993) The relationship between clinical activity and depression in rheumatoid arthritis. *Journal of Rheumatology* 20(12):2032–2037.

Wyke B (1981) The neurology of joints: a review of general principles. *Clinics in the Rheumatic Diseases* 7(1):223–239.

9 Fatigue and Sleep

C. WHITE
Mid Yorkshire Hospital Trust, West Yorkshire, UK

The aims of this chapter are to provide the nurse with an understanding of the relationship between fatigue and sleep in the rheumatic diseases, and to identify the role of the nurse in its management. After reading this chapter the reader should be able to:

- define fatigue and identify its causes;
- discuss the effects of rheumatic disease on fatigue;
- advise patients on how to minimise the effects of fatigue;
- define sleep and the benefits of restorative sleep;
- advise patients on ways to achieve a restful night's sleep.

FATIGUE

Fatigue is a major debilitating problem for patients with rheumatic illness and it is particularly associated with active disease. It can interfere with the patient's ability to function adequately and cope with everyday tasks. Consequently, it may lead to a reduction in work output, a predisposition to personal injury and cause an incremental loss of usable time, which culminates in:

- irritability with self and with others;
- frustration due to inability to complete a task;
- an overwhelming sense of helplessness and hopelessness;
- strained relationships with friends and family members due to lack of understanding of the nature and severity of fatigue;
- lack of personal control.

Fatigue can also lead to an inability to contribute to many aspects of normal family life. For instance, the fulfillment of the individual's role within the family may change and the ensuing financial consequences can be considerable. To manage fatigue, patients must recognise it as part of their disease and learn what causes it and what may help to alleviate it.

Rheumatology Nursing: A Creative Approach, 2nd edn. Edited by Jackie Hill.
Copyright 2006 by John Wiley & Sons, Ltd.

PERIPHERAL AND CENTRAL MUSCLE FATIGUE

It is important to differentiate between weakness and fatigue.

Weakness is defined as, 'an inability to produce the expected or desired force', whilst fatigue is defined as 'an inability to maintain the desired or expected force' (Edwards, 1981). A further distinction is usually made between central and peripheral fatigue (Table 9.1).

Central fatigue is when the impairment is located in the central nervous system. It is the lack of voluntary or nonvoluntary central drive, due for example, to poor motivation or the effects of anaemia.

Peripheral fatigue is when impairment is located in either the peripheral nerve, or contractile apparatus of the muscle. A voluntary muscular contraction involves a complex series of events. Weakness and fatigue can occur as a result of impairment at one or several links in the hierarchical neuromuscular chain, which links functions in the central nervous system to this contractile machinery.

Fatigue or dysfunction may result from defects in any of the commands in the chain of hierarchical physiological steps required to produce voluntary skeletal muscle contractions (Edwards, 1981). Patients with rheumatoid arthritis (RA) are highly susceptible to peripheral dysfunction, which includes:

- entrapment neuropathy;
- metabolic muscle wasting including steroid myopathy;
- intragenic muscle wasting;
- peripheral neuropathy;
- drug induced myasthenia;
- central dysfunction through pain or fear of pain.

OTHER DEFINITIONS AND CLASSIFICATIONS OF FATIGUE

Definitions of generalised fatigue

Generalised fatigue is also known as whole body fatigue. Fatigue has been defined by a number of authors. Smith Pigg et al. (1985) describes it as, 'a subjective complaint of weariness, exhaustion or lassitude, frequently associated with irritability, inefficiency, and decreased capacity for work'. Piper (1991) states that it is 'an overwhelming sustained sense of exhaustion and decreased capacity for physical and mental work'.

Classifications of fatigue

There are four classifications of fatigue:

- acute fatigue
- chronic fatigue

Table 9.1 Central and peripheral fatigue

	Site of fatigue	Cause of fatigue
Central	Brain	• Pain • Fear of pain • Anaemia • Poor motivation • Effects of drugs • Lack of energy due to disease activity (e.g., RA) • Psychological aspects including depression, anxiety, stress, boredom, responsibility and conflict • Environmental factors including social aspects, surroundings, noise, light and climate • Inadequate sleep or rest • Inadequate nutrition and obesity • Illness including drug therapy, physiological imbalance and surgery
	↓ Spinal column	Myelopathy (e.g., RA neck)
Peripheral	↓ Peripheral nerve	• Entrapment neuropathy • Peripheral neuropathy (e.g., in RA) • Radiculopathy
	↓ Neuromuscular junction	Penicillamine induced myasthenia
	↓ Muscle cell membrane	○ Steroid atrophy ○ Disuse atrophy
	↓ Transverse tubular system	○ Reflex inhibition atrophy ○ RA associated myositis
	↓ Calcium release	○ Other drugs ○ Inactivity
	↓ Actin-myosin activation	○ Exercise ○ Work
	↓ Myofibrillar cross bridge-formation	
	↓ Force generation	

• All of the rheumatic problems will cause the central effect.
○ All of these will cause increased perception of effort and will therefore increase central fatigue secondary to the peripheral problem.

(Adapted from Edward's Hierarchical Chain of Command [1981])

- subjective fatigue
- objective fatigue.

Acute fatigue is primarily induced by an excessive use of an organ or bodily system, and is usually of short duration and relieved by rest, sleep or a change in situation (Crosby, 1991).

Chronic fatigue is persistent, cumulative, not eliminated by rest and is usually associated with illness. Pronounced day-to-day fatigue may, eventually, lead to chronic fatigue (Crosby, 1991).

It is important to differentiate between fatigue which is chronic in nature and chronic fatigue syndrome. To qualify for the diagnosis of chronic fatigue syndrome a person must have debilitating fatigue that has lasted for more than six months, and no other medical or psychiatric condition that produces similar symptoms (Crosby, 1991).

A comparison of the distinguishing characteristics of acute and chronic fatigue is shown in Table 9.2.

Subjective fatigue is defined in Dorland's Medical Dictionary as 'perceptual, pertaining to or perceived only by the affected individual'.

Objective fatigue is something which is perceptible externally and may be physiological, biochemical or behavioural.

SYMPTOMS OF FATIGUE

Fatigue is used to describe a wide variety of signs and symptoms related to the failure to sustain some form of physical activity. It is a common experience in everyday life that limits our activities and horizons (Holder-Powell, 1990). In a healthy individual, fatigue may result from strenuous exercise, a busy day at work or emotional tension. Rest, relaxation or a change in activity usually brings relief. Both the fatigue and ensuing recovery period are normal experiences. Healthy people rarely consider fatigue as a serious problem because the duration of the condition is temporary and relief measures are effective (Tack, 1990). However, the symptoms of fatigue described by Hashimoto *et al.* (1975) are clearly felt by those afflicted and include:

- decrease of attention
- slow and impaired perception
- impairment of thinking
- decrease of motivation
- decrease of performance speed
- decrease of accuracy and an increase of errors
- decrease of performance capability for physical and mental activity.

Persons who are affected by fatigue exhibit the following symptoms:

- a general weakness in drive;
- loss of initiative;
- a tendency to depression which is associated with unmotivated worries;
- increased irritability and intolerance;
- occasional unsociable behaviour.

Table 9.2 Acute and chronic fatigue – distinguishing characteristics

Characteristics	Acute fatigue	Chronic fatigue
Purpose/Function	Protective	Unknown, may no longer be protective
Population at risk	Anybody	Primarily those suffering from some form of disease
Aetiology	Usually identifiable	May not be identifiable
	Usually involves a single mechanism or cause	Usually multiple causes
	Often experienced in relation to some form of activity or exertion	Often in experience with no relationship to activity or exertion
Perception	Normal	Abnormal
	Expected with specific activities	Excessive in comparison and disproportionate to past experience
	Primarily localised to specific body part or system	Generalised, physical and mental
	Pleasant or unpleasant	Unpleasant
Time to onset	Rapid	Insidious, gradual
		Cumulative
Duration	Short	Persistent
		More than one month
Method of relief	Usually alleviated by a good night's sleep, adequate rest, proper diet, exercise programme, or stress management techniques	Relief only partial or temporary with any method
		A combination of approaches may be needed
	Resolves quickly	Does not resolve quickly
Impact on activities of daily living and quality of life	Minimal	Major

(Adapted from Piper [1989])

FACTORS RELATED TO FATIGUE AND THE RHEUMATIC DISEASES

Although all rheumatic conditions can be implicated in fatigue, there is a particularly strong association with:

- rheumatoid arthritis
- systemic lupus erythematosus
- fibromyalgia
- myositis.

COMMON CAUSES OF FATIGUE

There are a number of factors which cause fatigue in rheumatic diseases. Some are directly associated with the diseases and their symptoms, such as disease activity and pain. Others are due to subsidiary circumstances, for instance, employment and environment. Findings by Schuman (1997) highlight the complex and multiple psychosocial determinants of fatigue.

Disease activity

Patients presenting with active inflammatory joint diseases generally feel unwell and tired and have painful, swollen joints. They also exhibit an increase in the duration of their morning stiffness and reduced grip strength. Laboratory investigations show an increase in the acute phase response, a fall in haemoglobin level and an increase in platelet count (Chapter 4). The combined effects of disease activity lead to:

- pain
- depression
- increasing fatigue.

Once treatment aimed at controlling the disease becomes effective, in theory fatigue should be substantially reduced. However, this does not always happen due to a number of other factors which can significantly affect function. One common contributor is cardio-respiratory unfitness.

Pain

Pain is a common feature of rheumatic disease and three of the more common causes are:

- inflammation;
- mechanical defects caused by joint destruction;
- overstressing affected muscles.

Patients complain that pain induces excess fatigue and that fatigue makes it more difficult to cope with pain. Many endure constant or chronic pain (Chapter 8), and this is very fatiguing.

Other factors pertaining to pain which affect fatigue include:

- intensity of pain
- nature of the pain
- duration of pain
- fear of pain
- location of pain
- patient expectations
- pain management.

If pain is managed effectively, it may help to increase the patient's activity, which will lead to a reduction in the peripheral element of fatigue which results from deconditioning and disuse atrophy. Consideration must also be given to the effects of pain control medication as this may also cause drowsiness (Chapter 8). Where possible, alternative pain control such as a TENS machine, heat and cold may be tried. These methods are discussed in Chapters 8 and 13.

Anaemia

Anaemia is an important indicator of disease activity in rheumatic disease and may add to the patient's disability by causing or increasing fatigue. The anaemia associated with systemic disease activity is an identifiable cause of fatigue brought about by the perception of increased effort. Appropriate treatment of anaemia can significantly reduce fatigue (Turnbull, 1987).

Muscle atrophy

Many rheumatological diseases result in muscle atrophy (wasting). This can be brought about either as a direct result of the disease and its treatment or as a result of disuse. When a muscle is atrophied, the remaining muscles are required to work harder in order to compensate which reduces endurance. A consequence of this is that fatigue occurs more rapidly. In addition, muscles do not adapt but remain the size and strength appropriate for the patient's ideal body weight (Newham et al., 1983). Consequently, if body weight is excessive, they are under greater stress than normal (Holder-Powell and Jones, 1990).

Physical activity

Disorder in the structure and function of the musculoskeletal system leads to physical limitation and the inability to exercise. These disruptions include inflammation of the:

- tendons
- joints
- muscles.

Regardless of the underlying cause, a dysfunctioning musculoskeletal system will have a direct effect on motor function thereby impairing the amount of physical activity performed. Increased physical activity can be a cause of fatigue in most individuals. However, people with arthritis require extra energy simply to undertake normal activity and this means that the amount of physical activity required to cause fatigue is much less than in a healthy person (Smith Pigg *et al.*, 1985). For instance, mechanical defects of the lower limbs caused by arthritis requires the patient to expend extra effort to mobilise; even walking short distances can be extremely fatiguing.

A frequent explanation by patients is that since they developed rheumatoid arthritis, they need to exert twice the effort and expend twice the energy in order to accomplish the same task (Crosby, 1991).

After a period of immobility most rheumatoid patients initially find exercise exhausting. This is due in part to unfamiliar sensations and inadequate cardiovascular and autonomic responses. These patients fatigue more easily after a period of inactivity and many, due to the nature of their disease, are forced to be less active (Holder-Powell and Jones, 1990).

Medication

Medications can be implicated in fatigue. Some cause drowsiness and others simply exacerbate the feeling of fatigue. Those implicated include:

- analgesia
- anticonvulsants
- antidepressants
- tranquilisers
- hypnotics
- antihistamines
- beta-blockers
- diabetic drugs
- diuretics
- hypotensives
- muscle relaxants
- cytotoxic agents.

Steroid-induced atrophy causes peripheral fatigue. This requires a greater expenditure of energy in order to maintain physical activity, which increases central fatigue. Medication such as steroids and cyclosporin can cause electrolyte imbalance, which can also cause fatigue.

Nutrition

Adequate nutrition is essential in the alleviation of fatigue (Chapter 10), but there are many problems which can make it difficult for the rheumatic patient to maintain adequate nutrition such as:

- The systemic nature of many rheumatic diseases causes an increase in energy expenditure for basic cellular function. For instance, low-grade fever will raise basal metabolic rate incurring an increased intake of nutrients.
- The painful nature of rheumatic diseases can lead to anorexia, due to the effects of disease on the person's physical or psychological functioning.
- Treatments such as nonsteroidal anti-inflammatory drugs may cause gastric side effects, and d-penicillamine, intramuscular gold and oral steroids can bring about changes in taste or cause mouth ulcers.
- Local pain in the temporomandibular joint may cause difficulty with chewing.
- Patients with scleroderma often find swallowing problematical.
- Sjögren's syndrome, associated with reduced tear formation and reduced salivary flow, induces a dry mouth, which can lead to difficulty in swallowing.
- Constipation is a side effect of some medication and this can cause loss of appetite.

It should be noted that alcohol and caffeine intake can contribute to fatigue.

Psychological aspects

Irritability, intolerance and unsociable behaviour are associated with fatigue. Increased fatigue should alert clinicians to assess changes of mood, reports of pain and stressful life events (Brandt, 1997). Patients with rheumatic disease are often depressed due to:

- chronicity of their disease
- pain
- uncertainty about the future.

Problems with relationships can occur because of the patient's inability to cope and from lack of understanding by others. Sexual relationships can become unsatisfactory because of fatigue, brought about by the cumulative effect of physical disability, disease activity and relationship problems (Chapter 6).

Patients often try to conceal their handicap, which can be stressful and debilitating. Stress, anxiety, conflict and responsibility are all contributors to fatigue. Boredom and monotony result in feelings of dullness and tiredness, and this quickly gives rise to daytime naps leading to poor sleep patterns.

Environmental factors

The environment in which the patient lives and works can have a profound effect on their fatigue. For instance, the size and type of the house, location and accessibility of rooms all have a bearing on the situation. If the bedroom and toilet facilities are upstairs and there is no ground floor toilet, the patient may need to climb the stairs a number of times each day, expending energy and adding to their fatigue. Poor kitchen design and lack of labour saving devices may also contribute.

Uncomfortable seating in the living area and an uncomfortable bed are not conducive to rest, neither is noise, unsatisfactory lighting, or excessive heat or cold. Some patients say that in hot weather they feel more exhausted and a room that is too hot is fatiguing.

Employment

Many patients find that performing daily activities of living particularly exhausting due to their pattern of morning stiffness. Morning stiffness is a problem when preparing for work; those with arthritis need to allow extra time in order to get ready. To get to work on time frequently involves patients getting out of bed long before they actually start. Work itself may be very exhausting and rest periods can be short. The time taken to complete a task may be much longer than previously and this leads to an increased workload. After work, preparation of meals, domestic chores, family and social commitments still have to be undertaken.

Lack of knowledge

Lack of knowledge may be a contributory factor that increases level of fatigue. Patients need to be taught how to conserve energy by:

- resting
- pacing and prioritising
- protecting their joints
- exercising.

Rest is important to restore supplies of energy. Short but frequent rest periods are essential, particularly when the patient is in an active phase of their disease. The value of planning and prioritising activities in order to conserve energy and reduce fatigue are invaluable. Protecting vulnerable joints, by wearing splints, using aids and altering the way in which tasks are undertaken can reduce pain which leads to reduction in fatigue. Exercise to maintain muscle tone and reduce atrophy also needs to be emphasised.

Offering written information to reinforce verbal teaching is essential as it has been shown that patients absorb only small amounts of information at one time.

ASSESSMENT OF FATIGUE

The multifocal dimensions of fatigue make assessment a difficult process. Assessing the patient's fatigue is an ongoing process as fatigue levels are not constant; they change with the patient's disease activity, treatments and rest. In addition, as patients undergo the process of education and learn how to manage their disease and fatigue, further variation will occur.

Assessment is usually by interview and it is necessary to obtain both subjective and objective information. Observation of the patient's behaviour and mood pattern, information about disease activity, laboratory findings, pain, work load, physical problems, coping mechanisms, drug history and diet should be noted. The rheumatology distress index is a valuable tool for measurement of fatigue and associated problems (Wolfe and Skevington, 2000).

Subjective assessment should include fatigue:

- severity
- duration
- time of onset (*e.g.*, morning or after work)
- effect of sleep
- effect of pain
- effect of stress.

MANAGEMENT

Recommendations to successfully help patients to manage their own fatigue include:

- adequate, though not excessive sleep;
- establishment or a work/rest cycle acceptable to the individual;
- elimination of excessive stress, anxiety, or boredom;
- range of movement exercises;
- a programme of activity compatible with the individual's capabilities;
- medication assessment/adjustment.

Effective use of disease-modifying drugs should help to reduce fatigue as the activity of the disease declines and pain, morning stiffness and anaemia lift. Environmental factors should be adjusted to reduce effort required to manage activities in order to allow for relaxation and adequate rest. The provision of aids to assist with activities should be considered and information about joint protection and energy preservation should be given. A structured and balanced exercise programme aimed at maintaining function, reducing pain and restoring muscle bulk, should be carefully planned with the physiotherapist.

The approach to management of fatigue is essentially multidisciplinary. Once the assessment is completed the nurse can identify the problems and refer to the appropriate member of the team for suitable intervention.

RECOMMENDED FATIGUE MANAGEMENT INTERVENTIONS FOR RHEUMATIC DISEASES

1. Complete fatigue assessment and initiate cause specific rehabilitation where applicable.
2. Develop a care plan and set realistic goals with the patient.
3. Assist with medical management including:
   - treatment of the disease to reduce disease activity;
   - treatment of anaemia if not directly related to the disease process;
   - correction of any chemical imbalance;
   - treatment of locally inflamed joints.
4. Arrange therapist intervention such as:
   - provision of and advice about convenient appliances;
   - corrective devices to reduce muscle fatigue, including insoles, foot raises, hand splints;
   - a safe exercise regime, modified regularly according to joint status.
5. Arrange social worker intervention if needed.
6. Educate patient which is the key to achieving optimal compliance, encouraging joint protection and energy conservation.
7. Encourage stress reduction and relaxation.
8. Introduce patient to support or peer groups which may be helpful, particularly if this is backed up by access to professionals.
9. Advise patient about telephone helpline service which makes patients feel less isolated and leads to identification of problems and an early resolution.
10. Assess patient's sleep pattern and advise on sleep management.

A fact sheet displaying hints that will help patients deal with their fatigue is shown in Appendix 9.A.

SLEEP

Sleep and rest are essential components of health and lack of either can affect well-being and quality of life. It is also an important element in recovery from illness, and sleep deprivation is a major impairment to recovery. In addition, sleep disruption makes coping with a chronic illness more difficult. The balance between activity and rest is important in the maintenance of health. However, the effects of rheumatic disease make this balance difficult to achieve and adds to the consequences of the disease. Activity promotes tissue growth and development whilst rest allows restoration and repair, as well as renewal of energies. Assisting patients to balance activity and rest can significantly reduce the effects of the disease and improve their quality of life.

Sleep is a natural process and is a compelling human need. However, for those affected by rheumatological disease, joint pain, stiffness and physical discomfort can significantly reduce the quality or amount of sleep achieved. Disturbed sleep exacerbates the adverse effects of disease and reduces the quality of life. This, in turn can feed back negatively, causing increased pain perception, fatigue, anxiety and depression, all of which adversely affect sleep. Sleep disturbances are thought to be both a cause and a consequence of various immune and autoimmune disorders (Lashley, 2003).

Rest and sleep are affected by the physical stresses a person experiences at a given time. The extent of illness will affect the need for sleep and rest. It is likely that the seriousness of the illness will increase the time needed for sleep and rest.

REST

Rest can be defined as a decrease or change in activity such that physical discomfort and psychological stress are reduced, allowing for renewal of energy. Napping, sleeping, relaxation, changing activity, or simply sitting and admiring the view, are forms of rest that help renew physical or mental energy. The type of relaxation required and its effect on restoring energy will vary from person to person.

Rest periods are important as they help patients to avoid becoming overtired or overstressed. Rheumatic diseases may cause a deficit in muscle mass, tone, and strength, making muscles less effective. This, combined with mechanical problems resulting from defective joints, requires an overexpenditure of energy. The physiological processes slow down during rest to allow for renewal of energy and rest prevents further exhaustion of already stressed muscles and joints. For this reason several short rest periods are more beneficial than one long one.

CONDITIONS NEEDED FOR SLEEP

Sleep occurs when a person loses conscious awareness of what is happening around them, reducing their ability to respond to environmental stimuli. Most rest occurs during sleep, with human beings spending an average of 7 out of 24 hours sleeping. The complex physiological processes of sleep and its effects are not fully understood but are thought to be both protective and restorative in nature. Sleep requires:

• absence of external stimuli
• suitable environment
• daily routine of bedtime
• relaxation of muscles
• comfortable bed.

There is an enormous variation in the individual habits adopted by people going to bed with the expectation of sleep. These habits are associated with routines and rituals, which the individual finds necessary to induce and maintain, sleep.

THE FUNCTIONS OF SLEEP

Oswald (1984) states, 'there are over 100 research reports showing that the protein synthesis and cell division for the renewal of tissue like the skin, bone marrow, gastric mucosa, bone and brain take place predominantly during that time of day devoted to rest and sleep'. Therefore adequate sleep is essential to those patients who have a chronic illness; sleep will help the healing process and lessen the psychological problems resulting from inadequate sleep.

The physical rest that occurs during sleep helps to conserve energy. The physiological functions of sleep are thought to be multifocal and include genetic, nutritional, and environmental components. Therefore it follows that the purpose of sleep is also multifocal.

NORMAL SLEEP

A good night's sleep and good daytime refreshed wakefulness are interrelated; each depend on the quality of the other. Sleep requirements are subjective and can vary enormously. If the sleeper is satisfied with its duration, continuity and architecture, then it may be considered normal. The average duration is about 7½ hours, but a range of 3–12 hours is considered normal (Johns, 1984). Some people are early risers, whilst others are more active in the evening and tend to go to bed late.

Factors affecting normal sleep

There are many factors affecting normal sleep including:

- age
- diet
- gender
- ambient temperature.

Sleep patterns are known to change with age. Young adults sleep for about eight hours and elderly individuals might sleep for only six hours. Anxiety and depression frequently interfere with sleep and this is common in patients with musculoskeletal disease due to uncertainties about the future, work and family tensions. It is easier to relax physically than mentally.

Chronic pain experienced by most patients with musculoskeletal disease represents a major problem affecting sleep. Dyspepsia and pain from gastric ulcers can increase in intensity at night. This is significant for patients taking medication with gastrointestinal side effects who are at greater risk of gastric problems (Chapter 12). The effects of diet are unclear but spicy foods late at night tend to disturb sleep. A milky night-time drink may promote somnolence in some.

Alcohol has a hypnotic effect, increasing Stage 2 sleep and reducing REM and short-wave sleep early in the night (Jaffe, 1980). Later in the night, following the metabolism of the alcohol, rebound effects occur with the increase in REMs, dreams and frequent awakenings. However, alcohol has considerable analgesic properties and may be used by many patients who experience chronic pain, to reduce pain and aid sleep. If it is used frequently and to excess, the overall effect will be to increase insomnia. Drinks containing caffeine should be avoided at night as they act as central nervous stimulants.

The structure of normal sleep

In adults, sleep consists of two different states which have different psychological mechanisms, and behavioural and neurophysiological markers. These two states are commonly known as:

- nonrapid eye movement (NREM) – believed to be necessary for tissue restoration and protein synthesis;
- rapid eye movement (REM) sleep – needed for psychological restoration, maintenance of orientation and emotional stability.

(Chuman, 1983)

NREM can be subdivided into four separate stages:

Stage 1 (drowsing)

This is the lightest stage of sleep, the subject usually feels drowsy and not fully alert. Daydreams may occur in this stage of sleep.

Stage 2 (light sleep)

This is a stage of altered consciousness when body movements begin to diminish and dreams involving a story line first appear. Dream recall on waking is less vivid than for REM sleep.

Stage 3 (slow wave sleep)

During this stage body movement continues to diminish, deep sleep occurs.

Stage 4 (slow wave sleep)

There is a high degree of immobility and intense external stimuli are required to arouse the subject who is now in the state of deep sleep. Large increase in the secretion of growth hormone occurs at this stage.

Traditionally, stages 3 and 4 are considered together and termed short-wave sleep (SWS).

During a night's sleep, both REM and all four stages of NREM sleep occur many times, usually in cyclic fashion with the NREM sleep periods becoming shorter and the REM sleep periods longer as the night progresses. Most REM sleep occurs during the last third of the night. REM is characterised by:

* dreaming
* muscular relaxation
* high levels of physiological arousal.

The blood pressure fluctuates, pulse and respiration rates increase and may become irregular and oxygen consumption increases. If subjects are awakened they frequently report that they have been dreaming. Consequently, REM sleep is frequently referred to as dreaming sleep.

INSOMNIA

Insomnia may be described as a persistent relative lack of sleep, inadequate quality of sleep or both and reflects poor sleep pattern and poor quality sleep for at least three weeks. Subjects may have difficulties with initiation or maintenance of sleep or with early wakening. Changes in diet, anxiety, sleeplessness phobia, levels of arousal, obsessive thoughts and environmental disturbances all disrupt initiation of sleep. Interrupted sleep can be random or cyclic. Random awakenings can be caused by pain, sleep apnoea, breath-lessness, coughing and nocturia. Waking early in the morning can often occur with depression.

EFFECTS OF LACK OF SLEEP

Lack of sleep:

* reduces motivation and willingness to perform tasks;
* impedes mobilisation and restricts self-care;
* reduces efficiency at work;
* decreases attention span;
* affects social and family relationships;
* potentiates the effects of muscle and joint pain and stiffness;
* increases anxiety and depression;
* has the potential to exacerbate the disease;
* impairs memory;
* causes day-time sleepiness;
* causes fatigue.

HOSPITALISATION AND SLEEP

Patients in hospital suffer from disturbed and less effective sleep than in their own environment. Frequent problems suffered by hospitalised patients include sleep latency, interrupted sleep, early awakening and a feeling of not being rested. Factors frequently identified with poor sleep in hospital include:

* noise
* anxiety about health
* separation from family and friends
* unfamiliar environment
* monitoring of vital signs
* administration of medication
* interruptions
* discomfort
* hunger.

Sleep disruption is often intensified by sleep pattern changes, health problems and unfamiliar clinical settings. Hospital routines also prevail over an individual's normal bedtime routine and this often results in disturbed sleep patterns. Evaluation of a patient's past and present sleep patterns, monitoring of sleep/wake behavior and implementation of nursing intervention to promote sleep are important when caring for patients in hospital. Sleep assessment should include:

- observation of the time it takes to fall asleep;
- restlessness during the night;
- number of arousals;
- patient's sense of having a good night's sleep.

The last point is important regardless of other observation.

Nurses should allow hospitalised patients to continue the pre-sleep activities and routines they use at home. Some patients have a night-time alcoholic beverage and if they are normally heavy drinkers they may suffer from withdrawal if they are not allowed an alcoholic drink prior to sleep. Worries regarding the illness, investigations and treatments, should be discussed. Realistic measures for sleep onset and maintenance should be set with the patient and evaluated for effectiveness with the appropriate changes made in order to maintain or improve the quality of sleep.

Position relates to habit and physical factors such as breathing, temperature and joint pain. Individual position varies greatly and depends on comfort of the joints and muscles but should be conducive to relaxation and lead to sleep. However, where possible good body alignment should be used to prevent undue stress on the muscles, ligaments and joints. Encouraging movement when awake may help to reduce stiffness.

Pain has been shown to correlate with sleep disturbances and adequate pain control should be achieved prior to the onset of sleep in order to ensure an adequate night's sleep. When related to musculoskeletal pain, nonsteroidal anti-inflammatory drugs may be more efficacious than opioids, but the two can be used together if necessary. Important aids to promote rest and sleep include:

- provision of physical comfort
- alleviation of psychological stresses
- structuring of daily activity schedules
- structuring of a restful environment
- appropriate choice and time of analgesic administration.

Good personal hygiene aids comfort and thus improves the quality of rest and sleep. Prior to going to bed, a warm bath to which essential oils have been added, can be relaxing and help to relieve joint and muscle pain. Massage can be comforting and may induce sleep.

Allowing patients the opportunity to discuss fears, anxieties and frustrations can alleviate psychological stress. Anxiety about not sleeping and trying too hard to get to sleep can further distress patients and prevent sleep. Quiet soothing music may help to create a relaxed atmosphere.

Hypnotic drugs such as barbiturates and benzodiazepines should be selected and controlled carefully, since they affect the quality of sleep.

SLEEP DISTURBANCES IN SPECIFIC RHEUMATOLOGICAL DISEASES

Rheumatoid arthritis

In RA fragmented sleep can be associated with exacerbation of illness, with patients experiencing increased fatigue, morning stiffness, joint and muscle pain and weakness. The increase in pain is consistent with findings that sleep deprivation reduces the pain threshold (Shapiro et al., 1993) and improved sleep may reduce arthritis pain (Davis, 2003).

The physical and psychological recuperative benefits of sleep are such that the patient with rheumatological conditions should be encouraged to maintain as regular a sleep pattern as the painful nature of the disease will allow. Undisturbed sleep depends on a number of factors such as control of pain and discomfort by use of analgesia, night resting splints and joint position. An exercise programme to maintain muscle strength, prevent joint stiffness and improve circulation can also contribute to effective sleep and maintenance of independence.

A study comparing patients with RA whose disease had flared with those whose disease was well controlled, showed reduced sleep times with fragmented and occasionally prolonged awakenings in patients with active disease. In addition, there was a significant relationship between the number of awakenings and pain. The researchers suggested that measures to reduce pain might improve the quality and quantity of sleep in those experiencing RA flares (Crosby, 1989). Studies have shown that a good night's sleep can significantly reduce stiffness in patients with RA (Sharma and Haslock, 1979; Baumgartner et al., 1988). However, these studies involved using pain control and it is possible that the improvement in stiffness was caused by the analgesia rather than by the improved quality of sleep.

In patients with RA, the more severe pain experienced before and during sleep, the more fragmented the sleep. Compared to controls, patients with arthritis have lower indices of sleep quality, less effective sleep, higher levels of activity during sleep and more sleep disturbances (Lavie et al., 1992). Sleep abnormalities are common in children with juvenile rheumatoid arthritis and are multidimensional (Bloom et al., 2002).

Fibromyalgia

Approximately 90% of patients with fibromyalgia describe moderate to severe fatigue with lack of energy, decreased exercise endurance, or the kind of exhaustion felt with the flu or lack of sleep. Often the fatigue is more troubling than pain and generally, people with fibromyalgia wake feeling tired even after sleeping throughout the night. Sleep studies have shown that people with fibromyalgia have an abnormal sleep pattern, especially an interruption in their deep sleep (Shapiro et al., 1993). They may be aware that their sleep has become lighter and that they wake up during the night. Moldofsky (1986) studied fibrositis syndrome in a group of patients who had reported severe emotional stress at the time symptoms began. The study found increases in muscle tenderness, pain and stiffness. This appeared to be associated with disturbances of sleep and with the development of alpha rhythms in NREM sleep. In normal subjects, sleep disturbances sometimes produce symptoms similar to those in the fibrositis group, including fatigue and musculoskeletal aches and pains. This happened when sleep disturbance occurred during Stage 4 sleep. The symptoms did not occur when sleep disturbances occurred during REM sleep. Studies have also shown that a wide variety of factors could affect non-articular rheumatism including psychological stress, physiological disturbances, environmental stimuli and altered central nervous system metabolism (Moldofsky, 1986).

Medication to promote sleep may help patients with fibromyalgia. These include amitriptyline, doxepin, cyclobenzaprine and related medications. Although normally used to treat depression, in people with fibromyalgia they are generally used in very low doses and only at bedtime. Thus they are not specifically used as antidepressants or tranquilisers, but may relieve pain and improve sleep.

Even a very gentle exercise programme is thought to improve the quality of sleep. As muscle repair takes place during the restorative phase of sleep, with the production of hormones required to promote repair of muscle, improved sleep is an essential part as part of a rational approach to management that should be considered (Bennett, 2002).

Ankylosing spondylitis

The effect of sleep on patients with ankylosing spondylitis was studied by Jameison *et al.* (1995). Patients with ankylosing spondylitis usually feel worse in the morning, their stiffness and general discomfort easing throughout the day. Good sleep is associated with less nocturnal movement and yet exercise is essential. The study showed that a good night's sleep correlated with increased stiffness, difficulty in awakening, feeling tired and clumsiness in the morning. Pain correlated with subjective measures; difficulty getting to sleep and a worse quality of sleep, but less well with objective measures of sleep disruption. The study showed that improved sleep integrity, with little nocturnal movement, was related to a decrease in lumbar flexibility. It is suggested that patients with ankylosing spondylitis may benefit from being awakened in the night and that their sleep differs from sleep in healthy people.

SLEEP MANAGEMENT

Recommendations to improve the quality of sleep include advice about routines that are conducive to sleep onset, maintenance of quality sleep and adequate duration of sleep. The advice given will depend on individualised assessment and care planning with the patient. In Appendix 9.A is a list of information for patients that includes many aspects of advice related to sleep.

Patients with rheumatic disease frequently have poor sleep patterns, due to pain, discomfort and the need for day time rest. The chronic diseases cause persistent problems that affect sleep on a long-term basis. Consequently, the nurse caring for such patients requires skills and knowledge to adequately assess sleep patterns and advise on sleep management. A restful night's sleep will significantly reduce disease related fatigue, aid recovery and help patients cope with the effects of their disease.

A patient advice sheet on how to get a restful night's sleep is shown in Appendix 9.B.

The traditional management of rheumatoid disease fails to acknowledge the importance of fatigue. As a result, patients may find it difficult to accept that the fatigue they feel is a consequence of the disease process. By helping them to understand that fatigue is an expected part of their disease, health-care professionals can improve patients' control and coping mechanisms. Fatigue is a complex multifactorial and multidimensional problem, with numerous causative factors that can be biological, physiological, social and personal in nature. Some of the causes of fatigue are related to everyday life and others to the disease process. Increased understanding of these causes should lead to management aimed at reducing the effects of fatigue.

Since fatigue can result from a variety of causes, acting singularly or in a variety of combinations, it is difficult to give clear cut rules for its control or prevention. The optimum intervention depends on careful, individual assessment by the nursing staff and involvement of the multidisciplinary team. To date, a physiological basis for fatigue has not been identified and the causes remain multifocal. However, by increasing understanding of the causes and accepting observed behaviour patterns we can start to teach patients and their relatives coping strategies aimed at improving the quality of their life.

ACTION POINTS FOR PRACTICE

- Identify the patients in your clinical area who suffer from fatigue. List the possible causes of their fatigue and the relief measures you suggest.
- In a group session reflect on the lack of sleep in patients with rheumatological conditions. Identify ways you can encourage patients to get a good night's sleep in your clinical area.
- Conduct a small scale research project into the causes of fragmented sleep in your clinical area. Make suggestions for change.
- Discuss the components needed to assess and manage fatigue and compile a standard for practice.

APPENDIX 9.A HINTS TO HELP THE PATIENT DEAL WITH FATIGUE

General

Plan your day and consider special events occurring during the week.

Set priorities, do only the things that are most important.

Do as much for yourself as possible, but take rests – a number of short rests are better than one long one.

Ask for help from family and friends.

Rest before you are tired.

Conserve your energy as much as possible.

Organise home and work so that tools are handy and plan ahead to minimise activity.

Try not to sit for more than 20 or 30 minutes before standing or walking about a little.

If possible sit down for any job that takes more than ten minutes.

Try to avoid projects like cooking a meal that can't be stopped at any time should you feel tired.

Avoid doing jobs that take a long time in one session. It is better to do several short sessions.

Use a wheeled trolley to transport items, thus cutting down on the need to carry objects.

An apron with a large pocket is useful for carrying small objects.

Store frequently used items between eye-level and knee-level to reduce the amount of bending and stretching required.

Do not stay in one position too long. Stop frequently when traveling by car.

Joint protection

Protect your joints as much as possible.

Slide objects rather than lift them.

Use your larger joints where possible.

Use as many joints as possible to distribute work load, e.g., hold a cup in both palms.

Use good posture.

Take advantage of as many assistive devises as possible, e.g., use a trolley to carry equipment.

A car with power-assisted steering is an advantage.

Exercise

Remember to balance exercise with rest.

Exercise slowly at first then gradually increase the amount of exercise you do.

Walking and swimming are good forms of exercise.

Do your range of movement exercises daily.

Gradually increase the amount of strengthening exercises.

Relaxation
Practice relaxation techniques.

Diet
Eat a healthy well-balanced diet.
Cut down on dairy products, caffeine and alcohol.

Sleep
Try to improve the quality of your sleep by following the guidelines on how to get a restful night.

APPENDIX 9.B ADVICE ON HOW TO GET A RESTFUL NIGHT'S SLEEP

Sleep is an essential component of health; and the physical and psychological benefits of sleep are important in the management of rheumatological problems.

- Make sure your bedroom is conducive to sleep. Keep it free of equipment and smells (*e.g.*, cooking) that remind you of daily activity.
- Ensure that the room is a comfortable temperature.
- The curtains should block out the light.
- The bed should be firm yet comfortable with covers that are light and suitable to maintain ambient body temperature.
- Create a restful pre-sleep environment. Listen to relaxing music, read suitable books or practice relaxation techniques before you get into bed.
- Avoid strenuous exercise before going to bed. This can speed up the metabolic rate and tell the brain that it is time to be awake and active. Late afternoon and early evening exercise is best. Avoid strenuous mental activity near bedtime.
- Relaxation and a specific rest/exercise programme may be beneficial and contribute towards maintaining independence.
- Avoid long daytime naps and periods of inactivity.
- Aim to go to sleep at the same time each day. This helps to regulate your internal clock to normal sleep/wake rhythms.
- Don't force yourself to sleep or watch the clock if you can't. It's better to get up and read or watch a TV show until you feel naturally sleepy.
- Snacks before bedtime should be light and fluid intake limited. A hot milky drink at bedtime may promote sleep.
- Avoid going to bed hungry or too full. Hunger pains will keep you awake. Overeating can cause gastric reflux resulting in heartburn.
- Do not have coffee, tea, cola or a nightcap after dinner. The stimulating effects of caffeine can linger in your body for up to six hours causing an

uneven night's sleep. Alcohol may make you sleepy initially, but disturbs sleep later on.
- A warm bath taken before bedtime may relax tired muscles, reduce pain and help promote sleep.
- Pain should be adequately controlled before going to bed, anti-inflammatory medication may be required as well as analgesia. Other methods of pain control should also be considered such as hot or cold pack, heat pad or massage.
- Ensure that the joints are in a comfortable position, correctly aligned in order not to stress the joints. Night resting splints may be required to rest joints in a comfortable position.
- Don't get into the habit of relying on sleeping tablets. Many people can use them on a short-term basis without ill effect but used on a regular basis they lose their effectiveness or become ineffective, they also change the structure of sleep which may be harmful in the long-term.
- Do not stay in bed if you can't go to sleep. Get out of bed and sit and relax in another room until you feel sleepy. Repeat as often as required until you fall asleep.

REFERENCES

Bennett RM (2002) The rational management of fibromyalgia patients. *Rheumatic Disease Clinics North America* 28(2):181–199.

Baumgartner H, Hohmeister R, Blumenberg-Novoselac N (1988) An observer-blind crossover study to compare the efficacies of flurbiprofen, indomethacin and naproxen given orally rectally in the relief of night pain and morning stiffness due to rheumatoid arthritis. *Journal International Medical Research* 16:189–196.

Bloom BJ, Owens JA, McGuinn M et al. (2002) Sleep and its relationship to pain, dysfunction, and disease activity in juvenile rheumatoid arthritis. *Journal Rheumatology* 29(1):169–173.

Brandt JC (1997) The relationship of psychobiological parameters to fatigue in patients with rheumatoid arthritis. *Dissertation Abstracts International: The science and engineering* 7(10-B):6639.

Chuman MA (1983) The neurological basis of sleep. *Heart Lung* 12:177–182.

Crosby LJ (1991) Factors which contribute to fatigue associated with rheumatoid arthritis. *Journal Advanced Nursing* 16(8):974–981.

Crosby LJ (1989) Fatigue, pain, depression, and sleep disturbances in rheumatoid arthritis patients key aspects of comfort. In: Funk et al. (eds) *Key Aspects of Comfort*, New York, Springer pp. 299–301.

Davis GC (2003) Improved sleep may reduce arthritis pain. *Holistic Nursing Practice* May-June 17(3):128–135.

Dorland (2003) *Dorland's Illustrated Medical Dictionary* 30th edn. London, Elsevier.

Edwards RH (1981) Human muscle function and fatigue. In: Porter R, Whelon J (eds), *Human Muscle Function*, Physiological Mechanics. London: Pitman Medical 1–18 (Ciba Foundation Symposium No 82).

Hashimoto K, Kagi K, Grandjean E (1975) *Methodology in Human Fatigue Assessment.* London, Taylor and Frances Ltd.

Holder-Powell HM, Jones DA (1990) Fatigue and muscular activity: a review. *Physiotherapy* 11:672–679.

Jaffe JH (1980) Drug addiction and drug abuse, In: AG Gilman (ed) *The Pharmacological Basis of Therapeutics.* New York, Macmillan pp. 494–534.

Jamieson AH, Alford CA, Bird HA *et al.* (1995) The effect of sleep and nocturnal movement on stiffness, pain, and psychomotor performance in ankylosing spondylitis. *Clinical Experimental Rheumatology* 13:73–78.

Johns MW (1984) Normal Sleep. In: Priest RG (ed) *Sleep: An International Monograph.* Update Books.

Lashley FR (2003) A review of sleep in selected immune and autoimmune disorders. *Holistic Nursing Practice*, March–April 17(2):65–80.

Lavie P, Epstein R, Tzischinsky O *et al.* (1992) Actigraphic measurements of sleep in rheumatoid arthritis: Comparison of patients with low back pain and healthy controls. *Journal Rheumatology* 19(3):362–365.

Moldofsky H (1986) Sleep and musculoskeletal pain. *American Journal Medicine* 81(3A):85–98.

Newham DJ, Mills KR, Quigley B *et al.* (1983) The strength, contractile properties and radiological density of skeletal muscle before and one year after gastroplasty. *Clinical Science* 74:79–83.

Oswald I (1984) Good, Poor and Disordered Sleep. In: Priest RG (ed) *Sleep: An International Monograph.* Update Books.

Piper BF (1989) Fatigue: Current bases for practice. In: Funk *et al.* (eds): *Key Aspects of Comfort.* New York, Springer 24:187–198.

Schuman CC (1997) Pain and depression as predictors of fatigue in fibromyalgia syndrome patients: An investigation with aggregated and disaggregated data. *Dissertation Abstracts International: Section B: The Science and Engineering.* 57(12-B):7742.

Shapiro CM, Goll CC, Cohen GR *et al.* (1993) Heat production during sleep. *Journal Applied Physiology*, 56:671–677.

Shapiro CM, Devins GM, Hussain MRG (1993) *Sleep problems in patients with medical illness. ABC of Sleep Disorders.* London, BMJ Publishing Group pp. 59–62.

Shatrma BK, Haslock I (1979) Night medication in rheumatoid arthritis. The use of Sudilac. *Current Medical Research Opinion* 10:592–595.

Smith Pigg J, Webb Driscoll P, Caniff R (1985) *Rheumatology Nursing – A Problem Orientated Approach.* New York, Wiley Medical.

Tack BB (1990) Fatigue in rheumatoid arthritis: Condition strategies and consequences. *Arthritis Care Research* 3(2):65–70.

Tack BB (1990) Self reported fatigue in rheumatoid arthritis. *Arthritis Care Research* 3(3):154–157.

Turnbull A (1987) Anaemia in Rheumatoid Arthritis does it matter? *Arthritis Rheumatism Council Collected Reports on Rheumatic Disease*, Chesterfield: Arthritis & Rheumatism Council.

Wolfe F, Skevington SM (2000) Measuring the epidemiology of distress: The rheumatology distress index. *Journal Rheumatology* 27(8):2000–2009.

10 The Skin and Nutrition

N. REAY
University of Leeds, West Yorkshire, UK

S. SMITH
Chapel Allerton Hospital, West Yorkshire, UK

J. BYRNE
Stepping Hill Hospital, Cheshire, UK

This chapter is intended to promote a holistic and individual approach to skin integrity and outline the role of a well-balanced diet in the management of the rheumatoid patient. It is also intended to provide an insight into the relationship between nutrition and the skin. After reading this chapter the reader should be able to:

- undertake an assessment of the patient's skin;
- describe primary and secondary skin lesions;
- summarise topical therapies;
- describe the effects of rheumatic disease on the skin;
- summarise the components of a healthy well-balanced diet;
- identify the role of education in skin integrity and nutrition.

THE SKIN

Skin lesions can be an indication of a systemic condition and may even be the first clinical sign that there is a problem for the patient. Examples in rheumatic diseases are systemic sclerosis (scleroderma), systemic lupus erythematosus (SLE) and psoriatic arthritis (PsA). For these patients a regular assessment of their skin is vital as it may be an indication of deterioration in an underlying pathology. Close links between rheumatology and dermatology departments are essential if patients are to be treated effectively. If the rheumatology nurse is to provide high quality care for these patients, s/he will need to have an understanding of the basic facts of:

Rheumatology Nursing: A Creative Approach, 2nd edn. Edited by Jackie Hill.
Copyright 2006 by John Wiley & Sons, Ltd.

- the function of the skin
- its assessment
- potential treatments.

THE FUNCTIONS OF THE SKIN

The skin is a large, complex structure that covers the human body and acts as a protection. It is one of the largest organs of the body with a surface area of $1.8\,m^2$. It constitutes approximately 16% of our total body weight (Mackie, 1994). The most important functional properties of the skin are to:

- protect from external injury
- hold the other organs together
- help to maintain fluid balance
- control temperature
- sensation
- absorb ultraviolet radiation
- metabolise Vitamin D
- synthesise epidermal lipids which are an important protective barrier
- cosmetic function.

ASSESSING THE SKIN

Taking a history from the patient is helpful in assessing a patient's skin condition and this can be divided into four areas:

- the presenting complaint
- past medical history
- drug history
- social and family history.

It is essential for the nurse to have good observational skills and attention to detail during examination of the skin, including the ability to describe accurately what is seen. The whole of the patient's skin needs to be examined, preferably in natural light. Gawkrodger (2002) suggests the following as an important pattern to follow:

- note the distribution and colour of the lesions;
- examine the morphology of individual lesions, their size, shape, border changes and spatial relationship (Palpation reveals the consistency of a lesion.);
- assess the nails, hair and mucous membranes, sometimes in combination with general examination;
- utilise special techniques (e.g., microscopy of scrapings or the use of Wood's ultraviolet light) where applicable.

PRIMARY AND SECONDARY SKIN LESIONS

Primary lesions

Primary lesions are the first to appear and are due to the disease, or abnormal state, which can be distinguished from secondary or induced lesions.
   Primary lesions can appear as a:

• macule – a flat, circumscribed area of altered skin colour;
• papule – a small circumscribed elevation of the skin;
• nodule – a solid, circumscribed elevation whose greater part lies beneath the skin surface;
• weal – a transparent, slightly raised lesion, characteristically with a pale centre and a pink margin;
• vesicle (blister) – a small (<5 mm in diameter) circumscribed, elevation containing fluid;
• bulla (blister) – similar to a vesicle but larger;
• pustule – a collection of pus;
• plaque – a flat-topped palpable lesion;
• purpura – visible collection of free red blood cells with the skin;
• telangectasia – dilated capillaries visible on the skin surface.

Secondary lesions

Secondary lesions are the natural evolution of primary lesions and include:

• scale – thickened, loose, readily detached fragments of stratum corneum;
• crust – dried exudates;
• excoriation – a shallow abrasion often caused by scratching;
• ulcer – an excavation due to loss of tissue including the epidermal surface;
• scar – a permanent lesion that results from the process of repair by replacement with connective tissue;
• lichenification – areas of increased epidermal thickness with accentuation of skin markings which develop in response to chronic rubbing.

The cutaneous lesions most often observed in rheumatic diseases are shown on Table 10.1.

TREATMENTS

Treatment is specific to the patient's skin condition and upon the individual patient's requirements. For many chronic skin diseases, topical treatment is the safest and most effective long-term use. The advantage of direct delivery

Table 10.1 Lesions commonly seen in rheumatic disease

Disease	Macules/papules	Papulonodular	Vesicular/bullous	Pustular	Ulcerating	Petechial/purpura
Rheumatoid arthritis	•	•			•	•
Psoriatic arthritis	•					
Systemic lupus erythematosus		•	•	•	•	•
Scleroderma		•				
Sjögren's syndrome	•	•			•	•
Dermatomyositis	•	•			•	•
Sarcoid	•					
Reiter's syndrome	•					•
Behçet's syndrome		•	•	•	•	
Wegener's granulomatosus	•	•	•	•	•	•

and reduced systemic toxicity make topical treatment an attractive therapeutic option. Topical medications used in rheumatology include:

- Antiseptics such as iodine, potassium permanganate and silver nitrate may be used for skin lesions.
- Coal tar which has anti-inflammatory and antiproliferative effects is used for eczema and psoriasis.
- Corticosteroids have anti-inflammatory and antiproliferative effects and are used for eczema, discoid lupus erythematous and psoriasis.
- Dithranol is an antiproliferative used for psoriasis.
- Keratolytics such as salicylic acid, tretinoin and benzoyl peroxides are used for scaly eczema.
- Vitamin D analogues inhibit keratinocyte and proliferation and are used for psoriasis.

VEHICLES FOR TOPICAL MEDICATIONS

These active ingredients (above) are added to a base so that the patient can apply it to their skin. There a variety of bases.

Cream

Cream is a semi-solid emulsion of oil in water, which contains a preservative to prevent overgrowth of micro-organisms. It is stabilised by an emulsifier and is mostly water so it evaporates. Aqueous cream is popular due to being nongreasy, enabling easier application and removal.

Ointment

Ointment is a semi-solid grease/oil, sometimes containing additional powder. Ointment contains little or no water. The active ingredient is suspended and usually no preservative is needed. Emulsifying ointments such as ointment/liquid paraffin 50:50 are more favourable for dry skin disorders as they have a thicker consistency and the ability to rehydrate and occlude. Unfortunately, patients often find them to be too greasy and difficult to remove.

Lotion

Lotion is a liquid vehicle, aqueous or alcohol based, which may contain a salt solution. Lotions evaporate to cool the inflamed/exudative skin. Calamine lotion is a good example.

Gel

Gel is a semi-solid transparent non-greasy emulsion such as doublebase.

Paste

Paste is an ointment with a high proportion of powder, which gives a stiff consistency. Pastes can be applied to well-demarcated lesions. Dithranol is a good example of a paste. Due to its ointment base it is difficult to remove, especially if the patient has painful hands as in rheumatoid arthritis (RA).

QUANTITIES REQUIRED FOR TOPICAL APPLICATION

A useful guide is the fingertip unit (FTU), which equals ½g. One fingertip unit is the amount of topical agent, which can be applied to the terminal phalanx of the index finger. The whole body requires 20–30 g of ointment per single dose (Gawkrodger, 2002) and the safe maximum amount varies with the strength of the drug, the length of treatment and the age of the patient. Quantities required for an adult are:

- face or neck – 1 g
- trunk (each side) – 3 g
- arm – 1½ g
- hand – ½ g
- leg – 3 g
- foot – 1 g

EMOLLIENTS

Emollients are essential for dry skin disorders such as eczema and psoriasis. They also promote suppleness in systemic sclerosis. Emollients establish the surface lipid layer and enhance rehydration of the epidermis. This results in a more comfortable sensation for the patient. All emollients are made up of varying proportions of water and lipids, giving them different consistencies and degrees of oiliness. They prevent excessive evaporation and water loss within the skin. By using an emollient the patient will be providing the skin with additional water, which then increases its pliability and elasticity, often allowing the patient to gain freedom of movement. They are often used in conjunction with other topical medications to provide an increased absorption rate. Common emollients include:

- *Emulsifying Ointment*
- *Emulsifying Ointment with Liquid Paraffin 50:50*
- *Diprobase*
- *Aqueous cream*
- *Unguentum Merck*
- *Dermol*

- *Hydromol*
- *E 45*
- *Ultrabase.*

APPLICATION OF TOPICAL TREATMENTS

Unlike some topical medications, there is no limitation to the amount and frequency when applying emollients. Usually, more is better, and they can be applied as often as required. The emollient should be applied thinly, with smooth downward strokes in the direction of the hair growth. If they are applied too thickly, they may trap heat in the skin making it itch. Rubbing or massaging them in can block the hair follicles. The dryness of the patient's skin will determine how often they need to use their emollient and whether a cream or a greasier ointment, which will last longer, is needed. Bath emollients such as bath oils and emollients rather than soaps, can also be used as they will rehydrate the skin whilst washing.

PHOTOTHERAPY AND PHOTOCHEMOTHERAPY

Whilst sunlight can help certain skin conditions, a number of dermatological problems are caused or aggravated by exposure to natural sunlight. These photosensitive conditions are systemic lupus erythematosus (SLE) and polymorphic light eruptions. Photosensitive drug eruptions may induce a porphyria-like skin fragility and blistering. For treatment purposes both ultraviolet B (UVB) and ultraviolet A (UVA) are used therapeutically. Both of these treatments are prescribed for a variety of dermatological conditions. Patients with rheumatological conditions who suffer with eczema and psoriasis may benefit from UVB, and UVA is beneficial to patients suffering with systemic sclerosis.

UVB treatment (290–320 nm) is given three times a week (Arndt and Bowers, 2002).

The initial dose is determined from the patient's skin type (Table 10.2) and with each visit the scheduled dosage is increased. The normal course is 10–30 treatments. The side effects include acute sunburn and an increased risk of skin cancer. UVB can be used in psoriasis and mycosis fungoides and occasionally atopic eczema and pityriasis rosea.

Table 10.2 Skin types reacting to sunlight

Type I – Very sensitive, always burns easily, goes very red in sunlight, never tans
Type II – Very sensitive, always burns, goes red after sunlight, minimal tan
Type III – Sensitive, burns moderately, goes red, gradual light tan
Type IV – Moderately sensitive, goes red, tans brown easily
Type V – Minimally sensitive, rarely burns, always goes dark brown
Type VI – Never burns, always deeply pigmented, black

UVA alone has minimal effect and is therefore used in combination with psoralen. This combination is known as PUVA. Patients have an option of taking psoralens systemically or topically. Oral 8 methoxypsoralen is taken two hours prior to the UVA treatment of 320–400 nm (Arndt and Bowers, 2002), and as with the UVB treatment, the initial dose of UVA is determined by skin type. The treatment is given two to three times a week for 15–25 treatments.

An alternative to the oral psoralens is bath PUVA, which requires the patient to soak their skin in a bath of diluted psoralen prior to the UVA treatment. Local PUVA, topical psoralen is an option for particular conditions affecting the hands and feet such as psoriasis and dermatitis. Side effects from PUVA can include:

- nausea
- pruritus
- erythema
- increased risk of skin cancer.

Psoralen is deposited in the lens of the eye and so patients must wear UVA protected sunglasses during their treatment and up to 24 hours afterwards. PUVA can be administered for:

- psoriasis
- mycosis fungoides
- topic eczema
- polymorphic light eruption
- vitiligo.

PUVA is occasionally given for scleroderma but the doses may be lowered for this condition.

SUN PROTECTION

Tolerance to sunlight depends on the amount of melanin in the skin and the individual's capacity to produce melanin following exposure to the sun. Sunscreen prevents:

- ultraviolet-induced DNA damage
- cutaneous immunosuppression
- generation of T suppressor cells.

The effect of sunscreen on the prevention and development of skin cancers is controversial (Arndt and Bowers, 2002). Sun protection factor (SPF) value is the ratio of the time required to produce erythema through a sunscreen product to the time required to produce the same degree of erythema without the sunscreen. The SPF usually ranges from 2 (minimal protection) to 15 or greater (ultra). SPF 2 gives 50% protection, SPF 15 gives 93% protection and SPF 34 gives 97% protection. The use of higher SPF sunscreens appears to increase the duration of recreational sun exposure and provide a false sense of security.

LIGHT AMPLIFICATION BY STIMULATED EMISSION OF RADIATION (LASER)

In this procedure, high intensity light energy is applied to the tissue. Laser surgery is a rapidly changing field and new types of lasers are constantly being introduced. Lasers vary from a continuous wave carbon dioxide laser to a short-pulsed pigment Q-switched ruby laser. Laser treatment is used for:

- port wine stain nevi
- viral warts
- tattoos
- tumours.

Pulsed dye laser treatment is an option for scleroderma patients with telangiectasia as it can obliterate the broken blood vessels. It can also be an option for treating persistent areas of calcinosis, depending on the size and location.

RHEUMATIC DISEASES AFFECTING THE SKIN

There are a number of diseases that affect the skin, including:

- systemic sclerosis
- SLE
- psoriatic arthritis
- Raynaud's phenomenon.

SYSTEMIC SCLEROSIS (SCLERODERMA)

This is the systemic form of a spectrum of autoimmune connective tissue disorders commonly known as scleroderma (meaning hard skin). It is a complex disease both in its diagnosis and management and has the highest mortality of all the rheumatic diseases (Denton and Black, 1999). Systemic sclerosis is subtyped into:

- diffuse systemic sclerosis
- limited systemic sclerosis (formally known as CREST).

Both of these subtypes affect the skin, and have underlying processes of inflammation and fibrosis which may affect internal organs and structures. The presenting symptoms are varied and until the classical hard skin is seen, the correct diagnosis may be illusive. A description of this condition and potential organ involvement is found in Chapter 2.

SKIN CARE

Assessment of the skin

It is important that the classic skin thickening and tightness seen in systemic sclerosis is assessed. The Modified Rodnan Skin Score is the most frequently used technique in systemic sclerosis assessment (Furst *et al.*, 1998). It is a pinch test of 17 areas of the skin and the scoring is:

- 0 – normal
- 1 – thickened
- 2 – can't pinch it
- 3 – can't move it.

The maximum possible score is 51. As it is a subjective technique, the same person should undertake the assessment on the same patient whenever possible. An increasing skin score or feeling of tightness of the skin may be a sign of increased disease activity and therefore should be a red flag toward review of the patient's management plan.

Interdisciplinary care

To maximise independence, physiotherapy, podiatry and occupational therapy referral are accepted as standard good practice for patients with systemic sclerosis. Physical therapy involves hand and facial exercises to maintain mobility of the affected areas. These should only be undertaken within patients' comfort levels. Hard evidence for these exercises is limited (Reay *et al.*, 2001), but anecdotally they do help, and at present are considered to be best practice.

Dryness

Patients with systemic sclerosis often have dry skin and are advised to use a simple moisturiser such as aqueous cream or E 45. It is applied over the dry patches of the body as often as possible, optimally four applications a day. This not only makes the patient's skin feel better, but encourages the patient to become familiar with their skin appearance, and to check for signs of change such as increased thickening or ulceration.

Itching

Itching is a frequent and very debilitating problem in those with systemic sclerosis. It can cause discomfort, lack of sleep and frustration. Patients often scratch to the point of breaking the skin. Treatment can be difficult and there is little research into effective therapies. However, anecdotally, aqueous cream with 1% menthol can be helpful to reduce itching.

Ulceration

Ulceration can be a frequent problem in patients with systemic sclerosis. Although it can appear anywhere, it is particularly seen in the extremities of the fingers and feet. The possible causes include:

- prolonged Raynaud's attacks
- vasculitis
- repetitive trauma from deformities of the digits (such as reabsorption of the terminal phalanx as seen in systemic sclerosis).

Advice about ulceration begins with methods of prevention such as avoidance or management of Raynaud' attacks. This should be reinforced by management of the underlying disease. The ulcer itself should be kept clean and dry, and patients often find a thin hydrocolloid such as granulfex is appropriate for noninfected digital ulcers.

Treatment of infected ulcers

Treat infected ulcers using the following procedure:

1. Begin with taking a swab for an assessment of culture and sensitivity to find which microbes are present.
2. Prescribe the appropriate antibiotics.
3. Assess the wound for size and depth. A photograph with a scale marker is ideal for this. Daily clean with a sterile saline preparation and apply a dressing covered with a non-adherent dressing. Review this plan of care regularly.
4. Ensure the patient has sufficient analgesia and is aware of the need to use it regularly.
5. Liaise with community staff such as the practice or district nurses if the patient or their carer is unable to dress the wound themselves.
6. Consider the need for hospital admission if the infection is not improving, or if there are other signs of worsening of the underlying disease. For example, ulceration caused by vasculitis may not improve without systemic dampening down of the underlying disease; ulcers triggered by Raynaud's may require a course of intravenous antibiotics combined with three to five days of an intravenous prostacylcin such as Iloprost.

Hyper/hypo pigmentation

Systemic sclerosis patients frequently have patches of altered pigmentation that gives the impression that they have a suntan. The cause of this is unclear, but it often leads to comments from others such as 'You're looking well.' or 'Have you just been on holiday?' which can become frustrating for patients who may feel far from well. This altered pigmentation may also present as a salt and pepper distribution in darker skins. There is no recognised treatment except the use of camouflage makeup on exposed areas.

Telangiectasia

Telangiectasia are dilated blood vessels which can be seen near the surface of the skin. They may be seen in patients with systemic sclerosis, and are also the 'T' in the CREST acronym, now known as limited systemic sclerosis. Although telangiectasia are usually physically painless, they can lead to great psychological distress as they frequently appear on the face and are not easily covered by commercial makeup. Two treatments can be useful: camouflage make-up and laser therapy.

Camouflage make-up is a conservative treatment which is a specialised make-up that is excellent at covering these lesions, but is only available on prescription. The prescription and application of camouflage make-up is a specialist service which is available in some areas through the NHS. If this is not a local provision, the British Red Cross offer an excellent service requiring medical referral. The patient will then have the appropriate camouflage makeup applied together with instruction on self-application. This is followed by a letter to the patient's GP with full details of their individual requirement.

Laser therapy can remove these lesions and many dermatology units now offer this treatment.

SYSTEMIC LUPUS ERYTHEMATOSUS (SLE)

SLE is an autoimmune disorder with patients classically presenting with a rash at some stage in their illness (Brown, 2003). Perhaps the most well-known feature is the photosensitive malar or butterfly rash that extends from the cheeks and over the bridge of the nose, sparing the nasolabial folds. Other common dermatological problems are:

- vasculitis
- alopecia
- Raynaud's phenomenon.

SUBACUTE LUPUS

The highly photosensitive rash of subacute lupus is commonly circular with a well-defined border and seen chiefly in exposed areas such as the upper chest. Subacute lupus is associated with antibodies to anti-Ro/SS-A (Brown, 2003).

DISCOID LUPUS

Discoid lupus affects a wider age group of people than SLE and is associated with (Hughes, 1994):

- erythema;
- hyperkeratosis and scaling;
- follicular plugging;
- telangiectasia and atrophy of skin appendages;
- inflammatory plaques on the face, arms and trunk;
- lesions also seen on the scalp and mucocutaneous areas;
- relatively small risk of developing systemic lupus erythematosus.

Skin protection

Skin protection is particularly important in SLE, as ultraviolet light (UVA and UVB) can damage circulating DNA leading to serious exacerbations of the disease (Wallace, 2000). Patients must be advised to use a high-factor sunscreen at all times. The minimum SF for SLE patients is 25. Sunscreen is available on prescription for these patients. Advice about clothing should also be given such as:

- wear long-sleeved tops;
- wear trousers or long skirts;
- use sun protection and reapply frequently;
- wear a wide-brimmed hat to protect the face.

Patients with SLE and scleroderma are often young women. Those who are mothers tend to feel inadequate as they don't have the energy or physical dexterity needed to support their children in school or in family life. Offering time and support is an essential part of the nursing care of these patients. Working with the patient in the context of their family, individually or collectively, may be appropriate. The holistic care required may come from a suitably trained and experienced nurse, or it may be necessary to refer the patient to an external agency such as a trained family counsellor. When working in these circumstances, the skill of the nurse lies in the correct timing and placing of such facilitation.

Management of the skin problems of SLE is essential and the nurse may also consider appropriate referral such as:

• dermatological input
• camouflage make-up
• possible peer support through local groups or charities, such as lupus UK.

This nursing care in combination with the two-pronged approach of tackling the underlying disease with medication, and the use of topical preventative measures are essential requirements for optimum care.

PSORIATIC ARTHRITIS (PsA)

This seronegative arthropathy is associated with psoriasis. The percentage of those with psoriasis who will go on to develop PsA ranges between 6% and 42% (Gladman et al., 1987). The classification criteria for PsA remains debatable (Mease et al., 2005; Helliwell and Taylor, 2005). Patients with PsA are unfortunate because in addition to experiencing the relapsing and remitting inflammatory arthritic disease activity, they are also subjected to the skin effects of psoriasis. This two-fold burden may cause profound psychological effects (Finlay and Kelly, 1987; Finlay and Coles, 1995). When managing PsA, the global approach outlined by Holdsworth (2003) should be taken:

• identify and relieve the symptoms of the disease;
• help the patient to understand and manage the disease;
• maintain the patient's normal lifestyle;
• maintain the patient's musculoskeletal function;
• suppress joint inflammation;
• prevent structural damage and disability.

Psoriasis is associated with scaling plaques which are well-circumscribed, circular, red papules with a silvery white appearance. They are typically seen in body folds, elbows, knees, scalp and the lumbosacral area.

Langley et al. (2005) has suggested that psoriasis may be further classified as:

• plaque psoriasis
• guttae psoriasis
• flexural (inverse) psoriasis
• erythroderma
• generalised pustular psoriasis
• palmoplantar pustulosis
• psoriatic nail disease.

MANAGEMENT

Worry and anxiety affect at least a third of patients with psoriasis, and when this is added to the physical and psychological effects, PsA may have an affect on many of the aspects which contribute toward their quality of life (QoL). This is reflected in the tools which are available to assess the psychological affects of PsA, many of which focus on the patient's QoL (Langley *et al.*, 2005; McKenna *et al.*, 2003). They include:

- Psoriasis Quality of Life Questionnaire Dermatology Utilities (McKenna *et al.*, 2003);
- Dermatology Quality of life Scales (deKorte *et al.*, 2002);
- Psoriatic Arthritis Specific Measure of Quality of Life (McKenna *et al.*, 2004);
- Psoriatic Arthritis Specific Measure of Quality of Life (McKenna *et al.*, 2003);
- Psoriasis Life Stress Inventory (Sampogna *et al.*, 2004);
- Impact of Psoriasis Questionnaire (Sampogna *et al.*, 2004);
- Psoriasis Disability Index (Finlay and Coles, 1995).

The regular use of assessment tools will enable the nurse to gain insight into the patient's perception of the effects of their skin disease. This will enable the nurse to target support and education appropriately. Liaison is an important aspect of this support, as family and friends are often affected by the effects of the disease such as:

- altered body image
- lowered self-confidence
- low self-esteem.

These problems may lead the patient to avoid going out, hence the risk of losing both social confidence and social outlets. There are also implications of having a skin condition and finding suitable employment (Helliwell and Wright, 1995), and this in turn can affect not only finance, but also relate back to lowered self-esteem and confidence.

RAYNAUD'S PHENOMENON

Raynaud's is commonly described as a phenomenon. However, its effects make it worthy of inclusion in this section. The condition often presents in the fingers and they go white, blue and then red. Pain is often present during the latter stage. The symptoms of Raynaud's are caused by episodic vasospasm. Raynaud's can also affect other areas such as the toes and the tip of the nose.

Raynaud's is subdivided into:

- primary Raynaud's
- secondary Raynaud's.

Primary Raynaud's is a standalone condition affecting nine times more women than men. Secondary Raynaud's is a relatively rare condition in which the Raynaud's is closely associated with a secondary pathology such as systemic sclerosis, SLE and RA. Severe cases of Raynaud's can result in digital ulceration and even necrosis.

DIAGNOSIS AND ASSESSMENT

In order to make the diagnosis of primary or secondary Raynaud's a comprehensive medical history is required making particular note of:

- age at onset of the Raynaud's;
- length of time the patient has had Raynaud's;
- duration of the attacks;
- if the attacks occur in summer as well as winter;
- any active ulcers or history of digital ulcers;
- migraine;
- any medication being taken (e.g. beta blockers);
- any signs or symptoms of a connective tissue disease.

MANAGEMENT

The management of Raynaud's is largely preventative. Cold triggers vasoconstriction and so information about the wearing of electrically heated gloves, thermal socks and gloves and chemical hand warmers is important. Drug therapy is discussed in Chapter 12.

WORK

Advice with regard to the work environment may be required, as a cold or damp work place may induce Raynaud's attacks. For instance, patients with Raynaud's should use protective gloves if their work involves restocking freezer cabinets or working outside in the colder months. Other environmental problems include:

- smoky atmospheres
- manual work with vibrating machinery
- unduly stressful work.

OTHER COMMON SKIN PROBLEMS

There are a number of other problems that affect the skin in the rheumatic diseases including:

- nodules
- gouty tophi
- calcinosis
- steroid therapy
- vasculitis
- leg ulcers.

NODULAR LESIONS

One of the extra-articular manifestations of RA is the development of nodules (Hill and Hale, 2004). These occur in 20% of patients with seropositive RA and tend to affect those with severe disease (Hollingworth, 1988; Matteson *et al.*, 1995).

Nodules are firm, subcutaneous, moveable lesions and are usually painless. They vary in size and have an inner core of necrotised collagen, fibrin and cell debris. They tend to develop over bony prominences such as the:

- elbows
- heels
- ischial and sacral prominences
- occipital scalp.

This citing makes them very susceptible to mechanical trauma. In some patients nodules may subside as improvement in disease activity occurs. Unfortunately, in some patients taking methotrexate, they may worsen even when disease activity improves.

GOUTY TOPHI

Gouty tophi are solid deposits of sodium urate that appear as irregular, firm nodular swellings (Jordan, 2004). They are yellow/white in colour and appear to shine through the overlying skin. If there is local inflammation the surrounding skin may become erythematous. They typically occur in the digits of the hands and feet, the ear and the olecranon bursa (Hill, 1999). They can become infected.

CALCINOSIS

Calcinosis is found in systemic sclerosis, polymyositis and dermatomyositis. Calcinosis occurs when calcium salts are deposited in the tissues. These deposits are palpable and intracutaneous, subcutaneous or facial sites are affected (Cushnaghan and McDowell, 1999). Calcinosis can be found on the:

- digits
- forearms
- knees
- shins
- thighs
- buttocks
- elbows.

They can ulcerate and a gritty toothpaste-like substance drains out (Cohen and Emmerson, 1995; Dieppe, 1995; Steen, 1995). If they ulcerate they can take many weeks to heal. However, regular soaking in an antiseptic solution, topical application of an antibiotic and an occlusive dressing may help.

STEROID THERAPY

Steroid therapy can cause the skin to bruise easily or even tear. This is due to the reduction of collagen and elastin, which leads to the loss of support for blood vessels which renders them fragile. Steroids can also cause retention of sodium which can cause oedema. The combination of oedematous ankles and legs with fragile skin can lead to the development of ulcers if the skin is damaged (Pigg et al., 1985).

A raised level of corticosteroid delays wound healing and increases susceptibility to infection as it suppresses the natural immune and inflammatory responses. The delay in wound healing is thought to occur only during the inflammatory and proliferative phases of the response. This may be due to the suppression of collagen synthesis and production of fibroblasts (Dunne and Robertson, 1992; Hinchliff and Montague, 1988; Morrison, 1992). If the skin breaks down, a wound develops leaving the patient susceptible to local infection that can rapidly spread (Griffiths and Jordan, 2002).

VASCULITIS

Vasculitis means inflammation of a vessel. It is relevant to skin care because of its manifestation in skin lesions. In some diseases such as SLE and RA, small vessel vasculitis may occur (Kumar and Clark, 1990). The initiating factor of a rheumatoid leg ulcer can be an underlying vasculitis. However its development and chronicity may be progressed by long-term use of glucocorticosteroid, arterial and/or venous insufficiency, dependent oedema and trauma (Matteson et al., 1995).

LEG AND FOOT ULCERS

Much emphasis has been placed on the occurrence of leg ulcers as they can have a great impact on the quality of the patient's life (Hildegard, 1995). Conversely, little prominence is placed on foot ulcers, which are anecdotally a common problem that can be seriously incapacitating.

Leg ulcers

Immobility plays a part in the development of leg ulcers. For patients with RA, contributing factors are:

- local vasculitis
- poor venous return due to immobility
- steroids therapy
- poor nutrition
- obesity
- oedema.

The causes, contributory factors, factors that delay healing and preventative measures are summarised in Table 10.3.

Patient concordance with the management of leg ulcers is crucial to successful healing (Moffatt, 2004). Factors that influence concordance include the patient's attitude to care and this is underpinned by their knowledge of their disease. Unfortunately many patients have little knowledge of their condition and little understanding of the effect of the underlying pathology of wound healing. Rheumatology nurses need to ensure that patients are aware of these factors.

Foot ulcers

Foot ulceration can present many problems to the patient including:

- pain
- restricted mobility
- susceptibility to infection
- reduced social interaction
- limitations on self-care
- poorer quality of life.

There are a number of risk factors associated with foot ulceration including:

- peripheral neuropathy;
- vasculitis;

- foot deformity such as callosities, metatarsal subluxation, valgus deformities;
- ill fitting footwear.

Management of foot ulceration follows the model:

- ensuring the patient has support and understands their management as foot ulceration can be painful, disabling and frightening;
- referral to Podiatry services;
- pressure relief (from orthotic designs such as a total contact inlay in order to redistribute pressure across the foot);
- pain relief;
- assessment of the ulcer – size, depth, site and stage (such as sloughy, clean, granulating, epithelising);
- appropriate dressing to the state of the ulcer (Examples are inadine if infected, intrasite or sorbsan if the ulcer is sloughy.)
- alert medical team for assessment of underlying disease status and management.

Table 10.3 Factors related to leg ulcers

Causes	Contributory factors	Factors delaying healing	Prevention
Arterial disease	Vasculitis	Immobility/reduced mobility	Early recognition of at-risk patients
Vascular disease (chronic venous hypotension)	Poor mobility/ immobility	Malnutrition	Planning of appropriate care
Diabetes mellitus	Oedema	Psychosocial issues/ problems	Promotion of mobility
Rheumatoid arthritis	Frailty	Leg oedema	Treatment of underlying causes
*Malignancy	Previous surgery	Multiple diagnosis (several medical problems).	Skin care
*Trauma	Smoking		Healthy diet
*Metabolic disorders			Recognition and action on psychosocial issues/problems
*Lymphoedema			Patient and carer education
*Blood disorders			Discouragement of smoking.
*Infection			

*less common causes

IMMOBILITY

One of the largest predisposing factors to the development of a pressure sore is immobility, as unrelieved pressure causes compression of the tissues against bony prominences (Morrison, 1992). Immobility is a major problem for patients with rheumatic diseases and can be caused by:

- pain
- stiffness
- joint contracture
- disorganisation of the joint
- fatigue
- depression.

It is important that the multidisciplinary team works toward maximum mobility for each patient. This may require a number of different modalities, for example the use of walking aids or electric chairs, physiotherapy or the prescription of effective analgesia.

The education of the patient, relatives and carers will promote mobility through greater understanding, allowing patients to set their own goals and make their own decisions (Benbow, 1996). Knowledge of drug therapy allows the patient to judge the most efficacious time to take their medication, so enhancing mobility (Hill, 1990; Hill, 1997).

RELIEVING PRESSURE

Positional changes are the key to pressure relief. The frequency at which this is undertaken will depend on the needs of individual patients, but a minimum of every two hours is recommended (Morrison, 1992).

Use of pressure-relieving mattresses and seat cushions is often indicated but these should be used as an adjunct to and not instead of positional changes. The range of mattresses and cushions is constantly being improved, and articles and up-to-date information are published regularly in the nursing press (Cowan, 1996; Cowan, 1997). Care should be taken to assess the research supporting the use of these products and the appropriateness of each to individual patients (Fletcher, 1997). Many rheumatology patients find the covers on products make them too hot and others do not like the sensation of the mattresses changing pressure. Patients often favour mattresses that appear no different to an ordinary mattress and some overlay-type mattresses meet these preferences. The appearance of normality can help to promote the patient's self-esteem and also acknowledges that they may share their bed with their partner!

DIET AND ARTHRITIS

Good nutrition is vital for good health and the Essence of Care initiative (NHS Modernisation Agency, 2003) is geared to improving nutritional services for patients (Davidson, 2004). Although patients are bombarded with information about diets from the media, the information is rarely evidence-based. This can lead patients to eat a nutritionally inadequate diet leading to malnutrition and the adverse effects of this can be:

• delayed wound healing
• impaired immune function
• depression
• muscle weakness
• respiratory difficulties.

Patients often have queries about diet such as 'Does it cause arthritis?' or 'What should I eat?' and these questions are usually addressed to the nursing staff. It is vital that nurses are sufficiently informed about diet and its effects so they can address these questions.

A NUTRITIONALLY BALANCED DIET

Pattison (2001) has described general healthy eating guidelines and states that a balanced diet should include:

• fresh food to increase vitamin and mineral content and reduce additive and preservative content;
• red meat two to three times per week to lessen the intake of saturated fat;
• frequent intake of fish, white meat, beans, nuts and pulses;
• oily fish such as trout, mackerel, salmon or herring two to three times a week (increasing the intake of Omega-3 polyunsaturated fats and vitamin D);
• increase in olive oil and rapeseed oil (poly and monounsaturated fats) and a decrease in butter and hard fats.

A healthy well-balanced diet will help the patient with arthritis to maintain optimum health. The skin is sensitive to changes in nutritional status, consequently the malnourished patient is susceptible to pressure sores, and vitamin A is known to be required to maintain the integrity of skin. A well-nourished body will recover more easily from the frequent flares of disease and episodes of ill health that rheumatic patients endure.

Dieticians define a healthy diet as one that incorporates all the essential nutrients such as:

- amino acids
- vitamins
- carbohydrates
- fibre
- fatty acids essential to cell function which maintain an optimum body weight.

Most foods contain some of these nutrients, but most are deficient in one way or another and so a variety of foods must be eaten to ensure that the diet is well-balanced (Thomas, 1994). All the essential nutrients can be found in animal products such as meat, fish, cheese, eggs and milk in combination with vegetables and fruit.

DIETARY PROTEIN AND AMINO ACIDS

The protein requirements of the body vary depending on the metabolic rate and health status. Pregnant and breastfeeding mothers need an increase in intake for growth in foetal and maternal tissue. Similarly, the rheumatic patient who has increased tissue damage, and so greater repair requirements, needs an adequate protein intake. Protein is constantly being broken down into amino acids and resynthesised. Some amino acids are lost early on in the process but many are reutilised to ensure adequate serum and tissue protein levels. This process is under hormonal and metabolic control, allowing the body to adjust to the health status of the tissues. For example in an acute inflammatory episode there is an increase in the utilisation of amino acids. Consequently the dietary source needs to be adequately maintained to meet the increased demand from the tissues. The body can cope with a temporary reduction in protein, but if it persists, a deficiency will result in detrimental effects on tissue healing and general health status.

In general, animal proteins such as fish, meat and dairy products are more readily digestible than vegetable proteins. However, a high-fibre diet can increase protein digestibility by as much as 10%.

PROTEIN SUPPLEMENTATION

In cases of hypoproteinaemia, protein supplementation may be indicated. If the patient is able to eat a normal diet, the regular consumption of foods rich in protein such as milk, eggs, meat, fish, vegetables and fruit may suffice. However, if the patient is systemically unwell and has anorexia, the addition of skimmed milk powders to drinks may be a better method. The dietician will be able to offer further advice about protein supplementation from the wide range of supplementary feeds available.

Patients with liver or renal dysfunction may experience impaired synthesis and/or excretion of protein and in these cases, manipulation of dietary protein must be managed with great care.

DIETARY FATS

Dietary fats comprise:

- triglycerides
- phospholipids
- cholesterol.

Triglycerides are the largest group and comprise about 95% of body fat. They consist of one molecule of glycerol combined with three fatty acid molecules. Fats are insoluble in water, and weight for weight yield more energy on combustion than carbohydrates. Consequently they are a very convenient form in which energy yielding molecules, the fatty acids, can be stored.

Phospholipids are important in the composition of some cell structures. They are structurally similar to triglycerides, but one of the three fatty acids is replaced by phosphoric acid.

Cholesterol is structurally different to typical fats but is insoluble in water and soluble in organic solvents.

FATTY ACIDS

Stearic acid is a typical fatty acid. It consists of a chain of carbon atoms to which hydrogen is attached (a hydrocarbon chain) and ends in the form of an acid carboxyl group. Each carbon atom has two hydrogen atoms bonded to it and this means there is a hydrogen atom at every possible site on the hydrocarbon chain. Fatty acids that have this feature are termed saturated fatty acids. Another common fatty acid, oleic acid, has a different structure. Here, there is a double bond between two of the carbon atoms in the middle of the chain. This means that two carbon atoms have only one site available for a hydrogen atom, and so the chain does not contain the maximum possible number of hydrogen atoms. This type of fatty acid is called an unsaturated fatty acid. There are 21 fatty acids found in the diet, the most common being:

- palmitic
- stearic
- oleic

- linoleic
- linolenic
- arachidonic.

ESSENTIAL FATTY ACIDS

The body is able to synthesise most fatty acids, but the unsaturated fatty acids linoleic, linolenic and arachidonic, all essential to tissue function, must be provided in the diet. These are known as the essential fatty acids and are precursors of prostaglandins, chemicals involved in the inflammatory process.

DIETARY EFFECTS OF SATURATED AND UNSATURATED FATS

Saturated fatty acids are known precursors of cardiovascular disease and a reduction in their intake may reduce heart disease. Obesity, lack of exercise, systemic illness and smoking are predisposing factors to heart disease. This places the rheumatic patient at potential risk because of:

- reduced ability to exercise
- impaired systemic health
- patients' smoke.

To reduce their risk patients should:

- substitute saturated fats with polyunsaturated fats;
- reduce excessive fat intake.

Polyunsaturated fats do not contain cholesterol and are a safer option as they reduce low density lipoprotein concentrations, the group of cholesterols that are associated with heart disease. Polyunsaturated fats are contained in some margarines and vegetable oils.

A high intake of fat can precipitate obesity, particularly detrimental to patients with joint damage. Obesity hinders mobility, lowers self-esteem and greatly increases the load carried by weight-bearing joints. As a guide women should have no more than 70 g/day and men no more than 90 g/day (Price, 2005).

CARBOHYDRATES

Carbohydrates are usually in the form of sugars and starches. Starches are carbohydrates derived from plants, and sugars can be described as their soluble form. They are classified according to their chemical complexity:

- monosaccharides – single units or molecules (glucose, fructose, galactose);
- disaccharides – two monosaccharide molecules (sucrose, maltose, and lactose);
- polysaccharides – large numbers of monosaccharide molecules (starches, glycogen, cellulose and dextrins).

The main functions of carbohydrates are to:

- provide a rapid source of energy and heat;
- store energy;
- spare protein.

Foods which supply carbohydrates include sugar, jams, bread, pasta, cereals fruit and vegetables. Carbohydrates are converted to glucose and absorbed into the blood. All bodily tissues, especially the brain, need carbohydrate as a vital fuel for their function. To meet these demands the body attempts to maintain a steady level of glucose in the bloodstream at all times (homeostasis). Under normal circumstances the blood glucose rises after eating if:

- There is a surplus of stored glucose in the liver or muscles.
- The level of carbohydrate exceeds that required to maintain blood glucose and glycogen levels, it is converted to fat for storage.

Once exercise is initiated these glycogen stores are released back into the bloodstream to maintain a steady level.

The normal blood glucose level is between 2.5 and 5.3 mmol/litre and maintenance is vital for normal bodily function. Homeostasis is maintained by insulin and glucagon acting in a complementary manner; blood glucose levels are increased by glucagons and reduced by insulin. If insulin function is abnormal the blood glucose level remains excessively high. If the level falls excessively, a feeling of hunger prevails, associated with a sense of agitation and depression. If the diet is tuned to maintain a steady glucose level, these peaks and troughs may be avoided.

More complex carbohydrates such as those found in potatoes, pasta and rice are digested at a slower rate. If they are eaten in their most natural form, for example potatoes with their skins, brown rice, wholemeal pasta, they are more likely to appease the appetite as they remain in the stomach longer and maintain a more stable blood sugar level.

DIETARY FIBRE

Dietary fibre is a complex mixture of carbohydrates that consists of plant cell walls. It is indigestible and therefore offers little value to nutrition. Its functions are to:

- provide bulk
- stimulate peristalsis
- attract water that softens and bulks the faeces
- prevent constipation
- prevent gastrointestinal disorders.

The recommended intake of fibre is 18–20 grams per day but in developed countries where a more refined diet is eaten, the average intake is 11–12 grams per day. There are a number of benefits to increasing fibre intake.

Satiation of appetite

For the overweight person extra fibre will help to satisfy the appetite and so can help in weight reduction. Fibre is a very natural slimming aid and also has the advantage of being cheap.

Relief of constipation

The increased bulk and water retention can help to regulate bowel habit. Analgesics, particularly those containing codeine, can cause severe constipation. Many rheumatic diseases cause pain, stiffness and debility which leads to immobility and lack of exercise. This can cause stasis of the bowel. Extra fibre will stimulate peristaltic action.

High-fibre diets also lower blood cholesterol and are thought to reduce the incidence of cancer of the large intestine.

VITAMINS

Vitamins are defined as any organic compound required by the body in small amounts for metabolism and health. They assist in the:

- formation of hormones
- blood cells
- nervous system chemicals
- genetic material
- skin integrity
- muscle regeneration
- recovery from acute episodes of inflammation.

Vitamins act as catalysts, combining with proteins to produce metabolically active enzymes that in turn produce hundreds of important chemical reactions throughout the body. There are thirteen well-defined vitamins and their sources, roles and reference nutritional intake has been described by Pattison (1998). The fat-soluble vitamins A, D, E and K are generally consumed along with fat containing foods and stored in body fat so they do not need to be consumed each day. The eight water-soluble B vitamins and vitamin C cannot be stored and must be replenished daily. The only vitamin that can be produced by the body is vitamin D. All others are derived from the diet.

Large sums of money are spent on vitamin supplements but dieticians suggest that a well-balanced diet will provide all thirteen vitamins in adequate amounts. Many patients with rheumatic diseases request advice regarding vitamin supplementation and it should not be assumed that they are able to provide themselves with a well-balanced diet.

Many patients eat what is easiest for them to manage or what their relatives or carers prepare. When assessing a patient's intake of vitamins it is useful to ask them to outline their daily diet. One way of doing this is to ask them to describe the meals they had the previous day and how they were prepared. If a broader picture is needed, request them to keep a diary of everything eaten during a week. This will enable specific vitamin deficiencies to be highlighted. If further specialised advice is needed, consult the dietician.

OBESITY IN THE RHEUMATOID PATIENT

Obesity has become almost an epidemic in the UK. Twenty-two percent of men and 23.5% of women are defined as being obese (DoH, 2004). Weight will remain stable if the dietary intake balances the energy expended by the body. However the patient with arthritis may have difficulty achieving this balance. Weight gain and subsequent obesity is a very common problem in disabled patients, particularly those with osteoarthritis. Many find it extremely difficult to exercise actively even when their disease is well-controlled. Factors influencing the extent to which patients can exercise include:

- joint pain
- stiffness
- muscle weakness
- muscle wasting.

Obviously the degree of joint pain and the level of disease activity varies between patients, but very few are able to sustain a programme of exercise that is vigorous or regular enough to burn off excess calories. The boredom and frustration of immobility compound the problem of weight gain and the temptation to indulge in comfort eating is understandable. Patients who are housebound also find themselves alone for long periods and derive solace from eating.

Chronic disability can degrade and demoralise a person and poor body image results in personal neglect. Medications such as steroids can induce weight gain and clothes do not look or feel good to wear.

The patient with weight problems needs to be treated with compassion. Advice must be practical and sensible. Literature should be made available regarding:

- sensible diets
- local slimming clubs
- exercise facilities that cater specifically for the disabled or less able patient.

Some local rheumatology units hold sessions for patients at their local pools, but it should be noted that swimming pools need to be about 10°F (6°C) warmer than usual to provide an environment more conducive with hydrotherapy.

For the patient with osteoarthritis of the weight-bearing joints, weight reduction is a therapeutic option. Walking can result in the knee experiencing an impulse loading of up to eight times body weight. Therefore joint pain and discomfort are very likely to be reduced if obese patients reduce their weight.

THE UNDERWEIGHT OR MALNOURISHED PATIENT

Acute and chronic inflammatory disease can result in an increased metabolic rate where energy expended exceeds dietary intake. The patient may eat normally but still lose weight. This in association with tiredness and malaise leads the patient to wonder whether they have an additional, more serious illness such as cancer. There are several points to consider:

- Has the patient actually lost weight?
- How much weight has the patient lost and over what time period?
- Has the weight loss been in parallel with the patient's disease activity?
- Does the patient have an adequate appetite?
- Is the patient's diet well-balanced?
- If the patient's diet and appetite are poor can they think of a reason why?

Practical difficulties may form part of the problem. For instance:

- The patient may not drink to avoid walking to the toilet.
- Food preparation may pose such great difficulties that it is easier not to eat.
- The patient may be too fatigued to bother to cook.
- Manual dexterity may inhibit food preparation.

If this is the case, referral to the occupational therapist for adapted cutlery and kitchen equipment can help. Rheumatic diseases are energy-depleting and fatigue may increase the demand for, but reduce the will to prepare a meal. Pain may also contribute to difficulties with nutrition; opening packets and jars, stirring or lifting pans can prove impossible for some patients. Medical review of medication and assistance from the occupational therapist and physiotherapist can be of great benefit (Arthur, 1994; Crosby, 1991; Ryan, 1995).

If weight loss is due to other medical problems an assessment of the general health of the patient should be undertaken.

GASTROINTESTINAL PROBLEMS

Disorders of the gastrointestinal tract can often result in weight loss and anorexia. Problems can be identified by asking patients:

- Do you have mouth ulcers or a sore mouth?
- Do you have a dry mouth?
- Is the process of chewing painful because of jaw pain?
- Do you have difficulty swallowing?
- Do you experience indigestion, heartburn or vomiting?
- Have you ever seen blood in the vomit?
- Have you any history of hiatus hernia, gastric ulceration?
- Is constipation and/or diarrhoea evident?
- Have you ever noticed blood in your stools? (If yes, do you have haemorrhoids? These can be the source of bleeding rather than a site higher up in the tract.)

Many of these problems can be addressed and treated by the nurse. For instance advice regarding mandibular pain, mouth care and mouth sprays for a dry mouth caused by Sjögren's syndrome. Advice about constipation and swallowing difficulties due to scleroderma can also be given. If the nurse can provide a concise patient history, this will aid the doctor to plan medical management and save the patient time.

FASTING AND RHEUMATOID ARTHRITIS

The suggestion that the gut may be involved in the immune-mediated process of RA suggests that elimination of antigenic material in the gut could result in a reduction of inflammatory symptoms. Fasting can be defined as the voluntary refraining from food for a limited period of time. Fasting causes a sudden and dramatic fall in exogenous energy that would normally be supplied by the diet. After a relatively short time the shortage of energy must be compensated to supply metabolic needs and this is achieved by release of endogenous energy from the liver glycogen, muscle protein and fat tissue (Landsberg and Young, 1976). When these compensatory changes occur, metabolic hormones are readjusted and it may be at this point that the inflammatory process of RA is influenced.

Fasting does appear to reduce disease activity in RA. However, the benefit is short-lived and deterioration is noted within several days of reintroduction of food (Skoldstam et al., 1983; Sundvist et al., 1982). Overall, there is no clinical evidence to support the promotion of fasting as an adjunct therapy in the management of RA.

FOOD INTOLERANCE

The immunological presentation of certain antigenic substances in the gut may be a precursor to an inflammatory process in RA. If foods likely to be antigenic are removed from the diet, improvement in disease activity may be expected. An elemental diet is a hypoallergenic protein-free diet that contains:

- amino acids
- glucose
- trace elements
- vitamins.

It provides food in its simplest form; protein as amino acids, carbohydrates as glucose and fat as medium-chain triglycerides (Kavanagh et al., 1995). The introduction of an elemental diet has dramatic immediate benefits. Unfortunately, the effects are short-lived and disappear rapidly after the reintroduction of food. Reintroduction of specific foods appears to produce a variety of individual responses. Some respond significantly to one food, whilst others respond to a lesser degree. It is concluded that allergy to diet is not a major causative factor contributing to the aetiology of RA (Kavanagh et al., 1995: Van de Laar and Van Der Korst, 1992; Panush, 1990; Beri et al., 1988; Felder et al., 1987; Darlington et al., 1986).

OMEGA THREE FATTY ACIDS

Essential fatty acids are derived from the diet and are divided into two groups:

- linoleic acid – omega-6 fatty acids found in corn, safflower, soy and other vegetable oils;
- alpha-linolenic acid – omega-3 fatty acids found in fatty fishes such as tuna, sardines, salmon and in certain plants such as the evening primrose.

Essential fatty acids provide energy and are an integral part of cell membranes. They are also the precursors of prostaglandins, thromboxanes and collectively termed eicosanoids. This group of chemicals is involved in the development and regulation of immunological and inflammatory processes (Sperling, 1991). When cells involved in immune reactions are stimulated, the body's existing store of essential fatty acids are mobilised from the phospholipid pools for synthesis of prostaglandins. The type of prostaglandins produced is dependent on the type of essential fatty acids present (Meade and Mertin, 1978). If the essential fatty acid store is rich in omega-3 fatty acids such as PGE3, prostaglandins that demonstrate beneficial anti-inflammatory properties will be produced. However, if the diet contains a majority from the omega six group, prostaglandins will be activated that promote the inflammatory process.

The British diet appears to be low in omega-3 fatty acids (Ruxton, 2004) and good sources include oily fish such as tuna, salmon and trout. However, tinned varieties, particularly tuna, lose much of their natural oils during processing. Research appears to support the anecdotal claims that the supplementation of omega-3 fatty acids results in a subjective improvement in symptoms in a percentage of patients (Cleland et al., 1988; Darlington, 1988). Several studies have demonstrated that high doses of fish oils can help patients with mild RA to reduce their NSAIDs (Cleland and James, 1997). Two meta-analyses have been undertaken (Fortin et al., 1995; Cleland et al., 2003). Both these reviews have demonstrated reductions in clinical indices but no effect on biochemical assessments for disease activity.

Fish and evening primrose oils have been shown to provide a safe and efficacious adjunct therapy in the management of RA and many patients believe in their efficacy. Neither fish oils nor evening primrose oil can be prescribed for RA, but the latter is available for psoriasis as gamolenic acid.

NUTRITION AND WOUND HEALING IN RA

Nutrition is a basic human requirement (Grieve and Finnie, 2002) and plays a central role in recovery from ill health. Patients with RA are prone to skin breakdown and leg ulcers are common place (Oien et al., 2001). Wound healing requires a good blood supply and a number of nutrients (Vickers, 2004). The nutrients of particular importance follow (Casey, 1998):

- Proteins are necessary for cell mytosis and migration, immune response, and synthesis and secretion of intracellular and extracellular proteins, particularly collagen.
- Carbohydrates metabolise into adenosine triphosphate which is needed for all cellular activity.
- Vitamins A and B are necessary for the maturation and strengthening of collagen.

- Vitamin C is necessary for cell mitosis and migration, collagen synthesis and function of the immune system.
- Zinc is necessary for cell mytosis, strengthening and maturation of collagen and protein synthesis.
- Iron is necessary for the delivery of oxygen to the wound bed.

DIET AND GOUT

Gout is the most common cause of inflammatory arthritis in men aged >40 years (Jordan, 2004). It is caused by high levels of uric acid (hyperuricaemia). This can be caused by either overproduction or underexcretion (Hill, 1999). Hyperuricaemia has both internal and external causes. Internal causes include cell breakdown, genetic factors hyperlipidaemia, hypertension, obesity and impaired renal function. Internal causes include alcohol intake, medication and dietary purines. A diet low in purines and the limitation of alcohol intake are important elements of disease control. Offal such as kidney, liver, sweetbreads and heart contain high levels of purine and must be avoided. Other culprits are pate, meat extracts such as Bovril and Oxo and yeast extract. Fish to be avoided are herring, mackerel, sardines and shellfish. Weight control is important. Patients who suffer from gout are usually overweight. However, it is important that patients do not try to reduce their weight immediately following an attack as this can precipitate another one.

OSTEOPOROSIS AND DIET

Osteoporosis has been discussed elsewhere, but a few sentences regarding the dietary intake of calcium and vitamin D (by exposure to sunlight) is appropriate here. Prevention of osteoporosis is an important part of care, and rheumatology patients should be assessed for risk factors. Burden and Allsworth (1997) have discussed risk factors, and at-risk patients can identified as those who:

- start the menopause aged 45 years or younger;
- have been on 7.5 mgs of steroid longer than 3 months;
- have reduced mobility;
- have an intake of calcium <400 mg/day;
- have been submitted to bed rest for six months or longer;
- suffer from malabsorption syndrome.

If calcium and vitamin D supplementation is required, they are most effective given in combination (Pattison, 1998).

ACTION POINTS FOR PRACTICE

- Develop two education programmes specifically relating to skin integrity. One should be suitable for your students and colleagues, another for your patients and carers.
- Produce an information package for your patients relating to the nutritional aspects of their care.
- Undertake a literature search on the effects of diet on arthritis and critique the findings.
- Choose a patient and complete a case study relating the influence of diet to their disease.

REFERENCES

Arndt KA, Bowers KE (2002) *Manual of Dermatological Therapeutics* 6th edn. Lippincott, Williams & Wilkins.

Arthur V (1994) Nursing care of patients with rheumatoid arthritis. *British Journal of Nursing* 3(7):325–331.

Benbow M (1996) Pressure sore guidelines: patient/carer involvement and education. *British Journal of Nursing* 5(3):182–187.

Beri D, Malaviya AN, Shandily A *et al.* (1988) Effects of dietary restrictions on disease activity in rheumatoid arthritis. *Annals of the Rheumatic Diseases* 47:69–72.

Brown S (2003) Systemic lupus erythematosus. *Nursing Times* 99(40):30–32.

Casey G (1998) The importance of nutrients in wound healing. *Nursing Standard* 13(3):51–54.

Burden J, Allsworth A (1997) Osteoporosis: do we take it seriously? *Journal of Orthopaedic Nursing* 1(2):97–102.

Cleland LG, French JK, Betts WH *et al.* (1988) Clinical and biochemical effects of dietary fish oil supplements in rheumatoid arthritis. *Journal of Rheumatology* 15:10.

Cleland LG, James MJ (1997) Rheumatoid arthritis and the balance of dietary N-6 and N-3 essential fatty acids. *Rheumatology* 36:513–515.

Cleland LG, Jamer MJ, Proudman SM (2003) The role of fish oils in the treatment of rheumatoid arthritis. *Drugs* 63(9):845–853.

Cohen MG, Emmerson BT (1995) Gout. In: Klippel JH, Dieppe PA (eds) *Practical Rheumatology*. London, Mosby, 25:255–262.

Cowan T (1996) Pressure relieving aids for community use. *Professional Nurse* 12(2):131–138.

Cowan T (1997) Pressure support systems for hospital use. *Professional Nurse* 12(7):511–520.

Crosby LJ (1991) Factors which contribute to fatigue associated with rheumatoid arthritis. *Journal of Advanced Nursing* 16:974–981.

Cushnaghan J, McDowell J (1999) Rheumatological Conditions. In: Ryan S (ed) *Drug Therapy in Rheumatology Nursing*. Gateshead, Whurr Publishers.

Darlington LG (1988) Do diets rich in polyunsaturated fatty acids affect disease activity in rheumatoid arthritis? *Annals of the Rheumatic Diseases* 47:169–172.

Darlington LG, Ramsey NW, Mansfield JR (1986) Placebo controlled blind study of dietary manipulation therapy in rheumatoid arthritis. *The Lancet* 1(8475): 236–238.

Davidson A (2004) Good nutrition is vital for good health. *Nursing Times* 100(18):49.

de Korte J, Mombers FM, Sprangers MA *et al.* (2002) The suitability of quality of life questionnaires for psoriasis research: a systematic literature review. *Archives of Dermatology* 139:1221–1227.

Denton C, Black C (1999) Systemic Sclerosis: an overview of pathogenesis and treatment. *Rheumatology* 1(1):33–39.

Department of Health (2004) *More information on obesity.* Fact Sheet. London, DoH.

Dieppe H (1995) Clinical features and diagnostic problems in osteoarthritis. In: Klippel JH, Dieppe PA (eds) *Practical Rheumatology.* London, Mosby 12:141–155.

Dunne C, Robertson J (1992) Wound healing in rheumatoid arthritis. *Wound Management* 2(4):13–14.

Felder M, De Blecourt ACE, Wuthrick B (1987) Food allergy in patients with rheumatoid arthritis. *Clinical Rheumatology* 6(2):181–184.

Finlay AY, Kelly SE (1987) Psoriasis – an index of disability. *Clinical Experimental Dermatology* 12:8–11.

Finlay AY, Coles EC (1995) The effect of severe psoriasis on the quality of life of 369 patients. *British Journal of Dermatology* 132:236–244.

Fletcher J (1997) Pressure relieving equipment: criteria and selection. *British Journal of Nursing* 6:6(suppl) Focus on pressure sore management.

Fortin PR, Lew RA, Liang MH *et al.* (1995) Validation of a meta-analysis: the effects of fish oil in rheumatoid arthritis. *Journal of Clinical Epidemiology* 48(11): 1379–1390.

Furst DE, Clements PJ, Steen VD *et al.* (1998) The modified Rodnan skin score: is an accurate reflection of skin biopsy thickness in systemic sclerosis? *Journal of Rheumatology* 25(1):84–88.

Gawkrodger DJ (2002) *Dermatology – An Illustrated Colour Text* 3rd edn. Edinburgh, Churchill Livingstone.

Gladman DD, Shukett R, Russell ML *et al.* (1987) Psoriatic Arthritis (PSA) – an analysis of 220 patients. *Quarterly Journal of Medicine* 62(238):127–141.

Grieve RJ, Finnie A (2002) Nutritional care: Implications and recommendations for nursing. *British Journal of Nursing* 11(7):432–437.

Griffiths H, Jordan S (2002) Corticosteroids: implications for nursing practice. *Nursing Standard* 17(12):43–53.

Helliwell PS, Taylor WJ (2005) Classification and diagnostic criteria for psoriatic arthritis. *Annals of the Rheumatic Diseases* 64(Supp 11):pii3–ii8.

Helliwell P, Wright V (1995) Clinical features of psoriatic arthritis. In: Klippel J, Dieppe P (eds) *Practical Rheumatology.* London, Mosby.

Hildegard C (1995) The impact of leg ulcers on patients' quality of life. *Professional Nurse* 10(9):571–574.

Hinchliff SM, Montague SE (1988) *Physiology for Nursing Practice.* London, Bailliere Tindall.

Hill J (1990) Patient education: what to teach patients with rheumatic disease. *Journal of the Royal Society of Health* 110(6):204–207.

Hill J (1997) A practical guide to patient education and information giving. *Ballière's Clinical Rheumatology* 11(1):109–127.

Hill J, Hale C (2004) Clinical skills: evidence-based care of people with rheumatoid arthritis. *British Journal of Nursing* 13(14):852–857.

Hill J (1999) Gout: its causes, symptoms and treatment. Nursing Times 24(95): 48–50.

Holdsworth J (2003) Psoriatic arthritis. *Nursing Standard* 18(5):47–52.

Hollingworth P (1988) *Rheumatology.* London, Heinemann.

Jordan KM (2004) An update on gout. *Reports on the Rheumatic Diseases Series 5, Topical Reviews* 4:1–8.

Hughes GRV (1994) *Connective Tissue Diseases* (4th edn). London, Blackwell Scientific Publications.

Jordan K (2004) An update on gout. *Topical Reviews.* Chesterfield, Arthritis Research Campaign.

Kavanagh R, Norkman E, Nash P *et al.* (1995) The effects of elemental diet and subsequent foods reintroduction on rheumatoid arthritis. *British Journal of Rheumatology* 34:270–273.

Kumar PJ, Clark ML (1990) *Clinical Medicine,* 2nd edn. London, Baillière Tindall.

Landsberg CS, Young JB (1976) Fasting, feeding and regulation of sympathetic nervous system. *New England Journal of Medicine* 298:1295.

Langley RGB, Krueger GG, Griffiths CEM (2005) Psoriasis: epidemiology, clinical features and quality of life. *Annals of the Rheumatic Diseases* 64(suppl. 11).

McKenna SP, Doward LC, Whalley D *et al.* (2004). Development of the PsAQoL: a quality of life instrument specific to psoriatic arthritis. *Annals of the Rheumatic Diseases* 63:162–169.

McKenna SP, Cook SA, Whalley D *et al.* (2003) Development of the PSORIQoL, a psoriasis-specific measure of quality of life designed for use in clinical practice and trials. *British Journal of Dermatology* 149(2):323–331.

Mackie RM (1994) *Clinical Dermatology – an Illustrated Text Book,* 3rd edn. Oxford, Oxford Medical Publications.

Matteson EL, Cohen MD, Conn DL (1995) Clinical features of rheumatoid arthritis: systemic involvement. In: Klippel JH, Dieppe PA (eds) *Practical Rheumatology.* London, Mosby, 16:183–190.

Meade CJ, Mertin J (1978) Fatty acids and immunity. *Advanced Lipid Research* 16:127–165.

Mease PJ, Gladman DD, Krueger GG (2005) Group for Research and Assessment of Psoriasis and Psoriatic Arthritis (GRAPPA). *Annals of the Rheumatic Diseases* 64(Supp 11): p ii1–ii2.

Moffatt C (2004) Understanding patient concordance in the management of leg ulcers. *Nursing Times* 100(32):58–60.

Morrison MJ (1992) *A Colour Guide to the Nursing Management of Wounds.* London, Wolfe Publishing.

NHS Modernisation Agency (2003) *Essence of Care: Patient Focused Benchmarks for Clinical Governance.* London: NHS, MA.

Oien RF, Hakansson A, Hansen BU (2001) Leg ulcers in the patient with rheumatoid arthritis – a prospective study of aetiology, wound healing and pain reduction after pinch grafting. *Rheumatology* 40:816–820.

Panush RS (1990) Food induced 'allergic' arthritis: clinical and serological studies. *Journal of Rheumatology* 17:3:351–361.

Pattison D (1998) Fed-up with nutrition? *Journal Orthopaedic Nursing* 2:105–115.

Pattison D (2001) Nutrition and musculoskeletal disorders. *BHPR Newsletter*, London, BHPR.

Pigg JS, Driscoll PW, Caniff R (1985) *Rheumatology Nursing: a Problem Oriented Approach*. New York, John Wiley.

Price S (2005) Understanding the importance to health of a balanced diet. *Nursing Times*, 101(1):30–31.

Reay N, Stevens R, Moreno P *et al.* (2001) Evaluation of hand and face exercises in patients with scleroderma. *Arthritis and Rheumatism* 44(supplement):S210.

Ruxton C (2004) Health benefits of omega-3 fatty acids. *Nursing Standard* 11(18): 38–42.

Ruxton CH, Reed SC, Simpson MJ *et al.* (2004) The health benefits of omega-3 poly-unsaturated fatty acids: a review of the evidence. *Journal of Human Nutrition and Dietetics*.

Ryan S (1995) Nutrition and the rheumatoid patient. *British Journal of Nursing* 4(3):132–136.

Sampogna F, Sera F, Abeni D (2004) Measures of clinical severity, quality of life and psychological distress in patients with psoriasis: a cluster analysis. *Journal Investigative Dermatology* 122:602–607.

Skoldstam L, Jorfelt L, Lindell B *et al.* (1983) Specific plasma protein as indices of inflammation during modified fast in patients with rheumatoid arthritis. *Scandinavian Journal of Rheumatology* 12:161–165.

Sperling RI (1991) Dietary omega three fatty acids: effects of lipid mediators of inflammation of rheumatoid arthritis. *Rheumatic Diseases Clinics of North America* 17:2.

Steen VD (1995) Systemic sclerosis. In: Klippel JH, Dieppe PA (ed) *Practical Rheumatology*. London, Mosby 34:343–350.

Sundvist T, Lindstrom F, Magnusson KE, Skoldstam L *et al.* (1982) Influence of fasting on intestinal permeability and disease activity in patients with rheumatoid arthritis. *Scandinavian Journal of Rheumatology* 1:33–35.

Thomas B (1994) *Manual of Dietetic Practice* (2nd edn). Oxford, Blackwell Scientific Press.

Van De Laar MAF, Van Der Korst JK (1992) Food intolerance in rheumatoid arthritis. A double blind, controlled trial of the clinical effects if elimination of milk allergens and azo dyes. *Annals of the Rheumatic Diseases* 51:298–302.

Vickers A (2004) Delayed wound healing in patients with rheumatoid arthritis. *Nursing Times* 100(14):61–63.

Wallace DJ (2000) *The Lupus Book – Guide for Patients and their Families*. Revised and Expanded Edition. New York, Oxford University Press.

III Therapeutic Interventions

11 Multidisciplinary Team Care of the Rheumatic Patient

P. FITZGERALD

Chapel Allerton Hospital, West Yorkshire, UK

The aim of this chapter is to explore the central role of the nurse within the multidisciplinary team (MDT), and describe how the team can enable patients to care for themselves and retain/regain optimum independence. Rehabilitation can maximise independence by providing the patient with the ability to exercise choice and regain control of their life (Hawkey and Williams, 2001). After reading this chapter the reader should be able to:

• understand the difficulties that rheumatic patients experience;
• identify the different skills of the MDT;
• understand how teamwork enhances patient care;
• appreciate the unique role of the rheumatology nurse within the MDT;
• describe the positive results of good communication.

Patients with rheumatic disease face a plethora of problems that no single profession can fully help the patient to overcome (Hill and Reay, 2002). The rheumatology community has therefore accepted that an MDT, working in a coordinated manner, can provide a better outcome for the patient (Davis *et al.*, 2000). Although each member of the MDT has their own roles and responsibilities, those roles and boundaries can overlap. To work successfully as an MDT, members have to be aware of each other's role and how they can act in a complementary manner (McGee and Ashford, 1996). Equally all members of the team have to respect, cultivate and promote professional autonomy and recognise when it is appropriate to refer to other MDT members (Carson *et al.*, 1997).

COMMUNICATION

Communication between members of the MDT and the patient is vitally important. MDT working is associated with joint decision-making, adaptation of care to patient's needs and changes in allocation of tasks between professionals. This approach can improve the quality of patient care and results in a reduced hospital stay for patients (Zwarenstein and Bryant, 2003). However, communication across professions can prove difficult whether it is in written or verbal format. Being interactive, encouraging teamwork and having MDT meetings are positive ways of improving communication (Fox, 2000).

The ability of the team to communicate with patients and their relatives is also an important aspect of care. Health professionals must recognise that meeting the needs of the family can be just as important as meeting the needs of the patient (Abraham, 2004). Written information in the form of patient leaflets can be used to assist with patient education, but this format is not a replacement of verbal discussions (Hill, 1997). The patients and significant others need to be able to ask questions and seek out explanations regarding their concerns. The nursing role encompasses spending time with patients, assessing their concerns, meeting their educational needs, and if their disease progresses and their medications are changed, revisiting these topics.

THE NURSING ROLE

Nurses play a pivotal role within the MDT that includes:

- acting as the patients' advocate;
- ensuring individualised plans of care reflect the patient's goals;
- coordinating the work of the MDT (Baldwin, 2003).

The RCN Rheumatology Nursing Forum has published a philosophy of care that provides clear guidelines on the beliefs that govern practice (RCN, 2001). The philosophy of care is an essential part of nursing and advocates:

- a therapeutic relationship with the patient that addresses physical, psychological, social and sexual needs within an MDT context;
- enabling the patient to achieve a state of adaptation;
- empowering, supporting and guiding the patient and their families when increased input from health professionals is necessary such as hospital admission, change in therapies, frequent hospital monitoring or a course of physiotherapy;
- providing effective researched-based practice.

In order to care for rheumatology patients effectively, whether it is in an inpatient, outpatient or community environment, a holistic model of care should be used. Holistic patient assessment should include:

- disease knowledge and management;
- self-care abilities;
- social and environmental factors.

White (1998) has used these topics to display the comprehensive needs of rheumatology patients. A comprehensive list of areas to be assessed are shown in Table 11.1. When used in combination with the standards of care produced by the RCN (2001) they also enable the nurse to appreciate good practice and apply this to their own care systems.

DISEASE KNOWLEDGE AND MANAGEMENT

Patients who display an in-depth knowledge of their disease and its management are better able to cope with everyday life (Hill, 2003), and this is discussed in depth in Chapter 15.

PAIN

Chronic severe pain is usually a result of joint inflammation, and patients find this symptom is more debilitating and intolerable than the disease process which caused it. Melzack and Wall (1996) describe chronic pain as a challenge for the patient who has to learn to live and cope with the pain, and for health-care professionals who seek every possible means to help the suffering patient. A multiprofessional team approach to pain management is essential and the team usually comprises a nurse, doctor, pharmacist, physiotherapist, occupational therapist. The patient, who is the only one who can feel the pain, must be encouraged to contribute by communicating information about their pain (McCaffery and Beebe, 1997).

Analgesia

By virtue of being a constant presence, particularly in the inpatient setting, nurses can observe the patient's response to their treatments. This enables the nurse to make recommendations about changes in analgesics and thera-

Table 11.1 Assessment of the rheumatology patient

Disease knowledge and management	Self-care abilities	Environmental and social
Pain	Hygiene and skin care	Occupation
Fatigue/pacing and planning	Dressing	Transport
Stiffness	Nutrition	Housing
Joint protection	Elimination	Social and family support
Exercise	Mobility	Financial
Complementary medicines	Psychological state	Leisure
Medication	Body image and sexuality	
Sleep		

pies. In order to gain an insight into the effectiveness of analgesia prescribed, the doctor must listen to the patient and other team members. The pharmacist will be able to advise on analgesic ladders and which drugs are most suitable for steping up or down (Figure 11.1).

If pain management is difficult and the patient continues to suffer despite the efforts of the immediate team, the patient can be referred to the chronic pain clinic where the pain syndrome itself can be examined and novel, imaginative approaches to pain control may be used.

NONPHARMACOLOGICAL THERAPIES

The physiotherapist can use thermotherapy to reduce pain, stiffness and muscle spasms (Hurley et al., 2002). Hot and cold packs have been found to be safe and effective (Hill and Hale, 2004) but heat is not recommended for active joints. These treatments are easy and convenient, which means the patient can continue to use them at home to gain short-term relief (Hurley et al., 2002; Helewa, 1996).

Transcutaneous Electrical Nerve Stimulation (TENS) has an analgesic effect and works by stimulating the production of endorphins (Chapter 8). TENS can be used in patients with osteoarthritis and rheumatoid arthritis, but it tends to be more effective in single than in multijoint diseases. The physiotherapist may have to trial the TENS device when the patient is at rest and when they are mobile to assess any response (Helewa, 1996). If effective, a TENS device can be used at home.

When rheumatoid pain is caused by muscle tension brought on by maintaining a rigid posture, relaxation techniques may be beneficial (Carroll and Seers, 1998; Kaplan et al., 1993). Relaxation can also help temporomandibular joint problems and muscle spasms (McCaffery and Beebe, 1997). The occupational therapist or specially trained nurse can teach the patient relaxation techniques. A relaxation tape is often the easiest way for patients to continue this therapy independently.

FATIGUE, PACING AND PLANNING

Another common problem particularly associated with rheumatoid arthritis and fibromyalgia is fatigue (Chapter 9). The occupational therapist can teach the patient energy conservation techniques so that patients learn to pace themselves throughout the day (Sandle, 1990). For patients who have fibromyalgia, pacing is essential because they can be left debilitated for days if they overexert themselves. It is important for the patient to understand the effect of fatigue on their physical and psychological functioning so they will understand the factors that contribute to their fatigue. The patient needs to appreciate their role in pacing and planning their daily activities, using energy conservation and allowing time for relaxation (RCN, 2001).

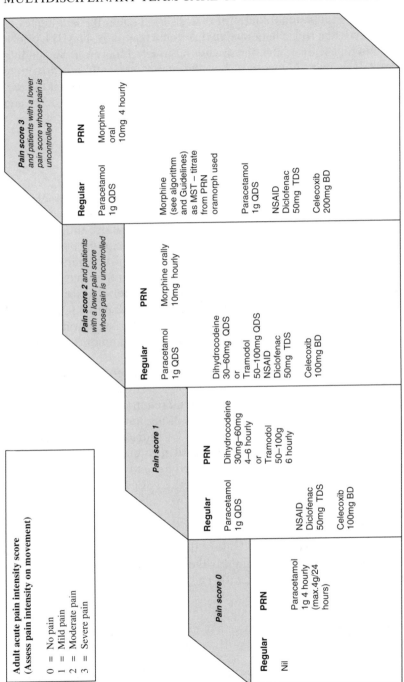

Adult acute pain intensity score
(Assess pain intensity on movement)

0 = No pain
1 = Mild pain
2 = Moderate pain
3 = Severe pain

Pain score 0

Regular
Nil

PRN
Paracetamol
1g 4 hourly
(max.4g/24
hours)

Pain score 1

Regular
Paracetamol
1g QDS

NSAID
Diclofenac
50mg TDS

Celecoxib
100mg BD

PRN
Dihydrocodeine
30mg–60mg
4–6 hourly
or
Tramodol
50–100g
6 hourly

Pain score 2 *and patients
with a lower pain score
whose pain is uncontrolled*

Regular
Paracetamol
1g QDS

Dihydrocodeine
30–60mg QDS
or
Tramodol
50–100mg QDS
NSAID
Diclofenac
50mg TDS

Celecoxib
100mg BD

PRN
Morphine orally
10mg hourly

Pain score 3
*and patients with a lower
pain score whose pain is
uncontrolled*

Regular
Paracetamol
1g QDS

Morphine
(see algorithm
and Guidelines)
as MST – titrate
from PRN
oramorph used

Paracetamol
1g QDS

NSAID
Diclofenac
50mg TDS

Celecoxib
200mg BD

PRN
Morphine
oral
10mg 4 hourly

Figure 11.1 Acute pain analgesic ladder for adult patients *(Adapted with permission from the Leeds Teaching Hospitals Pain Management Service)*.

Although the occupational therapist teaches the patient the techniques of pacing and planning and relaxation, energy conservation is an MDT effort. The physiotherapist prescribes therapeutic exercises tailored to suit individual patients (Helewa, 1996), as preserving muscle strength and providing cardiovascular conditioning can all assist the patient to cope with their fatigue. The nurse's role is to reinforce the importance of energy conservation and exercise and provide any additional information and support.

STIFFNESS

Stiffness which does not allow joints to travel through their full range of movement, or greatly reduces the extent to which movement is possible, can be a major disabling experience for patients with rheumatological conditions (RCN, 2001). Stiffness can also make it very painful to move the joints, and so adequate analgesia is required to enable patients to continue performing activities of daily living. As with pain, the physiotherapist or nurse may use hot or cold packs to relieve joint stiffness. The physiotherapist may also apply warm, melted paraffin wax to the patient's hands to relieve early morning stiffness (Helewa, 1996). This is often followed immediately by a series of hand exercises that can significantly improve the range of movement. This can produce positive psychological effects as pain and spasm are reduced (Smruti Riley, 1998).

The length of early-morning stiffness can be a helpful guide as to the extent of a patient's disease activity. When activity is low it can last for a few minutes, when activity is high it can last for many hours. Treatments may take the form of analgesics, nonsteroidal anti-inflammatory drugs, hot baths or showers and frequent changes of position (Arthur, 1998). The nurse needs to educate the patient on how and why the early morning stiffness occurs, so that they can take appropriate steps to relieve their symptoms and take control of their disease.

JOINT PROTECTION

Joint protection is often considered one of the main roles of the occupational therapist. Splinting of joints, particularly the hands and wrists, fall into three categories:

- resting
- functional
- correctional (Sandle, 1990).

The main objectives of using splints are to relieve pain, prevent development of contracture whilst supporting unstable structures, and also to protect from further damage. A commonly used wrist splints are shown in Figure 11.2.

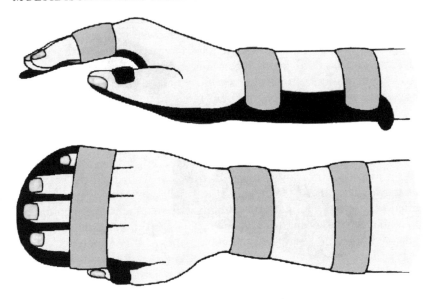

Figure 11.2 Resting splints.

The nursing role is to understand the principles of joint protection and to ensure that the patient appreciates the importance of their correct use.

The physiotherapist uses individualised exercise programmes to maintain the function of splinted joints. The exercises prescribed are intended to ensure that the body's own healing process does not become a source of difficulty through scarring, contractures or degenerative changes (Helewa, 1996).

Foot function and its protection is the domain of the podiatrist. Their aim is not only to check for callosities, hard skin and corns, but to establish the causes of abnormal foot function. The podiatrist can examine the patient's gait by investigating the biomechanical function of the feet. When a problem is diagnosed, the aim is to realign the foot with orthosis worn in the shoes (Figure 11.3). These supportive insoles help relieve pain by dissipating stresses and cushioning the forefoot and rear foot (Widdows, 1998). It is important to ensure the patient's footwear can accommodate insoles and/or foot deformities adequately. This may necessitate the involvement of the orthotist who can provide extra depth/width or custom-made foot wear.

EXERCISE

Muscle wasting is a common feature of patients with rheumatoid arthritis. This muscle atrophy is in part caused by disease process and part by disuse. Movement loss and immobility may also lead to fixed contractures. The aim

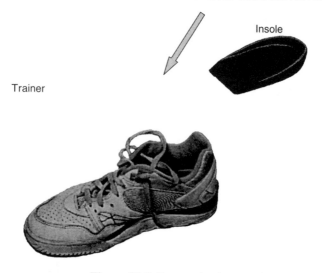

Insole

Trainer

Figure 11.3 Foot orthosis.

of exercise is to improve motor function, principally muscle strength, by repetitive muscle overloading. Dynamic exercise programmes for rheumatology patients were once thought to be harmful, exacerbating pain and disease activity. However, they are now believed to improve both physiological variables such as muscle strength, endurance and function, and psychological state in the form of self-efficacy and well-being (Hurley *et al.*, 2002). Therapeutic exercise for patients with rheumatological conditions serves many purposes, specifically it:

- preserves motion or restores lost motion
- increases muscle strength and endurance
- provides cardiovascular conditioning
- increases bone density
- enhances feelings of well-being
- provides active recreation (Helewa, 1996).

The physiotherapist can advise the patient on how to balance rest periods with exercise programmes in order to improve their physical well-being, particularly during a flare of their disease. They may also prescribe hydrotherapy as the buoyancy of the water reduces the effect of gravity and thus the loading on the joints. The warm water temperature also helps to relieve pain and so makes exercising easier. The nurse needs to be aware of the physical and psychological benefits of regular exercise. S/he is in an excellent position to encourage the patient to follow exercise programmes prescribed by the physiotherapist. S/he can also liaise with the physiotherapist and discuss any problems the patient may be experiencing, so ensuring patient adherence to their programmes.

COMPLEMENTARY MEDICINES

Complementary medicines and therapies are gaining popularity and finding a more substantive place in health care. It is important that the nurse ensures that the introduction of these therapies is always in the best interest of the patient (NMC, 1995), and before recommending any complementary therapy/ medicine must ensure they are working within the Nursing & Midwifery Council Code of Professional Conduct (NMC, 2002). Patients should not be encouraged to seek illusory cures or miracles through complementary therapies. Loss of independence can be extremely demoralising and can make people vulnerable (Lynn, 1996). However, patients need to accept their illness and be encouraged to discuss their thoughts and ideas with medical and nursing staff. This will allow for an objective and informed discussion to take place before patients invest their hopes and money in complementary therapies.

Some therapies are regularly offered within the National Health Service and these are usually accessed through the physiotherapist or occupational therapist. They include:

- acupuncture – fine needles inserted into selected points beneath the skin to relieve pain or induce analgesia;
- Alexander technique – development of awareness of balance, movement and posture;
- massage – treatment involving manipulation of soft tissue;
- Pilates – increasing strength, flexibility and body awareness (Robinson et al., 2001);
- meditation/relaxation – promoting self-control and reducing anxiety and tension (Hewitt, 1982).

Two alternative medications that rheumatology patients often wish to discuss are cod-liver oil capsules and glucosamine. Cod-liver oil is marketed as being able to relieve joint pains and helping to maintain a healthy body. Recent research conducted in Wales has suggested that cod-liver oil capsules can delay the onset of osteoarthritis (Arthritis Today, 2004). The same piece of research also showed a marked reduction in some of the enzymes that cause joint pain.

Glucosamine is widely available at health food shops and pharmacies where it is sold to relieve the pain of osteoarthritis, particularly in the large joints such as the hips and knees. The manufacturers suggest that by taking this supplement patients will assist the natural smooth working of the joints and help maintain connective tissue, and there is some evidence as to its effectiveness (Reginster et al., 2001). The pharmacist should be on hand to assist the patient in their decision making. For instance they will be able to advise of any interactions between the complementary medicines and the medicines prescribed by the doctor.

MEDICATION

The rheumatology nurse plays a central role in the education of patients; this includes information about their medications. The better informed the patient is about their drugs, the mode of action and potential side effects that may be experienced, the better their adherence (Byrne, 1999). A well-informed patient is able to weigh up the advantages of a drug against the potential side effects, enabling them to be an active participant, rather than a passive recipient, of care.

The nurse requires an in-depth understanding of drug therapies and their mode of action in order to inform the patient adequately. The drugs used to treat rheumatology patients can be categorised as:

• analgesics
• nonsteroidal anti-inflammatory drugs (NSAIDs)
• steroids
• disease-modifying antirheumatic drugs (DMARDs)

The chronicity of rheumatic diseases facilitates the development of a therapeutic relationship between the rheumatology nurse and his/her patient. This relationship places the nurse in an ideal position to act as the patient's advocate. Having cared for the patient over many months or years, the nurse should know the patient's past drug history and any side effects intimately. The nurse is therefore in a prime position to assist the medical staff when reviewing the patients' medications.

The pharmacist can provide the team with information on drug therapies and interactions and can also play a central role in ensuring the patient's adherence. Pharmacists are also involved in providing the patient with:

• information about their drugs;
• advice on how to take the medication;
• availability of the drugs to the patient on/after discharge from hospital.

Drug monitoring is an important aspect of rheumatology patient care. The rheumatology nurse plays a central role in ensuring that the patient remains well whilst taking their medications. The DMARDs taken can affect liver and renal function as well as suppress the immune system, causing a drop in numbers of white and red blood cells, whilst steroids can reduce white cell production and cause glucose intolerance, osteoporosis, peptic ulceration and atherosclerosis.

The nurse should make sure that patients have regular blood tests and that results are monitored. Haematological results together with knowledge about the patient's physical well-being are fed back to the doctor so medications can be reviewed appropriately. For further information regarding drug therapy and monitoring see Chapter 4.

SLEEP

Lack of sleep or disturbed sleep can have a negative impact on quality of life (Vennelle, 2000). The most common sleep complaint in rheumatology patients is insomnia, defined as the inability to sleep or to remain asleep throughout the night. The role of the nurse is to look at the causes of the patient's insomnia and aim to work together with the patient in order to resolve them. Underlying causes may include:

- pain
- depression
- stress
- uncomfortable positioning.

The nurse can educate the patient to improve their chances of getting a good night's sleep. This can include advice on:

- regular bed times;
- appropriately timed exercise;
- avoidance of alcohol and caffeine prior to retiring;
- ensuring the environment and bed is comfortable (Vennelle, 2000).

Positioning of joints during sleep and the use of resting splints, provided by the occupational therapist, may help to prevent pain and discomfort through the night.

The occupational therapist can teach relaxation techniques, which can be useful in decreasing stress and anxiety prior to sleep.

The nurse can advise the patient about taking adequate analgesia prior to retiring as this can ensure that pain does not prevent sleep or cause the patient to wake prematurely.

If the patient is depressed this may be linked to uncontrolled pain or stress about their illness/disability. These problems need to be addressed. The patient may benefit from being given the time to express their fears and anxieties, but the nurse must also recognise when help from other disciplines is required. The psychiatric team may need to be involved in order to help the patient cope with their depression.

The prescription of night sedation may be necessary, this can be discussed with the patient, the pharmacist and the doctor.

SELF-CARE ABILITIES

It is important that the patient maintains their maximum potential independence, and this can be aided by meticulous assessment in the following areas.

HYGIENE AND SKIN CARE

The rheumatology nurse needs to be aware that high standards of personal hygiene are very important for all patients. The rheumatology patient is particularly vulnerable because disease activity together with the side effects of drug therapies can make them susceptible to infections. When the nurse is assessing the patient, s/he needs to discuss each individual's personal hygiene requirements. The occupational therapist can address any problems with washing and dressing by supplying aids and adaptations that can assist independence. The nurse will need to assist the patient with any problems that cannot be solved in this way. For example the patient may be unable to wash and brush their hair because of decreased movement in the shoulders. Before discharge from hospital, dependence will need assessing and any shortfalls will need to be arranged in the community.

Observation of skin integrity of the rheumatology patient is also important. This is not just to maintain a positive body image, but to observe for areas of vasculitis that may develop (RCN, 2001). If skin breakdown does occur healing may be delayed, causing the patient increased pain and discomfort. The nurse can use the time spent assisting patients with hygiene and dressing to observe the skin and teach the patient what to look for. Patients should also be taught the importance of reporting any skin lesions as soon as they occur.

Mouth care is an essential aspect of care for rheumatology patients. Disease activity, side effects from medications and the dry mouth associated with Sjögren's syndrome can cause mouth ulcers which are not only painful and cause problems with eating, but are a potential site for infection (White, 2000). The role of the nurse is to teach the patient the importance of good oral hygiene and ensure mouth ulcers/sores are treated promptly (Rawlins, 2001). The patient needs to be aware that regular visits to their dentist are recommended so early detection of tooth erosions and potential sites for infection can be dealt with promptly.

Foot hygiene is also an important aspect of nursing care. The rheumatic patient is unfortunately prone to a high incidence of foot problems, and the podiatrist and orthotist will undoubtedly need to be involved in their care. The main objective for the whole team will be to keep the foot free from sores, and to detect calluses and deformities early. This way pain and discomfort can be kept to a minimum and the independence and mobility of the patient can be maintained.

DRESSING

The ability to be suitably groomed is essential in maintaining the patient's dignity and self-esteem. The ability to dress is only part of the equation of looking well-groomed. The nurse and the occupational therapist need to work together to identify where the patient may need help. There may be aids and adaptations that the occupational therapist can provide for the patient which will make dressing easier, for instance a reacher/grabber or shoe horn. Changing the routine of dressing may be necessary to make the task easier. For instance, sitting down to dress the lower half of the body and putting tops on without having to lift the arms over the head. The nurse needs to be aware of what the patient is being taught, so s/he can reinforce these methods in the patient's daily routines.

The maintenance of clothes should also be addressed when assessing the patient's ability to self-care. If patients cannot wash and iron their clothes then they may not be able to achieve their own personal standards, and this could be detrimental to their self-esteem. The assessment process undertaken by the occupational therapist should highlight areas where the patient needs assistance (Sandle, 1990). The occupational therapist can offer help by suggesting energy saving ways of caring for clothes, like sitting down to iron, or having the washing machine raised off the ground so the patient does not have to bend down. If the patient still remains unable to suitably care for their clothes, a referral to the medical social worker will need to be made so that help in the community can be arranged.

NUTRITION

The nutritional assessment of patients should go beyond their nutritional requirements and include their:

- ability to prepare the food
- desire to eat the food
- ability to eat independently
- ability to swallow.

In order to promote independence, quality of life and a healthy individual, the patient may need help in one or all of these areas (Eberhardie, 2004). The team approach to nutrition may include the occupational therapist, who will assess the patient's ability to prepare the food and discuss their needs in eating the food. They may offer aids and adaptations, but will also discuss labour-saving devises and tips. The dietician will look not only at the nutritional needs of the patient and offer supplements or alternate diets, but will also look at ability to swallow and offer tips on which foods are best suited to the patient's individual needs. The nurse can assist the patient to eat the food by:

- reinforcing information on how to use aids provided;
- ensuring diets provided are manageable;
- offering advice on fluid intake;
- offering advice about swallowing;
- liaise with the other disciplines to discuss any further needs of the patient.

If the patient still does not desire to eat, other sources of depressed appetite should be investigated, such as their medications. The pharmacist can offer advice on which medicines are likely to be causing the problem and this can then be discussed with the doctor. Alternative medication can often be tried in order to attempt to regain the patient's appetite. Encouraging the patient to maintain/regain good nutrition promotes a sense of well-being, reduces the risk of infections, and helps prevent osteoporosis and cardiac disease (Eberhardie, 2004).

ELIMINATION

When assessing the patient the nurse should establish their normal elimination routines, so that any changes to regular habits will be noticed early and can then be discussed and investigated. The most common problems are frequency/urgency of micturition and constipation.

Urinary problems

Urinary frequency/urgency is often caused by an infection. The rheumatology patient is susceptible to urinary infection due to immobility and the side effects of immunosuppressive drugs. The nurse should undertake a routine urinalysis to establish if there are signs of infection. If positive, a urine sample can be sent to the laboratory for culture and sensitivity. If an infection is diagnosed the doctor will prescribe a suitable antibiotic, and the nurse should also educate the patient regarding the importance of an adequate fluid intake.

Routine urinalysis can also detect protein in the urine. This can be an indication of infection but it can also signal renal problems which may be related to disease activity or drug toxicity. The doctor needs to be informed of results of regular urinalysis, whether positive or negative.

Constipation

Constipation can often be a side effect of analgesia. The nurse should encourage the patient to take a high-fibre diet and a good fluid intake in order to try and maintain regular bowel habits (McCaffery and Beebe, 1997). Regular exercise can also help maintain regular peristalsis, but this is often difficult for rheumatology patients. The doctor may need to prescribe regular laxatives to keep the faeces soft as well as encourage peristalsis of the intestines. Constipation needs to be avoided rather than treated once it occurs. If not controlled constipation can become as problematic as the patient's pain.

MOBILITY

Restricted mobility can cause a number of problems for the rheumatology patient including:

* breakdown of the skin – often caused by steroid therapy which causes delicate skin that tears or bruises easily (Cox, 1999);
* problems with manual handling (If patients are confined to bed because of a flare they can become reliant on staff to assist with changes of position.);
* generalised restricted joint movement caused by fatigue and general malaise (Patients can quickly lose muscle strength and joint mobility.);
* deep vein thrombosis;
* pulmonary embolism;
* chest infection;
* elimination problems.

The last four problems can develop in any bed-bound patient.

Intervention by the multidisciplinary team should be to maximise mobility and stabilise joints (RCN, 2001). The nurse needs to be aware of the causes and effects that disease activity can have on the patient's mobility, and also that mobility levels can alter throughout the day. S/he needs to assess the patient and plan care so that early morning stiffness and timing of pain relief coincide with self-care activities and exercise programmes.

The podiatrist and orthotist may need to asses the patient's feet, as biomechanical assessment of the feet can establish any correctable problems that are interfering with the patient's gait and mobility. The podiatrist can perform minor procedures on the feet to reduce pain from calluses and sores as well as ensuring nail care is maintained. The provision of padding and insoles to cushion the feet during mobility may also be necessary. The orthotist can assess the patient's footwear and provide extra width or custom-made shoes in order to accommodate foot deformities (Widdows, 1998).

Manual handling

The problems associated with manual handling are in relation to protection of all joints. Joint disease of the upper limbs can make it almost impossible for the patient to change position in bed, and the use of a monkey pole should be discouraged due to the risk of further damage (Cox, 1999). The nurse needs to ensure that a full assessment of the patient's manual handling needs are carried out and that the use of moving and handling equipment, appropriate to individual patient needs, are included in their plan of care. It is important to remember that long-term damage can be inflicted upon the nurse if s/he is exposed to repeatedly lifting and manually assisting the patient. Nurses have a duty to ensure that moving and handling equipment is used whenever appropriate (Mutch, 2004).

Walking aids and splints

The physiotherapist can assess the patient for the use of walking aids to reduce lower limb loading during mobilisation, and so relieve pain and improve mobility (Hurley *et al.*, 2002). In order to prevent increased pain and joint damage of the upper limbs, the use of specially designed walking aids such as fisher sticks (Figure 11.4) or gutter frames may be used. These aids redistribute the weight-bearing load on damaged joints.

Splints that provide joint support during self-care activities and mobilisation can be provided by the occupational therapist. S/he can also ensure that the patient will be safe when mobilising in their own home when climbing steps and stairs, accessing their property and driving (Sandle, 1990). When appropriate the occupational therapist may also assess the patient for the use

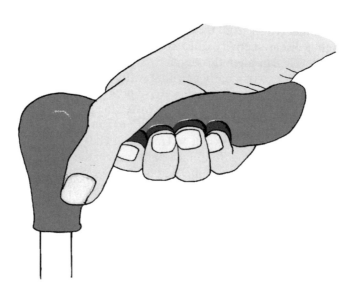

Figure 11.4 Fisher stick (Reproduced by kind permission from Geoff Hill [2000] *Rheumatology – A Handbook for Community Nurses.*)

of a wheel chair; this may be an assisted chair that someone else will propel, or an electric chair that the patient operates.

If the patient is unable to use public transport, the medical social worker can provide advice on claiming mobility allowance that will enable them to get out and about.

PSYCHOLOGICAL STATE

Chronic rheumatic conditions can have a profound impact on a person's psychological well-being (RCN, 2001). It is the role of the nurse to:

- encourage a therapeutic relationship
- enable patients to discuss their problems
- plan appropriate care
- encourage the patient to become an active participant in their care (Ryan, 1999).

Le Gallez (1993) has stated that living with a painful and disabling chronic illness can lead to a change in personality. The nurse can help the patient to adapt to their illness and come to terms with any changing personal relationships that they may experience. Once diagnosed, patients may go through stages similar to those of grieving, experiencing emotions such as shock, anger, grief and depression. By providing support and engaging the patient in education about their illness and treatments, the nurse can help to alleviate some of these anxieties (Ryan, 1998). An empowered patient who is able to take control of life is less likely to suffer from anxiety.

Depression is common place, particularly in rheumatoid arthritis (Chapter 5) and the nurse needs to be able to recognise the symptoms. They may include:

- loss of interest in life
- lack of motivation
- fatigue
- agitation and restlessness
- lost or increased appetite
- sleeplessness or excessive sleeping.

If the patient appears to be depressed this needs to be discussed with the medical staff who may prescribe an antidepressant or referral to the psychiatric team (Ryan, 1999).

If the depression is pain-related, this needs to be addressed. Reduction of pain will enable the patient to remain independent and this will help to maintain a feeling of well-being, and so help to alleviate depression.

The patient's family and friends may also be affected, and giving them support can help with their adjustment to living with a relative who has been diagnosed with a chronic illness (Le Gallez, 1993). Self-help groups and organisations can be particularly helpful to patients and their relatives, as they are receiving support from others with similar experiences.

BODY IMAGE AND SEXUALITY

Physical symptoms, caused by chronic, rheumatological illness and side effects from medications can profoundly influence attractiveness, resulting in a distorted body image and loss of self-esteem (Muir, 2000). Altered body image can have a devastating effect on self-esteem and personal attitude (Kibble, 2001).

Positive attitudes and realistic goal setting can help patients develop strategies for living with their arthritis. Helping patients to find areas and hobbies in their life in which they can succeed helps to support positive thinking (Leino-Kilpi et al., 1999). The nurse should offer constructive coping strategies for each individual problem. This may include:

- timing of activities
- balancing rest and activity
- use of hot baths/showers to ease joint stiffness.

Discussion with the patient about their appearance and dress sense, body image and feelings of sexual attractiveness and cultural differences related to sexuality and coping, can help the nurse to build up an accurate picture of the patient's feelings and expectations. This can then be used to develop a manageable plan of individualised care to assist the patient to address their personal needs (Malek and Brower, 1984).

Sexuality

Research reveals that patients with rheumatic disease do experience sexual problems (Hill et al., 2003; Hill, 2004), and nurses have not been proactive in assessing this area of care. It takes a good deal of courage for the patient to reveal their sexual problems and it is important that the nurse needs to be nonjudgemental and open-minded whilst listening to them. Being able to talk about their problems and share their emotions may be all the patient needs in order to understand their own feelings (Irwin, 2000).

The patient may require practical advice in order to achieve comfortable sexual intercourse. The nurses can advise the patient to:

- practise relaxation techniques to promote comfort;
- take a warm bath or shower before intercourse;
- rest after completion of bathing and grooming activities;
- position pillows under affected, painful limbs for support;

- schedule analgesia to be taken prior to intercourse if possible;
- explore alternative ways of sexual expression.

It is important that the nurse establishes whether the patient prefers to discuss their problems with or without their partner being present. Also the nurse should bear in mind that some partners may be overprotecting their spouse for fear of hurting them, and this can create an additional strain on the relationship (Malek and Brower, 1984). By broaching the subject of sexuality, the nurse is demonstrating that it is alright to discuss these problems. The nurse can reassure them that their feelings and responses are normal and that they can continue/resume a healthy physical relationship with their partner. The occupational therapist may be involved in addressing some of the physical self-help advice for patients.

ENVIRONMENT AND SOCIAL

Rheumatic diseases have the ability to affect all aspects of a patient's life including their working and social lives and consequently their finances. These areas are important elements of the holistic nursing assessment, and problem solving will necessitate the inclusion of other members of the MDT.

OCCUPATION

Keeping patients in employment should be a high priority in their care management. Unemployment will affect the patient's self-perception, role alteration and family finance (Ryan, 1999). Forty-two percent of people diagnosed with rheumatoid arthritis will cease working within one year of the onset of symptoms (Kibble, 2001). Given that the common time of onset of some rheumatic diseases is in the patient's 3rd and 4th decade of life, the ensuing boredom and sense of uselessness may affect the patient for many years. Nurses must be proactive, providing guidance and support for the family, but also ensuring that the patient has access to relevant support agencies. The occupational therapist can assist with work based assessments, suggesting adaptations to the workplace such as specialist seating, positioning of workstations, wrist supports and splints that may enable the patient to continue working. If the patient's occupation is detrimental to their disease, the disability employment advisor could recommend alternative employment utilising transferable skills or suggesting further training opportunities. If the patient would benefit by working reduced hours, the medical social worker may suggest the patient claims the disabled person's tax credit, or other benefits to which they may be entitled, to enable the patient to stop working altogether without putting financial strain on their family.

TRANSPORT

Access to suitable transport is important for maintaining independence, preventing social isolation or enabling patients to get to work (RCN, 2001). The occupational therapist can provide appropriate advice to facilitate safe driving, like advising individuals on the use of mirrors in cars if head or neck movements are difficult. The orange badge parking scheme allows people with walking difficulties to park nearer to shops and public buildings. Occupational therapists can refer patients to their local mobility centre where they can get advice on obtaining wheelchairs and scooters. Public transport is often difficult to use and alternatives are expensive. However, the medical social workers can advise patients about benefit agencies and the nurse can assist the patient to assess their own problems and work out solutions to resolve them. For example, if travelling causes an increase in pain the nurse can advise prophylactic analgesia be taken prior to the journey. The use of splints will reduce strain and pain in the hands and wrists whilst driving, and sharing the driving with a partner on long journeys, or stopping frequently to allow for movement of joints will help.

HOUSING

The main aim of the MDT in this context is to help the patient to maintain independent living in his or her own home. However, the house may need to be assessed to ensure it is a safe environment. The joint stiffness, pain and immobility associated with rheumatological conditions, together with general lethargy and fatigue can mean that individuals quickly find it difficult to mobilise around their own homes. Stairs and steps can create a particular hazard. The occupational therapist plays a vital role in assessing the patient's ability to manage simple tasks of independent living in the kitchen and bathroom. They can provide advice on:

- adaptations to the fabric of the home
- labour saving devices
- aids to independence
- links to other agencies that can provide equipment.

The physiotherapist can assist the patient at home by ensuring safe transfers between furniture and negotiation of stairs. The medical social worker can advise the patients about available grants from the local social services department to assist patients with the cost of home adaptations such as alterations to the bathroom, or the purchase of a stair lift. In some severe cases, patients may need to accept help from a home care agency. This may be in the form of meeting hygiene needs and/or assistance to prepare meals. The nurse may have to spend time listening to the patient to allow them to express their fears and anxieties about their changing life and help them to understand why the care is needed.

SOCIAL AND FAMILY SUPPORT

The impact of a severe chronic rheumatic illness raises psychological and social issues for the patient, their family and friends. The traditional roles to which people conform often have to change as a result of illness. Families will need support to accept this and learn to live together as a cohesive unit. Family units may be affected in one of four ways:

- brought closer together
- minimal role alteration
- minimal changes in responsibility
- negative effect on relationships within the family.

The individual responsibilities held within the family before the onset of illness may no longer be physically possible. For instance the patient may not be able to undertake gardening, cleaning, cooking and laundry (Ryan, 1999). The family needs educating about the patient's illness and treatments and this can help them to more fully understand the patient and their care needs. This knowledge will help them to provide support without taking control and demeaning the recipient. Although the nurse plays a vital role in this area, she also needs to be aware of appropriate agencies where patients can receive guidance and support. One such organisation would be support groups (White, 1998). There are many locally held support groups for individuals with rheumatological illnesses, and the nurse should be able to advise the patient on how to access them. Attending such group sessions can prevent social isolation, as well as providing contact with others who have the same, or similar illnesses. Often, members share stories and coping mechanism which help each other in their adaptation to new life styles (Tadman, 2004). Another means of support for patients would be through an expert patients programme which would complement the professional care patients receive. These agencies use the patient's perception as a starting point and examine how illness is affecting their daily life. They assist patients to take control of their life and condition rather than allowing themselves to be defined by it (Thomas, 2004).

One area that is sometimes overlooked is the patient's spiritual needs. Spirituality is a component of well-being, based on values of commitment, love and affection. This well-being is experienced through a sense of belonging, acceptance, respect and inner peace (Kissane, 2004). Ensuring a holistic approach to care and making sure patients have the opportunity to air their concerns and identify intervention areas to nurses, can only improve the care received (Edwards, 2001). Referring individuals to the appropriate chaplaincy service can help with specific needs and desires, thus bringing comfort, hope and meaning.

FINANCIAL

The disability caused by chronic illness can often lead to a loss of earnings. Unfortunately, this decrease in finances comes when increased expenditure is required for medications, extra heating, use of convenience foods, adaptations to the home and appliances to aid independent living (RCN, 2001). Some patients find discussions about finances difficult, but the nurse must ensure the patient has the relevant information and if necessary refer to the appropriate team members and agencies. The social worker is available to discuss relevant statutory benefits with patients and their carers. These include:

- statutory sick pay
- incapacity benefit
- severe disablement allowance
- disability living allowance
- disability working allowance
- invalid care allowance
- income support
- housing benefit.

By addressing the patient's financial needs the nurse is ensuring that neither the patient nor their family are exposed to an increase in the stress which could lead to a lifestyle that is not compatible with illness.

LEISURE

Pain and fatigue often stop patients going out with their partners and families. The nurse needs to persuade patients to continue to socialise with their spouse and stress that they need to consider their partner's needs as well as their own (Le Gallez, 1998). Prioritising activities and preserving energy will help patients to enjoy their leisure time. The occupational therapist may be able to offer advice on aids and adaptations, so individuals can continue to pursue their chosen hobby. The patient may need help or encouragement to find a new hobby or different pastime if they are no longer able to carry on with their usual one. Self-help groups may have information on suitable interest groups, and being part of a group and its related activities may be a first step to pursuing leisure activities and becoming socially active again.

This chapter demonstrates the pivotal role that the nurse plays within the MDT, and highlights the breadth of experience required by rheumatology nurses to facilitate the best package of care for their patients. It also emphasises the multitude of problems that the patient with a rheumatic disease faces and the challenges these problems pose to the MDT. Each member of the team has a unique role to play, but good team communication and an understanding of the role of each health professional is crucial for timely and effective care.

ACTION POINTS FOR PRACTICE

- Think about the ways that you work as an MDT in your own environment and then list ways that you could improve team working.
- Describe a holistic approach to assessment and care of a patient, remembering that many problems and needs overlap.
- A 60-year-old married female has severe, unremitting RA. Outline the roles, responsibilities and boundaries of the different members of the MDT.
- Discuss the role and the responsibilities of the patient and carer as a member of the MDT.

REFERENCES

Abraham A (2004) Lack of communication affects the care of patients and families. *Professional Nurse* 19(6):351–353.
Arthritis Today (2004) Cod-liver oil shown to be effective in slowing down joint destruction. Chesterfield, Arthritis Research Campaign, April:124–125.
Arthur V (1998) The role of the nurse specialist in rheumatology. In: Le Gallez (ed) *Rheumatology for Nurses: Patient Care*. London, Whurr Publishers Ltd, 12–45.
Baldwin MA (2003) Patient advocacy: a concept analysis. *Nursing Standard* 5(17)21:33–39.
Byrne J (1999) Rheumatology part 2: the role of medication. *Professional Nurse* 14(5):355–358.
Carroll D, Seers K (1998) Relaxation for the relief of chronic pain: a systemic review. *Journal of Advanced Nursing* 27(3):476–487.
Carson M, Williams T, Everett A *et al.* (1997) The nurse's role in the multidisciplinary team. *European Journal of Palliative Care* 4(3):96–98.
Cox M (1999) Rheumatology part 3: the role of surgery. *Professional Nurse* 14(6):427–430.
Davis RM, Wagner EG, Groves T (2000) Advances in managing chronic disease. Research, performance measurement, and quality improvement are key. *British Medical Journal* 320:525–526.

Eberhardie C (2004) Assessment and management of eating skills in the older adult. *Professional Nurse* 19(6):318–322.

Edwards M (2001) Improving psychosocial assessment in oncology. *Professional Nurse* 16(7):1223–1226.

Fox E (2000) An audit of inter–professional communication within a trauma and orthopaedic directorate. *Journal of Orthopaedic Nursing* 4:160–169.

Hawkey B, Williams J (2001) Rehabilitation: the nurse's role. *Journal of Orthopaedic Nursing* 5:81–88.

Helewa A (1996) Physical therapy management of patients with rheumatoid arthritis and other inflammatory conditions. In: Walker J, Helewa A (ed) *Physical Therapy in Arthritis*. London: W.B. Saunders.

Hewitt J (1982) *Relaxation East and West*. Essex: Anchor Press Ltd.

Hill J (2004) The impact of rheumatoid arthritis on patients' sex lives. *Nursing Times* 100(20):34–35.

Hill J (2003) An overview of education for patients with rheumatic diseases. *Nursing Times* 99(19):26–27.

Hill J (1997) A practical guide to information giving. In: Woolfe AD, Van Riel PLCM (eds) Early Rheumatoid Arthritis. *Baillière's Clinical Rheumatology* 11(1): 109–127.

Hill J, Hale C (2004) Clinical skills: evidence-based nursing care of people with rheumatoid arthritis. *British Journal of Nursing* 13(14):852–857.

Hill J, Bird H, Thorpe R (2003) Effects of rheumatoid arthritis on sexual activity and relationships. *Rheumatology* 42:280–286.

Hill J, Reay N (2002) The diagnosis, assessment and management of complex rheumatic disease. *Nursing Times* 98(9):41–44.

Hurley M, Dziedzic K, Bearne L et al. (2002) *The Clinical and Cost Effectiveness of Physiotherapy in the Management of Elderly People with Common Rheumatological Conditions*. London, Chartered Society of Physiotherapy.

Irwin R (2000) Treatments for patients with sexual problems. *Professional Nurse* 15(6):360–364.

Kaplan KH, Goldenberg DL, Galuin-Nadeau M (1993) The impact of meditation based stress reduction programme on fibromyalgia. *General Hospital Psychiatry* 15(5):284–289.

Kibble K (2001) Rheumatoid arthritis – support beyond the medical diagnosis. *Primary Health Care* 11(5):27–32.

Kissane C (2004) Spiritual nursing care of older adults. *Nurse 2 Nurse Magazine* 4(4):29–32.

Le Gallez P (1993) Rheumatoid arthritis: effects on the family. *Nursing Standard* 7(39):30–34.

Le Gallez P (1998) Patient education and self-management. In: Le Gallez P (ed), *Rheumatology for Nurses: Patient Care*. London, Whurr Publishers Ltd, 98–142.

Leino-Kilpi H, Maenpaa I, Katajisto J (1999) Nursing study of the significance of rheumatoid arthritis as perceived by patients using the concept of empowerment. *Journal of Orthopaedic Nursing* 3:138–145.

Lynn J (1996) The rising popularity of complementary therapies. *Professional Nurse* 11(4):266–268.

Malek C, Brower S (1984) Rheumatoid arthritis: how does it influence sexuality? *Rehabilitation Nursing* Nov–Dec, 26–28.

McCaffery M, Beebe A (1997) *Pain, Clinical Manual for Nursing Practice*. London: Mosby Press.

McGee P, Ashford R (1996) Nurse's perceptions of roles in multidisciplinary teams. *Nursing Standard* 10(45):34–36.

Melzack R, Wall P (1996) *The Challenge of Pain*. Middlesex: Penguin Books.

Muir A (2000) Counselling patients who have sexual difficulties. *Professional Nurse* 15(11):723–726.

Mutch K (2004) Changing manual-handling practice in a stroke rehabilitation unit. *Professional Nurse* 19(7):374–378.

NMC (2002) *Code of Professional Conduct*. London, Nursing and Midwifery Council.

NMC (1995) *Complementary Therapies, Position Statement*. London, Nursing and Midwifery Council.

Rawlins C (2001) Effective mouth care for seriously ill patients. *Professional Nurse* 16(4):1025–1028.

RCN (2001) *Standards for effective practice and audit in rheumatology nursing*. London, Royal College of Nursing.

Reginster JY, Deroisy R, Rovalti .lC et al. (2001) Long-term progression of glucosamine sulphate on osteoarthritis progression: a randomised, placebo-controlled trial. *Lancet* 357:251–356.

Robinson L, Fisher H, Knox J et al. (2001) *The Official Body Control Pilates Manual*. St Helens: The Book People.

Ryan S (1998) The essence of rheumatology nursing. *Nursing Standard* 13:13–15, 52–54.

Ryan S (1999) Rheumatology part 4: psychosocial issues. *Professional Nurse* 14(7):509–512.

Sandle L (1990) *OT in Rheumatology – A holistic approach*. London: Chapman & Hall.

Smruti Riley H (1998) The role of physiotherapy in rheumatology. In: Le Gallez (ed), *Rheumatology for Nurses: Patient Care*. London, Whurr Publishers Ltd, 186–222.

Tadman J (2004) Vasculitis: new hope? *Arthritis Today* 124:22–23.

Thomas S (2004) The role of health professionals in supporting expert patients schemes. *Professional Nurse* 19(8):442–445.

Vennelle M (2000) Sleep disorders. *Professional Nurse* 16(3):968–971.

Widdows C (1998) The role of the podiatrist in rheumatology. In: Legallez P (ed), *Rheumatology for Nurses: Patient Care*. London, Whurr Publishers Ltd, 244–256.

White C (1998) Rheumatolgy: care in the community. In: Legallez P (ed), *Rheumatology for Nurses: Patient Care*. London, Whurr Publishers Ltd, 68–97.

White R (2000) Nurse assessment of oral health: a review of practice and education. *British Journal of Nursing* 9(5):260–266.

Zwarenstein M, Bryant W (2003) Interventions to promote collaboration between nurses and doctors (Cochrane Review) in: *The Cochrane Library 4*, 2003. Chichester: John Wiley and Sons Ltd.

12 Medications in the Rheumatic Diseases

J. WHITE
Leeds General Infirmary, West Yorkshire, UK

D. BRYER
Chapel Allerton Hospital, West Yorkshire, UK

The aim of this chapter is to provide a clear understanding of medications used in the rheumatic diseases. Many medications have potential side effects. These side effects and the monitoring required to ensure effectiveness and safety are discussed. After reading this chapter the reader should be able to:

- describe current philosophy of medication management;
- outline the actions and indications of first- and second-line therapies;
- discuss the indications and potential adverse effects of steroid therapy;
- describe the indications and administration for biologic therapies;
- outline the safety monitoring necessary for potentially toxic drug therapy.

Drug therapy plays an important role in the management of rheumatic diseases and advances in treatments such as the biologics has revolutionised the potential outcome for some patients (Scott, 2002). The philosophy to treat diseases such as rheumatoid arthritis (RA) with disease-modifying anti-rheumatic drugs (DMARDs) at a much earlier stage in the disease process has also been shown to be effective (Emery *et al.*, 2002).

Medications are commonly classified as:

- first-line therapy
- second-line therapy
- biologics.

FIRST-LINE THERAPY

ANALGESIA

Pain can impact on all aspects of a patient's life and can have a profoundly detrimental physical and psychological effect. However, pain is a subjective

Rheumatology Nursing: A Creative Approach, 2nd edn. Edited by Jackie Hill.
Copyright 2006 by John Wiley & Sons, Ltd.

phenomenon and only those experiencing it can decide what an acceptable level is. Nurses giving the patient advice about pain management must recognise this concept. To provide optimum management the nurse must also have intimate knowledge of the aetiology of pain (see Chapter 8) and understand:

* different types of analgesia
* when analgesia should be used
* how it should be used
* potential adverse reactions
* how to avoid or reduce adverse reactions.

In the rheumatic diseases, analgesics are usually used in combination with a nonsteroidal anti-inflammatory drug (NSAID) and/or DMARDs. Analgesics can be divided into two main groups nonopioid analgesics and opioid analgesics.

Nonopioid analgesics

These drugs are used for mild to moderate pain relief and include paracetamol and low-dose aspirin. Aspirin taken at doses exceeding 3.6 g daily acts as an NSAID. Conversely, NSAIDs taken as a single dose act as analgesics.

Paracetamol can be purchased over the counter in most chemists and supermarkets, and because of this some patients feel it is too mild for the type of pain they experience. However, paracetamol can be effective in the management of pain in some situations. For instance it is the drug of choice for osteoarthritis (OA) as it does not cause gastric side effects. It is also useful for patients experiencing pyrexia during an acute flare of arthritis as its antipyretic qualities can help to relieve pain. The maximum dose is 4 g in 24 hours, usually taken as 1 g four times daily. Side effects are usually mild and patients often complain of constipation. One of the most serious side effects is liver damage if overdosage occurs.

Aspirin is sometimes used in the management of mild to moderate pain and pyrexia, but can cause gastrointestinal disturbances if taken over long periods of time.

Compound analgesics

Compound analgesics combine drugs such as aspirin and paracetamol with an opioid agent. Although they can bridge the gap between nonopioid and opioid analgesia, they also have the potential to cause the side effects of both agents.

Co-codamol is a combination of paracetamol (500 mg) and codeine phosphate (8 mg or 30 mg), and the 8/500 strength is available as an over the counter product. Since the maximum dose of paracetamol is included in these tablets, patients should be advised not to take additional paracetamol.

Co-proxamol comprises a combination of 32.5 mg of dextropropoxyphene with 325 mg of paracetamol. It is widely used for the treatment of mild to moderate pain, and the maximum dose is 8 tablets in 24 hours. Again, patients should be aware that they contain paracetamol.

Opioid analgesics

This group of drugs is considered when pain is severe and the maximum dose of other types of analgesia has been ineffective. However, the use of opioids in rheumatic diseases is controversial. This is because the long-term chronic pain that is so often present, means that opioids need to be used for the long term, and this can cause dependency. Some drugs are particularly effective in the management of acute flares of arthritis, and for patients with active disease waiting for joint replacement surgery. These drugs include:

- buprenorphine
- dihydrocodeine
- fentanyl
- tramadol.

Unfortunately opioids are prone to side effects including:

- drowsiness
- dizziness
- nausea
- vomiting
- constipation
- potential dependency.

An important part of the nursing role is to provide patient education and information about medication. This is particularly salient when patients have been prescribed an opioid, because of their side effects and potential for dependency.

NSAIDS

NSAIDs are commonly used in the management of inflammatory arthritis. Their function is to reduce the symptoms caused by inflammation of the joints including:

- pain
- stiffness

- swelling
- warmth.

NSAIds work by inhibiting the production of prostaglandins. Prostaglandins are fatty acids that provoke the inflammatory response causing pain, erythema, warmth and swelling. Cyclooxygenase is the enzyme that enables arachidonic acid to be converted into prostaglandins. NSAIds prevent the action of cyclooxygenase and so reduce the production of prostaglandins. There are two forms of cyclooxygenase and these are referred to as COX 1 and COX 2. COX 1 is responsible for the prostaglandins that protect tissues. COX 2 is involved in the inflammatory process.

Although prostaglandin suppression helps to relieve inflammatory symptoms, it is also responsible for the major adverse effects of NSAIds; namely gastrointestinal disturbances and the effects on kidney function. This is because the beneficial effects of COX 1 include inhibition of gastric acid production. This helps to protect the lining of the gastrointestinal tract. Unfortunately, NSAIds that inhibit all prostaglandin production suppress the protective effects as well. This problem has led to the introduction of a new family of NSAIds, the cyclooxygenase-2 (COX 2) inhibitors such as etorocoxib and celecoxib. They work by selectively inhibiting the production of cyclooxygenase 2, thought to be responsible for the synthesis of prostanoid mediators of pain, inflammation, and fever (Pharmacia, 2004). COX-2 inhibitors are thought to be a safer than other NSAIds for patients who have experienced gastrointestinal side effects. The National Institute for Clinical Excellence has reviewed the use of COX-2 selective inhibitors and provided guidance on their use (NICE, 2002). More recently, some COX-2 inhibitors have been withdrawn because of side effects. At the time of writing rofecoxib has been withdrawn because of an increased incidence of heart attacks and strokes (Merck, 2004), and valdecoxib has also been suspended. Further information can be obtained from the Medicines and Healthcare Products Regulatory Agency (www.mhra.gov.uk).

The wide variety of NSAIds available makes it difficult for the practitioner to know which one should be prescribed. If one NSAID proves to be ineffective, another one should be tried. There can be a variation in response even when the NSAIds come from the same family. The aim is to choose a drug with the greatest efficacy and lowest toxicity.

Administration of NSAIds

NSAIds are usually taken on a regular basis in conjunction with DMARDs, depending on the disease. They work within hours or days of commencement, but a recurrence of symptoms will occur if the medication is discontinued. There are several different routes for the administration of NSAIDs:

- oral
- intramuscular
- rectal
- transdermal.

Oral compounds are often prescribed in slow-release compounds, which are particularly effective for patients who experience significant early-morning stiffness. A few NSAIDs can be administered intramuscularly including diclofenac, ketoprofen and piroxicam. Intramuscular administration is used in acute episodes where pain and inflammation relief are needed quickly. The drug should be given by a deep intramuscular injection into the gluteal muscle.

Some NSAIDs can be given rectally as suppositories. They are often prescribed to reduce the gastrointestinal side effects but they can have an adverse affect on the rectal mucosa, causing rectal bleeding. Some patients may experience difficulty inserting suppositories, due to reduced manual dexterity.

Ibuprofen, ketoprofen and piroxicam can be administered topically. Patients using this method need to understand that doses must be adhered to, as the active drug component is absorbed into the bloodstream.

Whatever the chosen administration route, patients commencing on NSAIDs should be advised to:

- report any symptoms of gastrointestinal upset to their nurse or doctor;
- never exceed the stated dose;
- when purchasing over the counter medication tell the pharmacist they are taking an NSAID;
- consult the prescriber or nurse if the drug is not helping to control their symptoms.

Additionally, those taking oral NSAIDs should always take their drug with or after food to reduce the chances of gastrointestinal side effects.

Potential side effects of NSAIDs

NSAIDs can have adverse effects on many organs in the body including the:

- gastrointestinal tract
- kidney
- liver

- respiratory system
- skin
- central nervous system
- blood.

The gastrointestinal tract

The gastrointestinal tract is most commonly affected by NSAIDs. Patients may experience a variety of symptoms including dyspepsia, nausea and vomiting and epigastric pain. There is a high risk of gastric ulceration associated with NSAIDs and patients who have experienced a previous ulcer would not routinely be prescribed an NSAID. Many patients get indigestion while taking an NSAID and they may benefit from one with a combined gastric protector such as diclofenac and misoprostol. The use of proton pump inhibitors such as lansoprazole and omeprazole in conjunction with an NSAID can also reduce the likelihood of gastrointestinal side effects. COX 2 inhibitors are also of use in patients who have experienced previous gastrointestinal disturbance.

The kidney

Renal side effects are dose-related and more likely to occur in the elderly. NSAIDs can also cause hypertension and oedema in some patients because of the potential to decrease renal blood flow. Therefore, elderly patients taking NSAIDs should have their blood pressure checked intermittently whilst on therapy. NSAIDs can also induce nephritis, nephritic syndrome and renal capillary necrosis but this is rare (Griffiths and Emery, 1996).

The respiratory system

NSAIDs can cause bronchospasm in some patients with asthma due to the inhibition of cyclooxygenase. Some individuals may also experience increased incidence of asthma attacks.

The skin

NSAIDs can cause skin sensitivities and reactions such as itching, rash, urticaria and photosensitivity.

The central nervous system

Memory loss and inability to concentrate has been reported in older people using NSAIDs (Goodwin and Regan, 1982). Indomethacin may cause dizziness and headaches.

The blood

The most common problem is iron deficiency anaemia due to gastrointestinal blood loss from ulceration or erosion. NSAIDs can cause prolonged bleeding time in some patients due to inhibition of platelet aggregation. Neutropaenia, aplastic anaemia, thrombocytopenia and agranulocytosis have all been reported with NSAID use.

NSAIDs can also interact with numerous other medications, and careful consideration of their use should be undertaken in patients with polypharmacy. A detailed list is provided in the relevant section of the British National Formulary (BNF).

NSAIDs and pregnancy

NSAIDs should be avoided in pregnancy if possible as they can cause:

- premature closure of the ductus arteriosis;
- impaired foetal circulation;
- increased postpartum and neonatal bleeding.

CORTICOSTEROIDS AND STEROID THERAPY

Corticosteroids are an effective method of reducing inflammation, particularly in rheumatoid arthritis (Criswell *et al.*, 2004). One study has also shown a reduction in radiological damage in patients with RA who received prednisolone (7.5 mg daily) early in their treatment (Kirwan, 1995). Corticosteroids work by binding to specific intracellular receptors, blocking the production of key cytokines and inhibiting T-cell activation and proliferation. Unfortunately, long-term side effects such as those listed below often outweigh the benefits:

- hypertension
- diabetes
- osteoporosis
- muscle wasting
- decreased resistance to infection
- Cushing's syndrome
- growth suppression in children
- adrenal suppression
- psychosis.

In contemporary management, steroids are used to provide temporary relief of symptoms until a DMARD becomes effective, or as an adjunct to other therapies in aggressive disease (Brownfield and Ryan, 1999). Patients themselves have concerns about steroid therapy and the adverse effects, and this sometimes prevents treatment (Morrison *et al.*, 2003). This can present a challenge for the nurse as s/he endeavours to support and advise the patient appropriately.

Routes of administration

Steroids are administered:

- orally
- intramuscularly
- intravenously
- intra-articularly.

Oral route

Low-dose therapy (up to 15 mg) will often be sufficient for maintenance control of disease symptoms in RA and polymyalgia rheumatica. Conditions such as systemic lupus erythematosus (SLE), myositis and temporal arteritis will require higher doses (20 mg–60 mg). The optimum dose is the lowest that induces a response.

Patients treated with oral steroid should be given a steroid card which provides information about their treatment regimen and care. This is important because synthetic exogenous steroids suppress the production of the endogenous steroid by the adrenal cortex. If exogenous treatment stops suddenly, the adrenal cortex may not be able to produce steroid, resulting in hypertension, hypoglycaemia and electrolyte imbalance. Patients should be aware that sudden cessation of treatment may induce a potentially fatal adrenal crisis. Withdrawal of oral steroids can also lead to a flare of symptoms, and so a slow dosage reduction is recommended.

Intramuscular injections

Drugs such as IM Depomedrone (40–120 mg) are used to rapidly reduce the symptoms of a flare or to control symptoms whilst DMARD's are initiated in RA. It is given by deep intramuscular injection to prevent muscle atrophy.

Intravenous pulses

Although treatment regimes will vary according to local policy and disease severity, pulse therapy comprising a number of short courses of intravenous infusions, usually methylprednisolone (500 mg–1000 mg) is given over 30–60 minutes. This type of administration requires hospitalisation as side effects such as changes in blood pressure, cardiac arrhythmias, bronchospasm or anaphylaxis can occur.

Intra-articular injection (IAI)

Painful, inflamed joints can be effectively relieved by IAI of a steroid such as depomedrone (10–80 mg depending on the size of the joint). Best results are obtained if the joint is rested for 24–48 hours following injection, and can be effective for up to three months. Contraindication of joint injections include:

- local infection
- intra-articular fracture
- anticoagulant therapy
- bleeding disorders.

Many nurses have gained skills in IAI techniques and can administer them but are advised to adhere to the Royal College of Nursing Rheumatology Guidelines.

Other indications for steroid use

Corticosteroid injections are also of benefit in bursitis, tendonitis, or enthesitis (Doherty, 1992), and can be injected into tender points and rheumatoid nodules. They are also used to treat giant cell arteritis as they reduce systemic inflammation (Norberg and Norberg, 2004). Vasculitides also respond well to high dose steroid either orally or intravenously.

SECOND-LINE THERAPY

Disease-modifying antirheumatic drugs (DMARDs) are prescribed to suppress the disease activity in systemic inflammatory arthritis. They are used in addition to other medications such as NSAIDs, analgesics and steroids. They include:

- azathioprine
- cyclosporin
- cyclophosphamide
- gold compounds
- hydroxychloroquine
- leflunomide
- methotrexate (MTX)
- mycophenolate mofetil

- penicillamine
- sulphasalazine (SASP)

Many of these drugs are potentially toxic and so monitoring is an important aspect of nursing care. Each DMARD has specific monitoring and guidelines are available. All the monitoring quoted in this chapter are taken from the Yorkshire Rheumatology Regional Guidelines for the Monitoring of DMARDs (2003). These guidelines have been approved for use by the Consultant Rheumatologists within the Yorkshire region. The British Society of Rheumatology (BSR) guidelines are an alternative, and can be found at www.rheumatology.org.uk.

AZATHIOPRINE

Azathioprine is often used as an adjunct to aid the reduction of oral corticosteroid therapy whilst controlling the disease itself (Kirwan *et al.*, 1995). It is given orally in doses of 1–2.5 mg/kg body weight daily, depending on clinical response, and can take up to three months to work. It is used in:

- RA
- vasculitis
- SLE
- dermatomyositis and polymyositis
- Behçet's syndrome
- polymyalgia and giant cell arteritis
- inflammatory bowel disease.

Mode of action

Although the mode of action is not entirely clear, it is known to interfere with DNA production, inhibiting replication or death of cells involved in the inflammatory process (Ryan, 1999). Side effects are predominantly associated with gastrointestinal symptoms and severe bone marrow suppression (Clunie and Lennard, 2003).

Special precautions

Intolerance and hypersensitivy can occur, which often responds to dosage reduction. Careful monitoring is required for bone marrow suppression (platelets <120 × 10^9/l; WCC 3 × 10^9/l; neutrophils <2 × 10^9/l).

CYCLOSPORIN

Used extensively as an immunosuppressing agent in organ transplantation, Cyclosporin is now licensed for use in RA. However, toxicity and lack of long-term data on disease progression mean that cyclosporin is usually reserved for patients with resistant RA who have failed to respond to other DMARDs (Parkinson and Alldred, 2002). Unfortunately, abnormal renal function and hypertension are often seen in patients treated with cyclosporin (Kvien *et al.*, 2002). Dosing is usually in two divided doses of 2.5 mg/kg per day for the first six weeks, increasing to a maximum of 4 mg/kg per day.

Indications

Indications for use are:

- patients with resistant RA
- severe psoriasis
- Behçet's syndrome.

Mode of action

Cyclosporin is known to block the development and utilisation of interleukin-2 which is responsible for T cell growth factor.

Special precautions

Cyclosporin should not be given to patients with:

- renal impairment
- uncontrolled hypertension
- recurrent infections
- malignancy.

The concomitant use of NSAIDs, particularly diclofenac, may affect renal function.

Monitoring

Baseline recordings of blood pressure and creatinine clearance should be taken and checked two weekly thereafter until a stable dose is achieved for three months, then monthly.
It should be noted that:

- Grapefruit juice can increase the bio-availability of cyclosporin.
- Patients on digoxin may need close monitoring due to the potential of digoxin toxicity.
- Hyperlipidaemia is common.

Vegetarians may not wish to take cyclosporin capsules as the coating contains gelatine, the solution is recommended in this case.

CYCLOPHOSPHAMIDE

Cyclophosphamide is a potent immunosuppressive alkylating agent. It has been used since the 1940's for the treatment of malignant disease, but it is also an effective treatment for severely resistant inflammatory disease due to it's immunosuppressive effects (Parkinson and Alldred, 2002). Daily oral doses range between 50 mg and 200 mg, increasing to 250 mg for short courses in severe disease (Miller, 1996).

IV pulse therapy is usually given at a dose of 10–15/kg body weight.

Indications

Cyclophosphamide in combination with steroid therapy is regarded as the standard treatment for all types of vasculitis. Courses of treatment are used initially to induce inflammatory suppression, followed by maintenance therapy with either methotrexate (MTX) or azathioprine (Tadman, 2004).

When combined with prednisolone, it improves the clinical symptoms of systemic sclerosis and related alveolitis. It is thought that this is due to the reduction of the endothelial damage of microvascular structures (Apras et al., 2003). There is debate about its clinical effectiveness to treat neuropsychiatric symptoms in SLE (Trevisani et al., 2004), but is commonly used to treat associated glomerular renal disease.

Mode of action

This is not entirely clear. It is known that it interacts with DNA and stops replication of cells such as lymphocytes, causing the cell to die. Cyclophosphamide is metabolised in the liver, and its metabolites, particularly acrolein, are excreted in the urine. It is a potent immunosuppressive and requires cautious use.

Special precautions

Nurses administrating intravenous cyclophosphamide should haven proven competency for handing cytotoxic drugs. Special precautions for this drug include:

- A metabolite of cyclophosphamide, acrolein, may cause haemorrhagic cystitis and requires the prophylactic use of Mesna 400 mg given alongside the treatment to prevent urothelial damage. Further doses are required four and eight hours following infusion. The patient should also be advised to increase their oral fluid intake where possible or receive supplementary intravenous fluids on their treatment day.

- It can potentate the effect of oral hypoglycaemics.
- It should be withheld or the dose reduced in the presence of bone marrow suppression (platelets <120 × 10⁹/l; white cell count (WCC) <3 × 10⁹/l; neutrophils <2 × 10⁹/l), severe infection, renal failure (creatinine >120 μmol/l), or hepatic failure (bilirubin >17 μmol/l; Alanine transaminase/Alkaline phosphatase (ALT/ALP) > 2–3 times normal limit).
- Maximum effect on bone marrow occurs at 5–10 days post-treatment; therefore blood monitoring should be taken ten days post-dose. Recovery is usually seen at 10–14 days.
- Storage of eggs or sperm should be offered to the patient prior to treatment, as there is an increased risk of irreversible infertility.
- Contraception should be practiced as pregnancy and breastfeeding are not advised due to the mutagenic, teratogenic and carcinogenic potential of the drug, for at least three to six months following treatment.

GOLD COMPOUNDS

Gold compounds have been used in the treatment of active RA for many years, and are thought to have an immunosuppressive action on the lymphocytes, monocytes and their mediators (Scharf and Christophidis, 1995).

Sodium aurothiomalate

Although newer agents have superseded gold injections as a treatment option there is still a clinical need for its use in some patients. A recent study of UK consultants established intramuscular gold as a third choice of DMARD, following MTX and/or sulphasalazine (SASP) and leflunomide (Jobanputra *et al.*, 2004). Although treatment with intramuscular gold has been shown to significantly reduce disease progression (Kvien *et al.*, 2002), its toxicity remains a contraindication for use in some patients (Maetzel *et al.*, 2000). It is given by intramuscular injection (IMI) 20–50mg weekly, reducing to fortnightly or monthly as symptoms improve. Usually a cumulative dose of 500–800mg is required to demonstrate effectiveness. If there is no response by 1000mg, it should be discontinued. Guidelines for nurses administering gold injections have been produced by the Royal College of Nursing (Voyce, 1999).

Mode of action

Following injection, gold salts are absorbed and sent to the synovium where it binds to the inflamed tissues. Although it is rapidly excreted in the urine, it has been found in tissues up to 20 years after discontinuation (Ryan, 1999).

Special precautions

Monitoring is crucial to safety as can be seen below:

- Initial test dose, usually of 10 mg, is given as toxicity to injectable gold occurs in 30–40% of patients (Day, 1994).
- Vasomotor reactions such as dizziness, nausea, weakness and hypotension can immediately follow injection, therefore the patient should be observed for a short period of time following administration (Ryan, 1999).
- Urinalysis should be carried out before each dose to monitor for renal toxicity, especially increasing levels of protein urea (>1 g in 24 hours).
- A rash which may be erythematous or severely puritic with raised eosinophil levels may indicate toxicity (Elderman *et al.*, 1983).
- Exfoliating dermatitis can cause mouth ulcers and severe stomatitis.
- Progressive neutropaenia can occur $<2 \times 10^9/l$ with or without a fall in platelets $<120 \times 10^9/l$.
- Inflammatory lung disease has been noted which is often difficult to differentiate from the effects of the RA on lung tissue (Ryan, 1999).

Auranofin (oral gold)

Although less effective, oral gold is sometimes chosen due to the less toxic effect on the kidneys and bone marrow. The usual dose is 3 mg tablet twice daily.

Mode of action

Absorption is rapid, but only 20–25% of the drug is absorbed with most being excreted in the faeces.

Special precautions

Monitoring is the same as for injectable gold.

Diarrhoea is a common side effect as is nausea and vomiting. Bulking agents may be useful and the drug should be taken with meals.

HYDROXYCHLOROQUINE

Hydroxychloroquine is an antimalarial drug used to treat moderately active RA. It can also be effective for mild SLE, and there is some suggestion that it could be used for long-term prophylaxis in the treatment of patients with antiphospholipid syndrome (Khamashta, 1999).

Mode of action

Its action is not fully understood, but it is thought to interfere with the interleukin-1 production from monocytes, and inhibition of neutrophils superoxide release (Walker, 1998).

Administration

Initially, administer 400 mg orally daily in divided doses, then 200 mg–400 mg daily maintenance dose.

Special precautions

Manufacturers recommend regular opthalmological examination due to incidence of ocular toxicity. However, as the incidence rate is low, the Royal College of Ophthalmologists recommends questioning about any ocular symptoms or visual disturbances prior to commencement of treatment. Only if any impairment is noted should patients be referred for assessment by an optometrist, and any abnormality should then be referred to an ophthalmologist.

Hydroxychloroquine should not be given to patients with psoriatic arthritis, as it has been known to exacerbate psoriasis. It should also be used with caution in patients with hepatic or renal impairment (BNF, 2004).

Potential side effects

Side effects are uncommon but include:

- indigestion
- diarrhoea
- skin rashes
- headaches
- blurred vision.

Pregnancy and breastfeeding

Hydroxychloroquine seems to be safe in pregnancy if the rheumatic disease is well-controlled (BNF, 2004). However, it is present in breast milk and so should be avoided when breastfeeding.

LEFLUNOMIDE

The therapeutic effect of leflunomide usually starts after four to six weeks; but it may take longer. It acts on the immune system but its precise action is not fully understood.

Indications

Leflunomide is indicated for moderate to severe RA.

Administration

A three day loading dose of 100 mg daily, followed by a daily maintenance dose of 10–20 mg is recommended. The loading dose is sometimes omitted in cases where significant side effects may occur.

Special precautions

Leflunomide should not be used in patients with:

- previous hepatic or renal impairment (BNF, 2004);
- previous impaired bone marrow function including anaemia, leucopenia, thrombocytopenia;
- previous history of tuberculosis;
- serious infections, nephrotic syndrome or severe immunodeficiency states such as AIDS;
- an age under 18, as its safety and efficacy have not been studied in this group (Aventis, 2004).

Live vaccines should not be administered whilst the patient is taking the drug.

Potential side effects

Diarrhoea, nausea, vomiting, abdominal pain, rise in blood pressure, headache, dizziness, alopecia, dry skin, rash, pruritis and urticaria are all potential side effects.

Leflunomide has a half-life of one to four weeks and if serious toxicity or side effects occur a washout procedure is needed. After stopping leflunomide, cholestyramine 8 mg is administered three times daily for a period of eleven days. An alternative is 50 g of activated charcoal daily for eleven days (Aventis, 2004).

Pregnancy and breastfeeding

The active metabolite of leflunomide is teratogenic in rats and rabbits, and it may cause foetal harm in humans. The possibility of pregnancy must be excluded prior to commencement of leflunomide and reliable contraception must be used by both sexes. If the above washout procedures are not used, the manufacturer recommend pregnancy is avoided up to two years after cessation of treatment, or until a plasma concentration of less than 0.02 mg/l is achieved. Breastfeeding is contraindicated when taking leflunomide as its metabolites can pass into breast milk.

Monitoring

Baseline full blood count (FBC), urea and electrolytes (U&E), liver function tests (LFTs) and blood pressure (BP) are required. If renal function is in doubt then a 24-hour urine creatinine clearance should be performed. The FBC, LFTs and BP are repeated two weekly for two months, monthly for four months, and when the patient is on a stable dose, at two monthly intervals. If leflunomide is to be used in conjunction with other DMARDs, particularly methotrexate (MTX), monitoring should continue monthly for the duration of the combination of treatment.

Treatment should be stopped if the WCC falls below $4 \times 10^9/l$, neutrophils fall below $2 \times 10^9/l$, platelets fall below $150 \times 10^9/l$, or the AST/ALT are greater than three times the upper limit of normal.

Treatment should also be stopped if the patient develops pruritis, rash, abdominal pain, nausea, diarrhoea, weight loss or alopecia. In these cases an urgent washout procedure may be necessary.

METHOTREXATE (MTX) AND FOLIC ACID

MTX has been used as a DMARD since the 1950's, and was approved for use in the treatment of active RA in the USA in the late 1980's. It is the most popular first choice DMARD in the UK (Hitt, 2003), and recognised as the gold standard treatment for RA (Weinblatt et al., 1992; Furst, 1995).

Mode of action

MTX is a folic acid antagonist and is classified as an antimetabolite cytotoxic agent. Antifolate agents slow down the production of blood cells and inhibit connective cell tissue division. Folate is essential for the production of blood cells. The original use of MTX was for the treatment of childhood leukaemia, and it is still widely used in acute lymphoblastic leukaemia and menigococcal meningitis. MTX also has a powerful action on cells undergoing DNA synthesis. Cells most influenced are those in the gastrointestinal tract and the epidermis, which accounts for the potential side effects of nausea, vomiting and mouth ulcers.

Indications

Indications for MTX are:

- active RA
- psoriatic arthritis
- ankylosing spondylitis with peripheral joint involvement (Marshall and Kirwan, 2001).

Administration

Administer a weekly dose, usually starting at 7.5 mg, increasing at 2.5 mg increments every two weeks. The maximum dose is usually 25 mg weekly, but 30 mg weekly has been used in severe cases. MTX is usually given orally initially, up to maximum tolerated dose. However, subcutaneous MTX can be substituted if the response is poor or significant side effects occur (Arthur et al., 2002; Bingham et al., 2003a).

Patients can be taught to self-administer their injections, but consideration has to be given to cytotoxic issues and risk management. Comprehensive guidelines have been published by the Royal College of Nursing (RCN, 2004).

Special precautions

MTX should be used with caution in patients with previous hepatic or renal impairment (BNF, 2004), and pulmonary toxicity may be a problem in RA. Patients must be advised to seek immediate medical advice if they experience dyspnoea, fever or a cough. MTX should be discontinued if pneumonitis is suspected.

Live vaccines should not be administered.

Potential side effects

Side effects include nausea, vomiting, abdominal pain, headaches, alopecia and rash. Patients may have an increased susceptibility to the herpes zoster virus.

Pregnancy and breastfeeding

MTX should not be taken in pregnancy as it is teratogenic. Manufacturers advise that effective contraception needs to be used for at least three months after cessation of therapy for both men and women prior to conception, although six months is commonly recommended. MTX is contraindicated whilst breastfeeding.

Monitoring

Baseline FBC, U&E and LFTs should be taken. If renal function is in doubt, a 24-hour urine sample should be collected for creatinine clearance.

Repeat the FBC and LFTs two weekly for two months, monthly for four months, then three monthly once on a stable dose. If the dose changes, monitoring should revert back to two weekly until a maintenance dose is established.

Therapy should be discontinued if WCC is $<4 \times 10^9/l$, neutrophils fall below $2 \times 10^9/l$, platelets fall below $150 \times 10^9/l$, or AST/ALT are above three times normal range. If oral ulceration, unusual bruising, rash, fever cough or shortness of breath, nausea or alopecia occur, therapy should be stopped and the rheumatology department contacted.

Folic acid supplements

Folic acid is usually given in conjunction with MTX because of the latter's antifolate action. Although regimes vary widely, 5 mg daily, apart form the day the MTX is given, appears to be common.

MYCOPHENOLATE MOFETIL (MMF)

MMF has an immunosuppressive effect in autoimmune disease, especially in SLE nephritis (Gaubitz et al., 1999). Early indication suggests a dose range between 0.5 mg and 2 g per day with concomitant steroid therapy.

Indications

Gaubitz et al. (1999) have demonstrated positive results in RA, vasculitis and SLE nephritis for those who have failed conventional therapies. Karim et al. (2002) advocate the use of MMF in renal lupus to reduce disease activity and extend survival rates in those patients with moderate to severe disease.

Mode of action

Derived from mycophenolic acid, MMF is a weak organic acid produced by the fermentation of penicillin stoloniferum, which interferes with the synthesis of RNA and DNA. Although its exact action is debatable (Karim et al., 2002), MMF is thought to inhibit the proliferation of T and B lymphocytes thereby decreasing antibody production.

Special precautions

Precautions to take with MMF include:

- It is most effective if taken on an empty stomach and swallowed whole.
- The most common side effect is diarrhoea which settles with dose reduction.

- Leucopenia has been noted in some patients; therefore frequent blood tests are recommended weekly for the first month, twice monthly for the second and third months and monthly thereafter.

PENICILLAMINE

Penicillamine (DPA) is seldom used due to inefficacy and toxicity (Parkinson and Alldred, 2002). Dosage begins at 125 mg daily increasing monthly to 750 mg depending on clinical response.

Indications

Benefit has been demonstrated in the treatment of RA with associated extra-articular features such as nodules and lung disease.

Mode of action

It is thought to suppress the immune system but its action remains uncertain. Early studies suggested DPA prevented the action of T-helper cells in the inflammatory cascade (Lipsky and Ziff, 1980).

Special precautions

Precautions to take with DPA include:

- DPA should be taken on an empty stomach as it is a chelator that absorbs essential metals such as iron from the diet. Iron supplements should be taken two hours before or after dosage.
- Patients with known DPA allergy and previous intolerance to gold are at risk of mucocutaneous reaction.
- Stomatitis and anorexia can occur due to the metallic taste some patients experience.
- Thrombocytopenia, neutropaenia and aplastic anaemia are common.
- Renal involvement causing withdrawal of the drug include:
  ❖ proteinurea >1 g in 24 hours
  ❖ nephrotic syndrome
  ❖ glomerulonephritis
  ❖ drug-induced lupus.
- Myositis may occur.

SULPHASALAZINE (SASP)

SASP is a combination of 5-aminosalicylic acid and sulphapyridine. Its action is not fully understood, but is likely that it may inhibit the production of cytokines (Symmons *et al.*, 1988). It is thought to be comparable in efficacy to parenteral gold, but much better tolerated (Wood, 1999).

Indications

Indications for SASP use are:

- active RA
- ankylosing spondylitis.

Administration

Administer 500 mg daily for one week, 500 mg twice daily for one week, 500 mg three times daily for one week, then 1 g twice daily maintenance. In cases of partial effectiveness, the dose may be increased up to 1 g three times daily.

Special precautions

Precautions to take with SASP include:

- Caution should be exercised with patients who have experienced previous hepatic or renal problems.
- Sulphasalazine should not be given to patients with sensitivity to sulphona-mides or salicylates.
- Caution should also be exercised in patients who are antinuclear antibody (ANA) positive.
- Patients wearing soft contact lenses should be made aware that staining may occur.
- There are potential drug interactions with phenytoin, trimethoprim and septrin.
- Live vaccines should be avoided.

Potential side effects

Gastrointestinal disturbances and rashes may occur. Nausea is the most common side effect.

Pregnancy and breastfeeding

SASP is not recommended in pregnancy as its safety is unproven. As it is expressed in breast milk, breastfeeding is not recommended.

It can cause reversible oligospermia, so advice should be given to men wishing to start a family.

Monitoring

Baseline FBC, U&E and LFTs should be taken.

Repeat FBC and LFTs two weekly for two months, monthly for four months then three monthly when the dose is stable.

Treatment should be stopped if WCC is <4 × 10^9/l, neutrophils <2 × 10^9/l, platelets <150 × 10^9/l, or AST/ALT are over three times upper limit of normal. Treatment should also be stopped if the patient develops a sore throat, oral ulceration, fever or rash.

COMBINATION DMARDs

If monotherapy is only partially effective, DMARDs are commonly used in combination. Common combinations are:

- MTX and SASP
- MTX, SASP and hydroxychloroquine
- MTX and biologic therapy.

Administration

Administer up to the highest dose of each of the DMARDs used (for example 25 mg MTX weekly, with SASP 1 g twice daily).

Special precautions

Combination DMARD precautions are the same as with special precautions with each individual drugs, but toxicity is more prevalent in combination.

Monitoring

Monitoring should be as per the individual drugs with the exception of an MTX/leflunomide combination. This can be particularly toxic and so monitoring should be continued monthly for the duration of the combination treatment.

IMMUNOGLOBULINS

Information regarding the use of immunoglobulins in rheumatology has been based on uncontrolled clinical trials and therefore optimal doses are yet to be defined. Trials to date suggest there is a potential benefit to be derived form the use of immunoglobulins for the treatment of:

- dermatomyositis
- polymyositis
- connective tissue disease.

Improved muscle strength, cutaneous lesions and reduction in creatinine kinase have been noted (Cherin *et al.*, 1991; Gelfand *et al.*, 1989). Giannini *et al.* (1996), demonstrated an initial, positive response to immunoglobulin therapy in a small multicentre trial of patients with early polyarticular juvenile RA.

MISCELLANEOUS DRUGS

ILOPROST

Iloprost is a prostacyclin analogue which inhibits platelet aggregation and initiates vasodilation. It is used in connective tissue disease and Raynaud's phenomenon when conventional treatments with calcium channel blockers have failed to improve peripheral circulation. Zulian *et al.* (2004) suggests that Iloprost is an efficacious treatment for critical ischaemia affecting the digits in connective tissue disease. Studies indicate a reduction in the severity of attacks, pain, the number of lesions, and amputation due to gangrene. There is also an indication that nebulised Iloprost may improve pulmonary hypertension associated with advanced systemic sclerosis.

BISPHOSPHONATES

Bisphosphonates are potent inhibitors of osteoclastic bone resorption and are an important therapeutic intervention in the management of:

- Paget's disease
- multiple myeloma
- malignancy-associated hypercalcaemia
- bone metastasis
- osteoporosis.

Bisphosphonates, such as pamidronate, bind to bony surfaces and induce osteoclastic apoptosis and improve the pain associated with the above conditions. Following phagocytosis by osteoclasts, bisphosphonates impair the biochemical reactions that lead to osteoclastic apoptosis and modulation of cytokine concentrations. This exerts an anti-inflammatory response. Bisphosphonates are effective in several rheumatological conditions, including AS, hypertrophic osteoarthropathy, reflex sympathetic dystrophy, diabetic neuropathic arthropathy and the synovitis, acne, pustulosis, hyperostosis and osteitis (SAPHO) syndrome.

The treatments of choice for postmenopausal osteoporosis are:

- alendronic acid (sodium alendrolate) 70 mg once weekly
- risedronate sodium 35 mg once weekly.

Unfortunately, there is a high nonadherence rate with these drugs. This is mainly due to gastrointestinal disturbances which some patients find intolerable, and a weekly dosage regimen which is easy to forget.

BIOLOGIC THERAPIES

Recent advances in the genetically engineered treatment for rheumatic disease have revolutionised therapy for patients failing conventional treatment. Biologic therapies are described as biologic response modifiers or targeted therapies. Increased understanding of the inflammatory cascade, has led to the development of specific immunoglobulins which block or alter the pro-inflammatory cytokines TNFα and interleukin-1 (IL-1). These cytokines are responsible for the establishment and maintenance of inflammation in a variety of autoimmune diseases such as RA, AS, psoriatic arthritis (PsA) and Crohn's disease (Oliver and Mooney, 2002; Scott, 2002). Overproduction of TNFα and interleukin-1 cause the inflammatory response that damages articular bone, cartilage and soft tissue. Commonly used agents are:

- infliximab
- etanercept
- adalimumab
- anakinra.

Anderson (2004) has cited the therapeutic outcomes of treatment with TNFα to be:

- increased function
- reduction in pain
- reduction in early morning stiffness
- reduction in swollen joints
- reduction in fatigue
- induction and maintenance of remission.

Other improvements demonstrated by the American College of Rheumatology (ACR) response include:

- reduction in the progression of joint damage determined by radiographic image;
- decrease in c-reactive protein (CRP);
- fall in erythrocyte sedimentation rate (ESR);
- reduced disease activity score (DAS28).

Biologic therapies are at present used for severe inflammatory RA. They have a 70% success rate in patients with resistant RA whose previous therapy has included MTX plus one or more additional DMARD (Emery et al., 1999). However, they require careful assessment and monitoring for recurrent infections and more serious illness such as demyelination and tuberculosis (Table 12.1).

These drugs are expensive, but the overall healthcare costs are complex and have major resource implications (Scott, 2002). For instance, radiographic remission can be induced early, which could lessen the overall cost of RA and reduce the chance of long-term disability (Hulsmans et al., 2000). The British Society for Rheumatology (BSR) and the National Institute of Clinical Excellence (NICE) govern the use of biologic therapies and have set patient inclusion and exclusion criteria (BSR, 2002; BSR, 2003; NICE, 2002). The Royal College of Nursing (RCN) provides guidelines for their use (RCN, 2003). The Biologics Register is a rigorous data collection system, set up by the BSR to collate ongoing data six monthly for all patients receiving biologics. This provides information about the efficacy, adverse events and eventually, long-term effects of these treatments.

In addition to RA, infliximab and etanercept are licensed in the USA and Europe for use in AS and are awaiting NICE approval for this disease in the UK. The evidence in AS to date shows a reduction in the rate of joint damage and improved functional ability as measured by the Bath Ankylosing Spondylitis Indices (Calin, 2002; Irons and Jeffries, 2004). The biologics also show promising results in PsA and in 2003, etanercept was licensed for its treatment (Kyle et al., 2005). The data demonstrates that they may be even more effective in AS and PsA than in RA (Braun et al., 2003; Davis, 2003). Despite their success, work continues to determine why some patients fail to respond or achieve an adequate response to anti-TNFα.

WITHDRAWAL OF THERAPY

Patients should stop their biologic therapy in the event of a severe infection until they have recovered.

Patients receiving biologic treatment who are undergoing surgical procedures or teeth extraction are usually advised to withhold their treatment prior to and following surgery to reduce the risk of infection. If the surgery is extensive, or includes a major joint replacement, treatment should be stopped at least two weeks prior to the operation or longer if this is the surgeon's preference dependent upon local policy and guidelines.

INFLIXIMAB

Infliximab is a chimeric monoclonal antibody, combining mouse and human immunoglobulins, which binds to free and bound TNFα and neutralises its effects. Ongoing studies suggest that when a combination of infliximab and MTX is administered to patients who have had RA for less than six years,

Table 12.1 Adverse effects associated with biologic therapies

Adverse Effects	Infliximab	Etanercept	Adalimumab	Anakinra
Serious infections	Viral infection 35% Pneumonia 5% Abcess formation Sepsis Granulomatous lesions Conjunctivitis Urinary tract infections/ pyelonephritis	Upper respiratory tract/Sinusitis Bronchitis Urinary tract infections Skin infections	Upper respiratory tract Bronchitis Urinary tract infections	1.8% infections Cellulitis Pneumonia Bone/joint infection
Injection site reactions		Itching and rash Common in first month –30% of patients	20% of patients	71% in first month
Hypersensitivity reactions	During and within two hours of infusion Fever/chills Chest pain Dysnoea and bronchospasm Hypo/hypertension Dry skin	Angioedema Urticaria	Rash, puritis	
Formation of antibodies	Some patients develop (HACA) Human Anti Chimeric Antibodies Decreased half life and efficacy of drug	No reduction in on effectiveness	Small number of patients – reduced effectiveness	

Malignancies	Lymphoma Others Similar to general population	Breast; Lung Lymphoma No difference from general population	Benign skin cancers No difference from general population	No difference from general population
Neurologic events	Demyelinating disorders such as Multiple Sclerosis Neuropathies Seizure	Demyelinating disorders such as Multiple Sclerosis Optic neuritis Transverse myelitis	Headache, dizziness	
Haematologic events	Anaemias Leukopaenia Lymphocytosis Neutropaenia Thrombocytopaenia Abnormal liver function	Thrombocytopaenia Pancytopaenia Aplastic anaemia	LFT abnormalities Decreased haemoglobin	Neutropaenia 1–10%
Autoimmunity	Increased risk 52% of developing +ve ANA/DsDNA	Increased risk of developing positive +ve ANA/DsDNA	1 in 2334 lupus-like reaction	

they have the potential to inhibit the pro-inflammatory cascade before other cytokines are stimulated (Breedveld *et al.*, 2004).

Indications and dosing

Infliximab should be administered in 250 mls of sodium chloride (0.9%) and given intravenously over two hours, although studies have proven that with careful monitoring, infusion rates can decrease after repeated infusions (Buch *et al.*, 2004).

For RA give 3 mg/kg at weeks 0, 2, 6 and then 8 weekly. It is given in combination with weekly MTX to reduce risk of infliximab antibody (Human Anti Chimeric Antibody) production.

For AS and PsA give 5 mg/kg at weeks 0, 2, 6 and then 6–8 weekly. It may be used with or without MTX.

For Crohn's disease (severe active disease) a single infusion of 5 mg/kg.

For Fistulising disease give 5 mg/kg at 0, 2, 6 and then up to 14 weeks later if symptoms recur.

For psoriasis give 5 mg/kg with frequency determined by skin condition.

There are early indications that infliximab may be useful in the treatment of Behçet's syndrome, particularly for those patients with ocular involvement (Estrach *et al.*, 2003; Sfikakis, 2002), and for Wegener's granulomatosis when combined with standard treatments such as cyclophosphamide (Nolle *et al.*, 2002).

Contraindications

Contraindications are:

- active TB;
- moderate to severe heart failure class III/IV;
- hypersensitivity to mouse products.

Special precautions

Anaphylaxis may develop within seconds of commencing the infusion. Local policies should be followed and the infusion stopped immediately. Once symptoms have settled the infusion may be restarted.

Patients should be screened for active and inactive tuberculosis prior to treatment and monitored carefully during and after treatment. Inactive TB requires prophylactic antituberculosis treatment as per local guidelines.

Infliximab should be reconstituted aseptically following the drug company's instructions and administered using a special sterile, nonpyrogenic, low-protein binding filter (1.2 micrometer or less) attached to the giving set.

ETANERCEPT

Etanercept is a fusion protein consisting of p75-TNF receptor type II and Fc portion of human IgG, which inhibits the binding of TNFα to its cell surface receptor. It can be used as monotherapy or in combination with MTX. Dosage is 25 mg twice weekly or 50 mg weekly by subcutaneous injection.

Indications

Etanercept is licensed in the USA and Europe for the treatment of:

- refractory RA;
- PsA (elevated levels of TNFα are found in synovium and psoriatic plaques);
- polyarticular juvenile arthritis.

Contraindications

Contraindications are:

- moderate to severe heart failure class III/IV;
- severe or recurrent infections;
- blood dyscrasias – pancytopenia/ aplastic anaemia.

Special precautions

Once reconstituted the injections should be administered as soon as possible to avoid contamination.

Storage should be in a refrigerator between 2–8°C.

ADALIMUMAB

Adalimumab is a fully human monoclonal TNFα antibody. It is used as monotherapy, or in combination with MTX or other DMARD's. It provides a new therapeutic option for those patients who have failed on other agents, especially infliximab, due to the production of autoimmune antibodies to the drug itself. Dosage is 40 mg every two weeks given by subcutaneous injection.

Indications

Adalimumab is indicated for refractory RA.

Clinical trials are currently examining the use of adalimumab for patients with PsA (Mease, 2004) and those suffering from sciatica (Brennan et al., 2004).

Contraindications

Contraindications are:

- active TB
- moderate to severe heart failure class III/IV.

ANAKINRA

In RA, IL-1 is present in the joints and blood in excessive amounts and it increases inflammation and causes joint damage. Anakinra is a recombinant human interleukin-1 receptor antagonist that blocks the action of IL-1, thereby reducing inflammation and joint damage (ARC, 2003). Comorbid RA patients on concomitant therapy have responded well to anakinra and experience only limited side effects (Fleischmann, 2003). However, it has not yet been approved by NICE as the cost-effectiveness and clinical benefits in relation to the other available agents is unclear. Patients who remain on anakinra following clinical trials and continue to respond well, can continue their treatment until their consultant decides otherwise (NICE, 2003). Dosage is 100 mg daily by subcutaneous injection. It is given in combination with MTX.

Indications

Anakinra is indicated for refractory RA.

Special precautions

Anakinra should not be used in patients with impaired renal function (Creatinine clearance of <30 ml/minute).

Increased risk of infection exists for patients with history of asthma.

NEW THERAPIES

Further research into immune-mediated inflammatory diseases continues to identify new molecular targets and therapeutic agents. Determining how cytokine dysregulation influences specific inflammatory diseases will help target therapies to treat each stage of the disease. Recognition of the pathogenesis of lymphocytes and macrophages is crucial to this research, and studies are currently exploring the prevention of inflammatory cell migration and control of the activation of pathogenic T-cells.

ABATERCEPT

Early studies indicate that CTLA-4-immunoglobulin, which has been developed to inhibit T-cell stimulation by B7 family molecules on the surface of the cell, significantly reduces inflammation and induces an increased ACR20 response in patients with resistant RA.

RITUXIMAB

It is recognised that B cells have a role in producing auto-antibodies such as rheumatoid factor, and that limiting B cells interrupts the chain of events that leads to the symptoms of RA (ARC, 2002). Rituximab is an anti B cell mono-clonal antibody (anti-CD20), used to treat patients with severe, resistant RA (Bingham *et al.*, 2003b). Rituximab removes the B cells from the blood. Recent studies show that a high proportion of patients experience symptom improvement, 20% experiencing dramatic results (Edwards *et al.*, 2004). It is currently licensed for use in nonHodgkin's lymphoma.

BOSENTAN

Recent international reports describe encouraging results of studies exploring the role of the dual endothelin receptor antagonist bosentan in pulmonary arterial hypertension associated with scleroderma (Humbert and Cabane, 2003). The drug appears to be well-tolerated with few side effects noted in the first year of trials. Bosentan may offer a novel treatment for scleroderma patients suffering from associated lung disease as studies demonstrate decreased dyspnoea and pulmonary arterial hypertension, alongside improvement in cutaneous fibrosis and functional ability (Humbert and Cabane, 2003).

TGF-BETA

The transforming growth factor (TGF) β 1 gene is pivotal to the inflammatory processes of bone remodelling and fibrosis, repairing cartilage and bone damage. TGF β 1 has multiple effects on the suppression of T and B cells, with increased production inhibiting the autoimmune response of chronic inflammatory disease (Jaakkola *et al.*, 2003). TGF β 1 may influence the onset of fibrosis and ankylosis in AS. Ongoing studies indicate there may be a role for TGF β in determining the genetic susceptibility to systemic sclerosis and the degree of cutaneous fibrosis involved (Susol, 2000).

PATIENT EDUCATION AND INFORMATION

Patient education is of the utmost importance in the nursing care of rheumatic patients, particularly in relation to DMARDs. All DMARDs have poten-tially serious side effects that influence fertility and childbearing choices. The RCN RNF guidelines (2001), clearly state that for patients to participate fully in their own care, they need an adequate knowledge base. It is the role of nurses and other health care professionals to provide this knowledge.

In primary care, general practitioners should provide advice on the disease, potential drug interactions and side effects. More specific advice and education is then provided in secondary care by the rheumatologists and clinical nurse specialists. In-depth drug information is given by the specialist nurses.

ACTION POINTS FOR PRACTICE

- Patient A has been started on a combination of MTX and leflunomide and is being considered for biologic therapy due to ongoing active disease. What advice would you have given patient A regarding their DMARDs monitoring? If the patient is to commence biologic therapy, what considerations need to be taken into account? If biologics are started, what long-term monitoring will be required?
- Patient B has been admitted to a rheumatology ward. For the past seven years patient B has been having gold injections administered in the community and monitored by the GP. Patient B has recently developed an itchy, raised, red rash covering their entire body. S/he also has proteinurea. What would your intervention/advice comprise?
- Patient C is currently well on infliximab and MTX. S/he is scheduled for a routine total hip replacement within the next month. What advice would you give regarding their medications?
- Patient D is newly diagnosed with polymyalgia rheumatica, treated with high dose steroids. This patient is also a type II diabetic on metformin. What advice would you give this patient regarding their concurrent conditions?

REFERENCES

Anderson D (2004) TNF inhibitors: a new age in rheumatoid arthritis treatment: This class of biologic response modifiers inhibits the inflammatory process that underlies rheumatoid arthritis. But adverse effects may be severe. *American Journal of Nursing* 104(2):60–68.

Apras S, Ertenli I, Ozbalkan Z *et al.* (2003) Effects of oral cyclophosphamide and prednisolone therapy on the endothelial functions and clinical findings in patients with early diffuse Systemic Sclerosis. *Arthritis and Rheumatism* 48(8): 2256–2261.

Arthritis Research Campaign (2002) Factsheet: B-cells / rituximab (Mabthera). http://www.arc.org.uk/newsviews/press/oct2002/rituximab.htm (20 May 04).

Arthritis Research Campaign (2003) Drugs for arthritis: Anakinra an information sheet. http://www.arc.org.uk/about_arth/infosheets/6263/6263.htm (20 May 04).

Arthur V, Jubb R, Homer D (2002) A study of parenteral use of methotrexate in rheumatic conditions. *Journal of Clinical Nursing* 11:256–263.

Aventis (2004) Arava 10, 20, and 100mg Tablets. http://emc.medicines.org.uk/emc/assets/c/html/displayDocPrinterFriendly.asp?docum/url (25 September 04).

Bingham SJ, Buch MH, Lindsay S *et al.* (2003a) Parenteral methotrexate should be given before biological therapy. *Rheumatology* 40:387–392.

Bingham SJ, Buch MH, English A *et al.* (2003b) Recurrence of aggressive rheumatoid arthritis despite Rituximab induced complete B cell depletion. *Rheumatology* 42(212) Suppl 1:86.

Braun J, Brandt J, Listing J *et al.* (2002) Treatment of active ankylosing spondylitis with infliximab: a randomised controlled multicentre trial. *The Lancet* 359(9312): 1187–1193.

Breedveld FC, Emery P, Patel K *et al.* (2004) Infliximab in active early rheumatoid arthritis. *Annals of the Rheumatic Diseases* 63(2):149–155.

Brennan S, Vanharanta H, Keenan A *et al.* (2004) *Treating sciatica with adalimumab: a pilot study.* SAT0146 http://mcic3.textor.com/cgi-bin/mc/printabs.pl?APP=eular2004SCIE-abstract&TEMPLATE=&keyf=1333&showHide=show&client (26 June 04).

British National Formulary (2004) www.bnf.org (20 May 2004).

British Society for Rheumatology (2002) *Guidelines for prescribing TNF-alpha blockers in adult RA.* www.rheumatology.org.uk (15 April 2004).

British Society for Rheumatology (2003) Reviewed guidelines for prescribing TNF-alpha blockers in adult RA. www.rheumatology.org.uk (15 April 2004).

Brownfield A, Ryan S (1999) Use of steroids in the treatment of rheumatoid arthritis. In: Ryan S (ed) *Drug Therapy in Rheumatology Nursing.* London, Whurr Publishers. 2:113–122.

Buch MH, Lindsay S, Bryer D *et al.* (2004) *Incidence of infusion-related reactions in patients receiving infliximab: recommendations for administration.* FR1022 http://mcic3.textor.com/cgi-bin/mc/printabs.pl?APP=eular2004SCIE-abstract&TEMPLATE=&keyf=1159&showHide=show&client (26 June 04).

Calin A (2002) Defining outcome in ankylosing spondylitis. Where have we been, where are we and where do we go from here? *Joint Bone Spine* 69:101–104.

Cherin P, Herson S, Wechsler B (1991) Efficacy of intravenous gammaglobulin therapy in chronic refractory polymyositis and dermatomyositis: an open study with 20 adult patients. *American Journal of Medicine* 91:162–168.

Clunie GPR, Lennard L (2003) Relevance of thiopurine methyltransferase status in rheumatology patients receiving azathioprine. *Rheumatology* 43(1):13–18.

Criswell LA, Saag G, Sems KM *et al.* (2004) Moderate-term, low-dose corticosteroids for rheumatoid arthritis (Cochrane Review). In: *The Cochrane Library,* Issue 1, 2004. Chichester, UK, John Wiley & Sons Ltd.

Davis JC (2003) Recombinant human tissue necrosis factor receptor (Etanercept) for treating ankylosing spondylitis: a randomised, controlled trial. *Arthritis and Rheumatism* 48(11):3230–3235.

Day R (1994) Pharmacologic approaches: SAARDI. In: Klippel J, Dieppe P (eds) *Rheumatology.* London, Mosby Year Book Europe.

Doherty M (1992) *Rheumatology Examination and Injection Techniques.* London, WB Saunders.

Edwards JCW, Szczepanski L, Szechinski J *et al.* (2004) Efficacy of B-Cell Targeted Therapy with Rituximab in Patients with Rheumatoid Arthritis. *New England Journal of Medicine* 350(25):2572–2581.

Elderman J, Davis P, Owen ET (1983) Prevalence of eosinophilia during gold therapy for rheumatoid arthritis. *Journal of Rheumatology* 10:121–123.

Emery P, Panayi G, Sturrock R (1999) Targeted therapies in rheumatoid arthritis: the need for action. *Rheumatology* 38:911–912.

Emery P, Breedveld FC, Dougados M *et al.* (2002) Early referral recommendation for newly diagnosed rheumatoid arthritis: evidence based development of a clinical guide. *Annals of the Rheumatic Diseases* 61:290–297.

Estrach C, Mpofu S, Moots RJ (2003) Behcets Syndrome and Anti-Tumour Necrosis Factor Treatment. Effectivity and Tolerability in 6 Patients. *Rheumatology* 42(Suppl 1):92.

Fleischmann RM (2003) Addressing the safety of anakinra in patients with rheumatoid arthritis. *Rheumatology* 42(Suppl 2):29–35.

Furst DE (1995) Practical clinical pharmacology and drug interactions of low dose methotrexate therapy in rheumatoid arthritis. *British Journal of Rheumatology* 34(Suppl 2):20–25.

Gaubitz M, Schorat A, Schotte H *et al.* (1999) Mycophenalate mofetil for the treatment of systemic lupus erthyematosus: an open pilot trial. *Lupus* 8:731–736.

Gelfand EW (1989) The use of intravenous immune globulin in collagen vascular disorders: a potentially new modality of therapy. *Journal of Allergy and Clinical Immunology* 84:613–615.

Giannini EH, Lovell DJ, Silverman ED *et al.* (1996) Intravenous immunoglobulin in the treatment of polyarticular juvenile rheumatoid arthritis: a phase I/II study. Paediatric Rheumatology Collaborative Study Group. *Journal of Rheumatology* 23(5):919–924.

Goodwin JS, Regan M (1982) Cognitive dysfunction associated with naproxen and ibuprofen in the elderly. *Arthritis and Rheumatism* 25:1013–1015.

Griffiths B, Emery P (1996) Today's management of rheumatoid arthritis. *Prescriber* 5th July, 31–43.

Hitt E (2003) Methotrexate replaces sulphasalazine as most popular first-choice disease modifying anti-rheumatic drug in UK. Rheumatology. http://www.docguide.com/news/content.nsf/NewsPrint/8525697700573E1885256D95.htm (24 September 04).

Hulsmans HMJ, Jacobs JWG, van der Heijde DMFM *et al.* (2000) The course of radiologic damage during the first six years of rheumatoid arthritis. *Arthritis and Rheumatism* 43:1927–1940.

Humbert M, Cabane J (2003) Successful treatment of systemic sclerosis digital ulcers and pulmonary arterial hypertension with endothelin receptor antagonist bosentan. *Rheumatology* 42:191–193.

Irons K, Jeffries C (2004) *The Bath Indices: Outcome Measures for use with Ankylosing Spondylitis Patients.* East Sussex, NASS.

Jaakkola E, Crane AM, Laiho K, Herzberg I *et al.* (2003) The effect of transforming growth factor B1 gene polymorphisms in ankylosing spondylitis. *Rheumatology* 43(1):32–38.

Jobanputra P, Wilson J, Douglas K *et al.* (2004) A survey of British rheumatologists' DMARD preferences for rheumatoid arthritis. *Rheumatology* 43(2):206–210.

Karim M, Alba P, Cuadrado MJ *et al.* (2002) Mycophenalate mofetil for systemic lupus erthyematosus refractory to other immunosuppressive agents. *Rheumatology* 41:876–882.

Khamashta M (1999) Management of the antiphospholipid syndrome. Continuing Professional Development. *Rheumatology* 1(1):22–26.

Kirwan JR and the Arthritis and Rheumatism Council Low Dose Glucocorticoid Study Group (1995) The effects of glucocorticoid steroid on joint destruction in RA. *New England Journal of Medicine* 333:142–146.

Kvien TK, Zeidler HK, Hannonen P *et al.* (2002) Long term efficacy and safety of cyclosporin versus parenteral gold in early rheumatoid arthritis: a three year study of radiological progression, renal function, and arterial hypertension. *Annals of the Rheumatic Diseases* 61(6):511–516.

Kyle S, Chandler D, Griffiths CEM *et al.* (2005) Guidelines for anti-TNF-α therapy in psoriatic arthritis. *Rheumatology* 44:390–397.

Lipsky PE, Ziff M (1980) Inhibition of human helper T cell function in vitro by D-Penicillamine and copper sulphate. *Journal of Clinical Investigations* 65:1069.

Maetzel A, Wong A, Strand V *et al.* (2000) Meta-analysis of treatment termination rates among rheumatoid arthritis patients receiving disease-modifying anti-rheumatic drugs. *Rheumatology* 39:975–981.

Marshall R, Kirwan J (2001) Methotrexate in the treatment of ankylosing spondylitis. *Scandinavian Journal of Rheumatology* 30:313–314.

Merck (2004) Merck announces voluntary worldwide withdrawal of vioxx. Available at: http://vioxx.com/rofecoxib/vioxx/hcp/hcp_notification_physicians.jsp [06.11.04].

Mease P (2004) TNFα therapy in psoriatic arthritis and psoriasis. *Annals of the Rheumatic Diseases* 63(7):755–758.

Miller DR (1996) Pharmacological interventions. In: Wegener ST, Belza BL, Gall EP (eds) Clinical Care in the Rheumatic Diseases. Atlanta, American College of Rheumatology 11:68–69.

Morrison E, Crosbie D, Capell HA (2003) Attitude of rheumatoid arthritis patients to treatment with oral corticosteroids. *Rheumatology* 42(10):1247–1250.

National Institute of Clinical Excellence (2002) *Guidance on the use of Cyclo-oxygenase (COX) 11 selective inhibitors, celecoxib, refecoxib, meloxicam and etodolac for osteoarthritis and rheumatoid arthritis.* London, NICE.

National Institute of Clinical Excellence (2002) Guidance on the use of etanercept and infliximab for the treatment of rheumatoid arthritis. *Technology Appraisal 36.* www.nice.org.uk/pdf/TA036guidance.pdf (05 April 04).

National Institute of Clinical Excellence (2003) Anakinra for rheumatoid arthritis. *Technology Appraisal 72.* http://www.nice.org.uk/pdf/TA072guidance. pdf (26 June 04).

Nolle B, Heller M, Lamprecht P *et al.* (2002) Effectiveness of TNF-a blockade with infliximab in refractory Wegener's granulomatosis. *Rheumatology* 41(11): 1303–1307.

Norberg E, Norberg C (2004) Giant cell arteritis: strategies in diagnosis and treatment. *Current Opinion in Rheumatology* 16(1):25–30.

Oliver S, Mooney J (2002) Targeted therapies for patients with rheumatoid arthritis. *Professional Nurse* 17(12):716–720.

Parkinson S, Alldred A (2002) Drug regimens for rheumatoid arthritis. *Hospital Pharmacist* 9:11–15.

Pharmacia (2004) Celebrex 100mg & 200mg http://emc.medicines.org.up.emc.assets/ c/html/displayDocPrinterFriendly.asp?docum.htm (27 September 04).

Royal College of Nursing (2001) *Standards for effective practice and audit in rheumatology nursing – Guidance for nurses*. London, RCN.

Royal College of Nursing (2003) *Assessing, managing and monitoring biologic therapies for inflammatory arthritis: Guidance for rheumatology practitioners*. London, RCN.

Royal College of Nursing (2004) *Administering subcutaneous methotrexate for inflammatory arthritis*. London, RCN.

Ryan S (1999) The role of the rheumatology nurse. In: Ryan S (ed) *Drug Therapy in Rheumatology Nursing*. London, Whurr Publishers.

Scott DL (2002) Advances in the medical management of rheumatoid arthritis. *Hospital Medicine* 63(5):294–297.

Scharf SL, Christophidis N (1995) Second line agents for rheumatoid arthritis. *Medical Journal of Australia* 63(21):215–218.

Sfikakis PP (2002) Behcet's disease: a new target for anti-tumour necrosis factor treatment. *Annals of the Rheumatic Diseases* 61(Suppl II):51–53.

Susol E (2000) Association of markers for TGFß3, TGFß2 and TIMP1 with systemic sclerosis. *Rheumatology* 39:1332–1336.

Symmons D, Salmon M, Farr M (1988) Sulphasalazine treatment and lymphocyte function in patients with rheumatoid arthritis. *Journal of Rheumatology* 15:575.

Tadman J (2004) Vasculitis: new hope? *Arthritis Today* 124:22–23.

Trevisani VFM, Castro AA, Neves Neto JF *et al*. (2004) Cyclophosphamide versus methylprednisolone for treating neuropsychiatric involvement in systemic lupus erythematosus (Cochrane Review). In: *The Cochrane Library, Issue 1*, Chichester, UK, John Wiley and Sons, Ltd.

Voyce MA (1999) The role of the community team in drug therapy. Appendix: Guidelines for nurses on the use and administration of sodium aurothiomalate in rheumatoid arthritis. 284–287. In: Ryan S (ed) *Drug Therapy in Rheumatology Nursing*. London, Whurr Publishers.

Walker G (1998) *ABPI – Compendium of Data Sheets and Summaries of Product Characteristics*. London, Datapharm Publications Ltd.

Weinblatt ME, Weissman BN, Holdsworth DE (1992) Long term prospective study of methotrexate in the treatment of rheumatoid arthritis: eighty four month update. *Arthritis and Rheumatism* 35:138–145.

Wood J (1999) (4) Rheumatoid arthritis; management with DMARDs. Pharmecutical Journal. 263:162–167 [online]. http://pharmj.com/Editorial/19990731/education/dmards.html (25 September 04).

Yorkshire Rheumatology Regional Guidelines for the Monitoring of Patients on Disease Modifying Drugs (DMARDs) (2003) 2nd edn.

Zulian F, Corona F, Gerloni V *et al*. (2004) Safety and efficacy of illoprost fro the treatment of ischaemic digits in paediatric connective tissue diseases. *Rheumatology* 43(2):229–233.

13 Complementary Interventions

A. CAWTHORN
University of Manchester, Manchester, UK

P. MACKERETH
Salford University, Manchester, UK

The aim of this chapter is to critically appraise the role of complementary and alternative medicine (CAM) in rheumatology and to evaluate its potential for use with patients and carers in the light of evidence-based practice. After reading this chapter the reader should be able to:

- evaluate the popularity of CAM for patients and healthcare professionals;
- describe the definitions of CAM;
- understand how individual therapies work and evaluate the evidence base for these therapies;
- critically appraise the issues surrounding the integration of therapies into practice.

The demand for complementary therapies by the general population has increased over the past two decades and patients with rheumatological disorders are no exception. As medicine struggles to fully alleviate the symptoms of disabling rheumatological conditions, nurses and other healthcare professionals (HCP) are exploring whether the use of complementary and alternative therapies (CAM) can assist in the alleviation of the stress and disabling symptoms associated with these diseases. However, the extent to which CAM impacts on individual practice varies depending upon the nurse's commitment to it. Nonetheless, there is evidence that complementary therapies are gradually being integrated into practice with variations ranging from nurses who are now training in simple-to-use techniques, to others who are developing and coordinating a range of CAM services for patients, as well as leading evaluation and research work in the field of supportive care.

Growing numbers of patients with rheumatological disorders are using (CAM) on their own initiative and increasingly, they are seeking the views of HCPs on its:

Rheumatology Nursing: A Creative Approach, 2nd edn. Edited by Jackie Hill.
Copyright 2006 by John Wiley & Sons, Ltd.

- use
- efficacy
- availability
- safety.

Although the aim of CAM is to complement their care, patients may be using therapies that do not necessarily achieve this, making it essential that HCPs have a clear understanding of the benefits and contraindications of using the therapies in certain situations.

Because of its growing importance and prevalence, it is essential that nurses keep themselves well-informed about all aspects of CAM and to that end this chapter examines the key issues regarding its use. These include:

- definitions and models of CAM
- reasons for its increasing popularity
- evidence base for its use
- legal situation regarding the integration of CAM into clinical practice.

DEFINITIONS OF COMPLEMENTARY AND ALTERNATIVE MEDICINE

The umbrella term 'CAM' represents a bewilderingly wide range of therapeutic and diagnostic methods that have little in common (Ernst, 2004) and as the range of therapies increases, it is important to clarify what they are and what part they play in healthcare.

Tavares (2003) used the term 'complementary' to describe all therapies used alongside conventional healthcare. A more comprehensive definition of CAM is: 'any diagnosis, treatment and/or prevention which complements mainstream medicine by contributing to a common whole, by satisfying a demand not met by orthodoxy or by diversifying the conceptual framework of medicine' (Ernst *et al.*, 1995). *The Supportive and Palliative Care Manual* (NICE, 2004) defines complementary therapies as encompassing a diverse range of interventions that can include physical, psychological and pharmacological therapies, to help with symptom control and to enhance well-being.

HISTORY OF COMPLEMENTARY AND ALTERNATIVE MEDICINE

Complementary therapies in healthcare are not new and the use of herbs, oils and laying on of hands or other forms of energy treatments, have existed in some form for thousands of years (Rankin and McVey 2001). Massage was practised and taught by nurses in the first half of the 20th century and widely used in orthopaedics and rheumatology (Goldstone, 1999). Goldstone considers massage to be an orthodox therapy and suggests that linking it with aromatherapy, which does not have the same pedigree, has confused the experience of massage in nursing, with the lack of experience in providing aromatherapy.

The recent upsurge in the popularity of CAM has lead nurses and other HCPs to review their utility in relation to modern healthcare. Over the past 20 years there has been much discussion surrounding the modern use and definitions of CAM leading to publication of several reports which have offered definitions of CAM, debated their popularity with the general public, their use by health professionals, regulation of therapies and their evidence base (British Medical Association, 1993; Foundation for Integrated Medicine, 1997; House of Lords, 2000).

The Foundation of Integrated Medicine (FIM), established by HRH the Prince of Wales, produced a discussion document on Integrated Healthcare (Foundation of Integrated Medicine, 1997). This document examined practical ways for conventional and complementary therapists to work in partnership. Their findings suggest that the best way forward would be to combine the best of conventional and complementary medicine in order to offer safe integrated care.

The recent *National Guidelines for the Use of Complementary Therapies in Supportive and Palliative Care* were compiled as a result of collaboration of experts in the field of CAM who explored the provision and availability of complementary therapies for patients suffering from long-term or chronic illness. (Tavares, 2003) They explored the provision and availability of complementary therapies and evaluated examples of best practice in the UK. The document is recommended for all practitioners in this field as it provides invaluable information in relation to safe use of individual therapies. It includes information relating to clinical governance, regulation and training of therapists and audit and evaluation.

POPULARITY OF COMPLEMENTARY AND ALTERNATIVE MEDICINE

Complementary and alternative therapies are gaining in popularity (Ernst and White, 2000). Surveys in the UK and Australia suggest that between 25% and 50% of the general population use CAM regularly, often at their own expense (Corner and Harewood, 2004; Ernst, 2003). The Foundation for Integrated Health examined consumer use and preference of CAM (Ong and Banks, 2003). They found that the most commonly used therapies were:

- acupuncture
- aromatherapy
- chiropractic

- homeopathy
- hypnotherapy
- herbal medicine
- osteopathy
- reflexology.

This work also highlighted an enormous increase in uptake of over-the-counter remedies such as herbal and homeopathic remedies, aromatherapy oils and self-help classes such as yoga, relaxation and meditation. The report concluded that the most frequent use of CAM is for illnesses of more than one year duration, the most common being for musculoskeletal problems and back and neck pain.

CAM IN HEALTHCARE

Much of the literature suggests that CAM is now finding a more substantial place within healthcare. A study of the provision of CAM within general practice found that 39% of general practitioner partnerships in England provided some form of complementary therapies through the National Health Service (Thomas et al., 2001). In rheumatology, Ernst (1998) found growing evidence of its use, but that there remains some scepticism about its usefulness amongst more senior medical colleagues. However, this scepticism did not apply to acupuncture, which enjoyed the best level of acceptance.

The Royal College of Nursing (RCN, 2003) reviewed the position of complementary therapies in relation to nursing practice and identified that the therapies offered most frequently by nurses were massage, aromatherapy and reflexology. Reiki healing was gaining in popularity, with acupuncture and acupuncture techniques beginning to be used by a number of respondents.

Patients appear to be motivated to use alternative therapies in the belief that CAM has the potential to offer positive benefits. Holdcroft et al. (2000) suggest that rheumatology patients, especially those with disorders that have generally unsatisfactory treatment options such as fibromyalgia syndrome (FMS), are high users of CAM. In one survey, 63% of patients with rheumatological disorders other than FMS, and 91% of those with FMS were currently using some form of CAM (Pioro-Boisset et al., 1996). In the USA, Astin (1998) found arthritis to be the most frequently cited health problem treated with CAM.

Ernst (1998) evaluated fourteen surveys of the use of CAM by rheumatology patients and concluded that the most popular treatment modalities were:

- massage
- acupuncture
- chiropractic.

Two further studies of patients with rheumatic diseases found that CAM used to be highly prevalent, with homeopathy being one of the most popular treatments (Visser *et al.*, 1992; Dimmock *et al.*, 1996).

The RCN has recognised the growth in this area and has developed guidelines for the safe integration of therapies into nursing practice (RCN, 2003). However, despite a greater consensus regarding the integration of therapies into healthcare, confusion still exists about how therapies are defined and why they are chosen.

MODELS DEFINING CAM

Over the years different models have been proposed that have attempted to categorise the broad range of therapies available. The House of Lords Report (2000) on complementary and alternative medicine divided therapies into three areas.

PROFESSIONALLY ORGANISED ALTERNATIVE THERAPIES

This area includes:

- acupuncture
- homeopathy
- herbal medicine
- chiropractic
- osteopathy.

COMPLEMENTARY THERAPIES

This area includes:

- aromatherapy
- bodywork therapies
- mind-body therapies
- reflexology.

ALTERNATIVE DISCIPLINES

This area includes:

- Ayurvedic medicine (traditional)
- Chinese herbal medicine (traditional)
- Eastern medicine (traditional)

- crystal healing (alternative)
- iridology (alternative)
- kinesiology (alternative).

In the USA, the National Center for Complementary and Alternative Medicine (NCCAM) categorised CAM therapies, dividing them into five broad types:

- alternative medical systems
- biologically based therapies
- energy therapies
- manipulative and body based methods
- mind-body interventions.

Whilst these models help governments and organisations to categories therapies, they are often less useful to those wanting a model that relates directly to clinical practice. Given that many nurses now acknowledge that complementary interventions have the potential to enhance care, it is important to develop a model that safely integrates CAM into healthcare.

THE INTEGRATIVE MODEL OF HOLISTIC CARE

The Integrative Model of Holistic Care (IMHC) is a way of conceptualising the use of CAM within healthcare and is applied here to rheumatology. The IMHC was influenced by the work of Kearney (2000), a palliative care consultant, and developed further by Cawthorn (2002) through her work as a nurse in rheumatology and rehabilitation and later in cancer and palliative care. The model involves offering CAM therapies, alongside medical care, to work with the person on their own healing journey (Cawthorn, 2004). It is shown diagrammatically in Figure 13.1.

The aim of the model is to offer an integrative approach to care, which acknowledges the medical management that the patient may be receiving (left side of diagram) and offers an approach that, through integration of CAM techniques (right side of the diagram) can enhance the care the patient receives. The three core components which link the two sides, offer a way of working that provides individualised, holistic care.

The first core aspect of the IMHC aims to work with the whole person (mind, body and soul) in supporting them through their unique response to their illness. (Molassiotis et al., 2004). Rheumatology patients frequently need support to cope with their diagnosis, prognosis and subsequent treatments and in adjusting to a life-limiting illness that often threatens their sense of self. This is facilitated by the development of a therapeutic relationship, through which the patient is invited to work in partnership with the nurse or therapist.

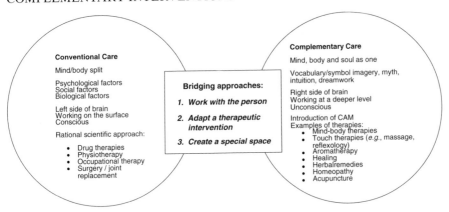

Figure 13.1 Integrative model of holistic care (IMHC).

The second aspect of the core model involves adapting therapeutic interventions to suit the patient's needs. This can involve a range of interventions to suit the patient's needs. Through close links with the multidisciplinary team, therapies are then introduced which are in the best interest and safety of the patient (RCN, 2003). The benefit to the CAM therapist from working in this way is that they have knowledge of treatment regimes and any contraindications for the particular therapy.

The third element at the core of IMHC is the creation of a special space, a holding environment where one person can attune to the other's needs. This space can be created anywhere, even in a busy ward or outpatient department. It is about the nurse or therapist learning how to create an invisible protective bubble around themselves and the patient, in which the patient feels sufficiently safe to share their concerns or needs and then, where possible, having these needs met. It is similar to a definition of containment given by Bions (1962), which entails being there with another to support them through their suffering.

Healthcare practice that offers interventions only from the left side of Figure 13.1 may leave the nurse feeling ill-equipped to deal with the psychological problems that patients present with. By utilising techniques from the right side of the diagram the nurse or therapist is able to support patients at a deeper level. This can prove therapeutic to patients who are struggling to come to terms with a disabling illness or who are attempting to cope with difficult symptoms such as pain, fatigue and altered body image. Tavares (2003) suggests that evidence is now emerging which demonstrates that CAM, used alongside conventional care, has an important role in helping to reduce the side effects of treatments. Often supportive techniques such as touch, massage, visualisation or relaxation can help create special spaces within clinical environments.

CHOOSING A COMPLEMENTARY THERAPY WITHIN A HEALTHCARE SETTING

Choosing a complementary therapy that will enhance patient care entails thorough investigation of potential benefits along with critical evaluation of the available research. The evidence base for complementary therapies needs to be considered by managers and clinicians, as well as commissioners and providers of care (Tavares, 2003).

It is sometimes argued that at present the evidence of effectiveness for most CAM therapies is minimal or nonexistent (Molassiotis *et al.*, 2004). However, Tavares (2003) takes a broader view and whilst acknowledging that the evidence base is greater for some therapies than others, argues that 'lack of evidence is not necessarily evidence of a lack of effectiveness'. Many would defend this position, whilst also calling for more research in this field.

Each therapy should be considered in relation to their application to practice and their evidence base and commonly used are discussed in the context which follows.

TOUCH AND BODYWORK INTERVENTIONS

The use of touch in human relationships is complex and plays an important role in our survival and security (Autton, 1989). Touch is a frequent activity within nursing and (Verity, 1996) suggests that it is used to:

- signal caring
- achieve nursing goals
- provide comfort.

Touch can be both an intentional and an intuitive act. The holistic practitioner will always attempt to combine the two, so that the maximum information and benefit can be obtained. Patients that have received a combined approach, recognise when the nurse is providing only instrumental touch, such as when giving an injection without intuitively acknowledging what the experience is like for the patient. An example where both intentional and intuitive touch are combined is during massage, where the therapist might palpate soft tissue, provide effleurage (stroking) and be noticing the patient's breathing as a possible indicator of enjoyment or discomfort with treatment.

SUPPORTIVE EMPATHIC TOUCH

This form of touch can be simply taught to nurses, as the aim is to communicate empathic understanding. Intention is a key issue in relation to touch and in the past, nursing practice has been criticised for being largely task-orientated in its touching behaviours. Supportive empathic touch works on a physical and intuitive level and provides comfort that is a physical expression of being there and with the patient. It is a familiar and valued nursing skill that requires sensitivity and time, but is a simple activity that can be profound in its humanising effects and is often moving for both the patient and the nurse. Nurses who are overburdened and time-deprived may avoid this intimate act, unsure of their capacity to be in the moment and open to be really present for another.

CONCERNS ABOUT TOUCH

The manipulation of soft tissue, in the form of massage, reflexology or aromatherapy has many possible benefits, some not yet fully understood or evaluated within healthcare. The work of the Touch Research Institutes (www.miami.edu/touch-research) and others has helped to clarify the benefits of massage for people with chronic diseases including fibromyalgia and cancer, and to diminish any concerns. Using a number of validated physiological and psychological measures, massage has been demonstrated to reduce cortisol levels, anxiety and pain (Field, 2000). Many arthritic problems respond well to massage, especially if it is gentle and avoids pressure on swollen joints. Touch therapies such as reflexology and foot massage could be an ideal non-pharmacological way of managing difficult symptoms, such as pain and nausea, as well as reducing stress and limiting anxiety (Stephenson and Weinrich, 2000).

MASSAGE

Massage combines both intentional and intuitive touch. It is a skill, used and taught by nurses in the past, but which fell out of favour until fairly recently. Ernst (2004) cites a Cochrane review of the use of massage in rheumatology, concluding that whilst massage does have some potential for this patient group, more research is needed because its evidence base is limited. Despite this, the use of massage in rheumatology is currently experiencing a revival. It is also widely used in supportive and palliative care where more evidence is emerging to support its effectiveness (Tavares, 2003).

Massage can vary from an easily taught, simple stroking to more complex techniques, requiring lengthy training. Therapeutic massage involves manipulation of the soft tissues of the body and can relieve tension and increase relaxation. A massage has the effect of calming the mind, soothing the nerves and relaxing the body. Massage can:

- reduce pain and stiffness by relaxing tight, aching muscles;
- reduce pain by stimulating large diameter fibres, which has an effect on the gate control mechanism in the spinal cord (Chapter 8);

- nourish tissues and assist in the removal of waste, through increases in blood and lymphatic circulation;
- lower the blood pressure, pulse and respiration rates;
- promote relaxation, if the massage is slow and soothing;
- increase a feeling of well-being and help with symptoms such as fatigue and depression, especially if the massage is slightly more stimulating.

In addition to the formalised use of touch which is practised using massage, nurses are being taught much simpler ways of offering touch which do not require an in-depth massage course (Cawthorn and Carter, 2000). The use of light massage using holding techniques and stroking can have a very relaxing, calming effect on patients. It can be taught simply, as the aim is to communicate empathic understanding. This form of touch can be described as supportive empathic touch.

REFLEXOLOGY

Reflexology is based on the principle that there are reflex areas in the feet and hands, which correspond to all the glands, organs and parts of the body (National Occupational Standards for Reflexology, 2005). It has been called an ancient healing art with a variety of techniques and philosophical approaches to its practice. Schools of thought regarding how reflexology works (Tiran, 1996), include:

- Eastern theory, in which treatment areas relate to acupuncture meridians and 'chi' energy flow;
- Western theory, that helping the recipient to relax and destress supports their innate ability to self-heal.

Dougans and Ellis (1996) believe reflexology is a branch of Chinese medicine, with the reflex areas being part of meridian systems similar to the mapping of acupuncture points. Many reflexology texts refer to an Egyptian wall painting discovered in 1897 in a tomb at Saqqara. The painting depicts a form of healing work demonstrating pressure and manipulation of the hands and feet and dated around 2250 BC.

Modern reflexologists do not claim to cure illnesses; rather they believe that reflexology can help in symptom management (Kunz and Kunz, 1993). In a Department of Health document aimed at informing primary care groups about complementary therapies, reflexology was described as the application of pressure to the feet and/or hands in order to assess the health of the patient and promote well-being (DoH et al., 2000).

Reflexology, in common with other CAM interventions, is usually carried out on a one-to-one basis. Typically, sessions are weekly and involve hands-on treatment lasting between 35 and 50 minutes. Patients are usually advised to attend a minimum of six sessions, as benefits are believed to be cumulative (Norman, 1992). It is not uncommon for patients who claim to experience benefit to continue attending, but usually on a fortnightly or monthly basis. The vast majority of reflexology treatments are carried out in the community, in either private clinics or in a patient's own home. Patients sometimes do not tell their general practitioner (GP) that they are receiving reflexology, possibly fearing that it might not be met with approval. However, increasingly, GPs and other health care practitioners are endorsing reflexology (Rankin-Box, 1997; Trevelyan, 1996).

Regulation of reflexologists

Consumers and providers of complementary therapies require competent and accountable practitioners. The education and regulation of CAM practitioners has been the focus of much criticism amongst healthcare professionals (British Medical Association, 1993; Foundation for Integrated Medicine, 1997). A survey of professional reflexology associations suggests there are in excess of 12,000 reflexologists currently operating in the UK (Mills and Budd, 2000), represented by over sixteen bodies, each with different requirements for training and ongoing registration. The majority of these groups are now working together as the Reflexology Forum to develop a standard curriculum for reflexology schools and recommendations for regulation and the continuing education of practitioners (Mills and Budd, 2000).

Reflexology research

Much of the growing research in reflexology has been conducted within palliative care, with reports of reduction in anxiety and pain (Stephenson and Weinrich, 2000) and improvements in well-being and relief from tension (Wright et al., 2002). Poole et al. (2001) in a study of patients (n = 243) with chronic low back pain compared reflexology with relaxation. The finding identified the main effect as statistically significant pain reduction, irrespective of group. Conversely, analysis of data from interviews with a subset of 22 participants showed greater reduction in pain, increased relaxation and an enhanced ability to cope following the reflexology. The case study below typifies the subtle improvements noticed by patients who use reflexology to manage chronic health problems.

Reflexology case study

Joan, aged 52, has rheumatoid arthritis and sought reflexology rather than massage as she found it uncomfortable to lay on a massage couch. The reflexologist gently worked both her feet and her hands, using cream rather than talcum powder. All the reflex points for stress were noticeably tender and after four sessions, Joan reported noticeable improvements in the quality and duration of sleep and less pain in her joints. In particular, her feet and hands felt looser. Joan described her feet as being 'spongy and soft' after the treatment, making walking a little easier for a few days each time. She continued to take her existing medications, using reflexology every two weeks to maintain the improved sleeping and mobility levels that had been achieved by week four.

AROMATHERAPY

Aromatherapy is an ancient healing art that has gained in popularity, to become one of the most popular therapies both for nurses and patients. It involves the controlled use of essential oils, manufactured from plant materials, to promote healing and relaxation of the body, mind and emotions. The oils have a balancing effect on the mind and body. In the UK, the practice of aromatherapy is still in its infancy, whereas in continental Europe it is more widely accepted by doctors and much more research has been undertaken.

Cooke and Ernst (2000) undertook a systematic review of the use of aromatherapy massage to reduce anxiety in healthcare settings. The six studies that met their inclusion criteria were undertaken in the field of cancer and supportive care. All these studies demonstrated a short-term reduction of the patients' anxiety levels. (Tavares, 2003)

Aromatherapy can be used in a variety of ways:

• massage
• baths
• compresses and irrigation
• creams
• inhalations
• mouthwashes.

Aromatherapy massage

Aromatherapy massage involves using a carrier oil, such as grapeseed or sweet almond, to which the essential oil is added. Concentrations of essential oils vary, but the lower dose recommended by Price and Price (1995), of 1%–1.5%, (2–3 drops in 10 mls of oil), is probably best suited to patients with rheumatic disease. The choice of essential oil is agreed between the patient and the nurse, based on a number of factors. Oils, which have proved useful for arthritis are:

• lavender (*Lavendula angustafolia*)
• Roman chamomile (*Anthemis nobilis*)

- lemon (*Citrus limonu*)
- ginger (*Zingiber officinale*)
- marjoram (*Origanum majorana*)
- juniper berry (*Juniperus communis*)
- black pepper (*Piper nigrum*)
- rosemary (*Rosmarinus officinalis*)
- eucalyptus (*Eucalyptus globulus*).

Baths

Essential oils can be useful in bathing, either in addition to massage or as an alternative, when massage is not appropriate. Appropriate essential oils are those previously stated as being useful for arthritis. Alternatively, lavender, marjoram, Roman chamomile or sandalwood could be chosen to help with sleep problems (Price and Price, 1995). Tavares (2003) recommends that to avoid skin reactions, the oils are diluted in a safe medium, such as milk before adding to the water.

Compress/irrigation

A compress is particularly useful where massage is not suitable, but where an inflamed joint or area of skin could benefit from the effects of the compress combined with the therapeutic effects of the oils. Two oils that have proved useful, either individually or combined, due to their anti-inflammatory properties are lavender and Roman chamomile (Buckle, 1997). A patch test, involving a small application of the oil mix, usually 1–2% dilution to a visible area of skin (*e.g.*, the forearm) is recommended first (Buckle, 1997). If there is no adverse reaction then two or three drops of oils either singularly or in combination can be added to 500 ml of either warm or cold water. This solution can also be used to irrigate an infected wound, which is useful as essentials oils are reported to have antibiotic, antiviral and antifungal properties (Buckle, 1997).

Creams

Creams are particularly useful where a skin condition is evident. Some skin conditions may be secondary to the disease, such as psoriasis or the butterfly rash associated with systemic lupus erythematosus. Others may be related to conditions such as athletes' foot. An aqueous cream is used as the base and two or three drops of essential oils, as prescribed by an aromatherapist (there is a wide range of oils that might be useful), added to each 10 mls of cream. Another effective medium for the essential oils is aloe vera gel, which is also beneficial when used alone.

Inhalation

Inhalation is a simple, but effective way of using aromatherapy. The oils are absorbed through the nose and travel via the olfactory system to the limbic system in the brain. Inhalation can be used in one of two ways. One or two drops of essential oil on a tissue can be placed on the pillow or alternatively, three to six drops of essential oil or oils, (again an aromatherapist would need to be consulted) can be placed in a bowl of hot water or a vapouriser. Caution must be taken if the patient, or others in the vicinity, has respiratory problems such as asthma. Electric vapourisers should not be used in the presence of oxygen and health and safety procedures must be followed in relation to the use of burners (Tavares, 2003).

Mouthwash

Mouthwash is useful either to freshen the mouth or when there is an infection of the mouth, gums or throat. In the latter case, antifungal/antibacterial oils such as lemon, tea tree (*Melaleuca alternifolia*) or peppermint should be used. Half fill a cup with warm water and add two or three drops of essential oils.

Aromatherapy case study 1

Jean was a 44-year-old woman with long standing psoriatic arthritis. The psoriasis was over most of her body but it was particularly problematic in the hairline where it had a tendency to bleed. Baths using lavender and Roman chamomile took away the irritation from the body. Aqueous cream with the same oils dramatically improved the hairline.

Aromatherapy case study 2

Sometimes, it is useful to use a variety of methods, as illustrated by the following case study.

Linda was a 30-year-old woman who had a five year history of systemic lupus erythematosus. Her main problems were pain, fatigue, tension, anxiety, sleep issues, poor circulation, photosensitivity and a very marked butterfly rash.

A variety of treatments were used. Aqueous cream with two drops of lavender and one drop of Roman chamomile to 10 mls of cream was applied daily to the rash. This allowed Linda to stop using her steroid cream. Weekly or fortnightly massage was given to back, arms and legs, to help relieve pain, tension and circulatory problems. The essential oils chosen were eucalyptus, lavender, ylang ylang (*Canango odorata*), marjoram, sandalwood, black pepper and ginger. Their use varied over time, and a maximum of three were used together. To help with anxiety and to support her whilst her beta-blockers were being reduced, neroli oil (*Citrus aurantium*) an anxiolytic oil was used. Between treatments, to support her at home and to help her sleep, Linda was recommended to use essential oils in the bath.

This regime proved very effective and both her rheumatologist and her GP were happy with the result. Before Linda received these treatments she experienced much pain and tension. Following them she required less analgesia and her quality of life was greatly improved.

HEALING AND ENERGY THERAPIES

Belief in the human potential for transmitting energies is not new. Some societies take healing for granted, whilst in others, such as in the UK it is not as well accepted. When discussing these therapies the nurse needs to make clear how they work since the term 'healing' could be misunderstood by the patient to mean 'cure'. Most evidence on the use of healing and energy therapies is from the field of supportive and palliative care. Tavares (2003) states that these therapies have the potential to:

- contribute to pain relief
- promote relaxation
- improve sleep patterns
- reduce tension, stress and anxiety
- provide emotional or spiritual support
- contribute to a sense of well-being.

The three most popular energy therapies are:

- therapeutic touch
- Reiki
- spiritual healing.

Whilst these techniques vary slightly, they have many similarities. In each, the patient is fully clothed and is either lying on a couch or bed, or alternatively, sitting on a chair. The technique is noninvasive, involving either light touch or holding techniques. Alternatively the practitioner can work without touching the patient, with their hands hovering over the patient.

THERAPEUTIC TOUCH

Therapeutic touch emerged in the 1970s, introduced into mainstream nursing education in New York by Delores Krieger, a professor of nursing. Sayer-Adams and Wright (2001), who teach therapeutic touch in England, see it as a contemporary interpretation of ancient healing practices. They describe it as a consciously directed process of energy exchange, during which the practitioner uses the hands as a focus to facilitate healing, its success being dependent upon the healer's ability to channel these energies. Any imbalance in energies can be assessed and the therapist works towards clearing these areas in order to promote a feeling of harmony and wholeness. Sayer-Adams and Wright (2001) present a comprehensive an overview and analysis of the evidence base.

REIKI

Reiki is an ancient form of healing which Dr Mikao Uswi rediscovered in the nineteenth century in Japan. Its uses are similar to those of therapeutic touch and a treatment takes between 20 minutes and one hour. Although evidence is beginning to emerge, the evidence base for Reiki is somewhat limited. However, anecdotal evidence suggests that it is gaining popularity in the field of supportive and palliative care, with nurses being trained up to level 2, which is practitioner level, and level 3, master/teacher practitioner level (Tavares, 2003).

SPIRITUAL HEALING

Spiritual healing is an ancient therapy, which has been used throughout recorded history. It is often referred to simply as healing and is a process that promotes better health by the channelling of healing energies through the healer to the patient (National Federation of Spiritual Healers, 1998). Ernst (2004) reports that there have been numerous forms of randomised controlled trials (RCT) published, on various forms of spiritual healing, but that it is still unclear whether it alleviates arthritic pain more than placebo.

HOMEOPATHY

Homeopathy is considered to be a complete system of healing (Pietroni, 1995). It has gained acceptance in the UK, where it is one of the few complementary therapies available through the NHS. Dr Samuel Hanemann, the founder of modern homeopathy, observed that many of the treatments given to treat disease, actually cause symptoms similar to those produced by the disease itself. This is based on the principle that 'like cures like'. The homeopathic remedies are obtained from animal, mineral or plant extracts and are preserved in an alcohol solution, which is then called 'the mother tincture'.

Research into homeopathy has not been sufficiently conclusive to satisfy some sceptics, who attribute its results purely to the placebo effect. However, this does not fully explain the results achieved by homeopathic veterinary surgeons, who successfully treat cattle with mastitis by adding remedies to their feed, or laboratory results which show the prevention of recurrent abortions in pigs (Pietroni, 1995).

Long and Ernst (2001) undertook a systematic review of homeopathic remedies for osteoarthritis. They concluded that there is evidence of efficacy in the treatment of OA, but that due to the paucity of rigorous studies conducted to date, further research is warranted. However, Tavares (2003) whilst acknowledging the limitations of the research, suggests that there is sufficient evidence to support its use in supportive care for:

- fatigue
- pain, including joint pain and muscle spasm
- anxiety and stress
- depression
- improve quality of life.

HERBAL MEDICINES

Herbal medicines, which utilize the healing properties of plant substances, have a long history of use by patients. Some of the more common herbal medicines are beginning to be integrated into rheumatology, either by patients alone or in conjunction with their rheumatologist. Two of the most common are fish oils for rheumatoid arthritis and glucosamine for osteoarthritis. Ariza-Ariza et al. (1998) reviewed RCTs of fish oil medication, finding it to be more clinically effective than placebo and leading to a significant reduction in long-term use of nonsteroidal anti-inflammatory drugs (NSAIDs). Ernst (2004) also supports the use of fish oil medications, confirming that they have a place as an adjunctive treatment for rheumatoid arthritis.

Ernst (2004) reports on the effect of glucosamine, which occurs naturally in the body, referring to it as the building block of substances found in the articular cartilage. It is now commonly marketed for osteoarthritis. He undertook two meta-analyses of studies of its use and concluded that it was superior to placebo. However, he went on to criticise the validity of the studies because of various methodological problems.

An important aspect of herbal medicines is safety and in particular whether they interact with other prescribed medications. Hypericum (St John's Wort) is a prime example. Whilst it has an excellent safety profile for use in mild to moderate depression, many patients and some nurses and other HCPs may be unaware of its potential interaction with other medications such as anticoagulants, oral contraceptives and antiviral agents, altering the therapeutic effect of these drugs in different ways.

MIND-BODY THERAPIES

Over the past three decades there has been an increasing interest in mind-body interactions in modern medicine. Psychoneuroimmunology (PNI) research studies the interrelationships between the brain, behaviour and the immune system and how our state of mind affects our health. Watkins (1997) suggests that as a result of PNI research, there is hard scientific data providing evidence that the central nervous system controls nearly all the body's defence systems.

Therapies included in this group are:

- relaxation
- visualisation
- meditation
- guided imagery
- biofeedback
- self-help management which involves stress and anxiety management
- counselling
- psychotherapy including hypnotherapy and cognitive behavioural therapy;
- bodywork.

Ancient healing systems have always recognised the link between the mind and the body. Kearney (2000) reminds us of the role of the shaman in providing physical, psychological and spiritual care. Ayurvedic Medicine, a holistic healing system of the Indian subcontinent used since 2500 BC, has as its guiding principle, that the mind influences the body (Arthritis Care, 2002). Much of the research into mind-body medicine is in the field of cancer care, although the principles are easily transferable to rheumatology.

RELAXATION

Ryman (1994) describes relaxation techniques as 'planned and structured activities leading to peace of mind and enhanced quality of life'. Carroll and Seers (1998) undertook a systematic review of all types of relaxation for chronic pain and arrived at cautiously positive conclusions in favour of its use. Relaxation produces a feeling of peace enabling the patient to release tension and to reduce feelings of anxiety and fear. It is one of the easier therapies for nurses to learn and integrate into their practice. This can be done either through reading a script or through use of audiotapes. Relaxation can be used on its own, or before moving on to visualisation or imagery.

VISUALISATION

Visualisation helps to develop a sense of well-being by using the mind to change negative images into positive ones. We all have a storehouse of positive memories, which if accessed can be used in difficult situations. It helps patients cope with their treatments and to manage the numerous invasive investigations, by allowing them to switch their thoughts and access pleasant memories. An example of this would be to teach patients to access memories of a pleasant experience such as a beach, or a personal achievement, whilst they are having an MRI scan or a joint injection.

IMAGERY

Imagery is a flow of thoughts you can see, hear, feel smell, or taste. It is a way that your mind codes, stores, and expresses information (Rossman, 2000). Imagery involves working with the unconscious, accessing the right side of the brain, which involves the use of symbol, myth, memories, daydreams and dreams and involves working with the deeper self.

At its simplest level it can be used to turn unwanted or negative images into positive ones. It can assist in the management of distressing symptoms such as pain, anxiety, nausea and body image (Cawthorn, 2004). Giedt (1997) uses guided imagery based on PNI principles as a nursing intervention, working on the basis that pain can cause both a physical sensation and a mental image. For example, in the case of a severe headache, by paying attention to the metaphors used by a patient to describe both the pain sensation and the headache, the nurse can help to change their perception and the headache. If they describe the headache as being like having their head in a vice, the nurse would work with them, first to imagine the vice and then to imagine releasing it. Another example would be to encourage a patient to imagine a cool fluid, which will reduce heat and so relieve a burning sensation.

ACUPUNCTURE

Traditional acupuncture

The word acupuncture derives from the Latin acus meaning needle and puncture, to puncture the skin. Acupuncture originated in China approximately 4000 years ago and has developed into an intricate holistic approach to healing. It is a treatment that aims to diagnose illness, as well as assisting the body to restore a balance, which in turn promotes health. According to traditional Chinese medicine, everything in the universe, including human beings, shares a motivating energy called 'Qi' (pronounced chee) which circulates between the organs along channels called meridians. Health is achieved by maintaining a balance between the yin and yang, the equal and opposite qualities of the Qi. Aspects of life can upset this balance and disturb the flow of Qi, causing disease or disharmony. The main aim of traditional acupuncture treatment is to restore the flow of the Qi and the balance between yin and yang.

Western approach to acupuncture

Many conventional HCPs who practise acupuncture reject the traditional theories of yin-yang, Qi and meridians. Current theory suggests that acupuncture points correspond to physiological and anatomical features such as peripheral nerve junctions and diagnosis is made in purely conventional terms. It is also thought that trigger points correspond to acupuncture points. (Vickers et al., 2002).

Acupuncture is now one of the most commonly used complementary medicines in both private and NHS practice (Vickers et al., 2002), with an estimated 7% of the population having received it (Thomas et al., 2001).

CARING FOR CARERS

The burden of caring for people with advanced chronic health problems usually falls on partners, family and friends. Witnessing a loved one being investigated, diagnosed and treated can be stressful and exhausting. Research in the USA evaluated the provision of massage to thirteen carers (Oregon Hospice Association and East-West College of Healing Arts, 1998) and identified a number of benefits. Following six massages, 85% reported reduced emotional and physical stress levels, 77% reduced physical pain and 54% much improved sleep patterns. In the UK a study involving focus groups, reported that a massage service for family members of patients receiving palliative care was well evaluated by participants (Penson, 1998). More recently, a service providing chair massage for carers in an acute cancer setting, has reported improvements in well-being, sleep and stress following single fifteen-minute massage sessions provided in ward settings (Mackereth et al., 2003).

LEGAL CONCERNS

The legal concept of 'duty of care' requires practitioners to always treat patients with due skill and care (Stone, 2002). Currently, complementary therapies are not generally perceived as a core healthcare service; but nevertheless, when provided, these interventions must be delivered by skilled and accountable practitioners. If the activity is delegated, those making referrals need assurance that it is beneficial and safe. Because complementary therapies often involve touch, the civil action of battery, or trespass to the person, which upholds respect for the patient's bodily autonomy, is of great importance. Informed consent is required, since battery occurs if touch is given to a patient, without first obtaining their permission. The case study below exemplifies poor ethical and professional practice.

LEGAL CONCERNS CASE STUDY

Staff Nurse Roberts has just completed a massage course at a local college. To obtain experience, she decides to carry out a full body massage on a patient in her care, who has fibromyalgia and depression. Prior to treating the patient, the nurse did not approach the patient's family, the consultant or ward manager to seek their support. The patient tells another nurse about the treatment, saying that although she enjoyed having her hands and feet massaged, it hurt in places on her back and she felt embarrassed about taking her clothes off.

MANAGERIAL ISSUES

The fictitious case study above may discourage managers from considering developing complementary therapy services. In addition to the potential for litigation, the intervention was clearly inappropriate and was carried out with no formal protocols in place to safeguard patient care. Rather than treating it as a learning experience, a skilled and accountable practitioner would have prepared thoroughly before providing services to patients. To provide safe and therapeutic interventions, policies and protocols must be agreed and practitioners equipped to adapt their skills to the individual.

An important starting point is the establishment of a complementary therapy committee, to carry out this work. This committee should have representation from practitioners, management and, if possible, service users. Alternatively, policy and practice committees could fulfil this role. A number of UK Trusts have been proactive in this area and can be approached for advice and copies of protocols and policies (Rankin-Box and McVey, 2001). *Guidelines for the use of Complementary Therapies in Supportive and Palliative Care* (Tavares, 2003) is a valuable resource for any team establishing complementary therapy services. It includes examples of protocols, referral documentation and a review of the evidence for a variety of therapies, as well as an extensive resource list. An important recommendation is the adoption of a coordinator/practitioner role to:

• facilitate service development
• recruit and manage volunteers and paid therapists
• act as a resource for healthcare staff and patients
• audit existing or piloted services.

This activity, along with evidence from literature reviews, can reinforce applications for future funding as a core service.

PRACTICAL CONSIDERATIONS

In practice, developing a complementary therapy service presents a number of challenges. Integration has been slow, with delivery often on an ad hoc basis, sometimes provided by interested nurses and allied health professionals as part of their role development or as a research project. In some centres, volunteer therapists, supervised by clinical staff, visit wards and departments to provide short treatments to patients. Individual patients can also request private treatment by self-employed therapists. It is essential that the patient and their consultant give prior consent to any interventions offered. The consent should be documented and a note of treatment sessions kept in the patient's records.

Because of potential problems with training standards and regulation, it is important for all parties to be assured of the competence of practitioners, their adherence to a code of conduct and that there is appropriate insurance cover. On a practical level, the therapist must be able and willing to adapt treatment to the individual. This may require further training and support from skilled mentors. Importantly, reflective practice and clinical supervision can help to sustain and develop therapeutic skills, safeguarding professional and accountable practice and supporting quality care (Mackereth, 2000).

Working in hospital environments can be very different from private practice. Finding a mutually convenient time for treatment is an example, with a need to avoid offering treatment at mealtimes, during ward rounds or at peak visiting times. Dryden *et al.* (1999) reported that the favoured time for treatment was early afternoon when the ward had a rest period and there were few visitors. Key points for practice are listed in Table 13.1.

CONCLUSION

Many patients are looking to CAM as a means of managing some of the symptoms of rheumatological diseases. The safe integration of CAM has been demonstrated in the field of supportive and palliative care and the models developed there provide an excellent example that can be replicated in rheumatology. Although the evidence base for therapies needs further development, there is sufficient evidence to demonstrate that an experienced therapist using appropriate therapies has the potential to help patients cope with difficult symptoms and improve their quality of life.

Research evidence for complementary therapies is increasing, but future research needs to adopt more rigorous and appropriate methodology. Issues relating to integration of therapies into healthcare must be noted especially as models of good practice are now available.

ACTION POINTS FOR PRACTICE

- Assess the evidence base for the therapies used in your practice area.
- Evaluate the use of touch and consider what therapies primarily use touch.

Table 13.1 Practice points for nurses using complementary therapies (CTs)

Preparation

- Ensure you have consent from the patient, their consultant and the departmental head nurse.
- Encourage the patient to inform their family and/or partner that they are considering receiving CTs.
- Ensure you have made a workable contract with the patient. For example, identify how they might like to feel at the end of the session (e.g., energised, relaxed or more comfortable, but not a substitute for prescribed pain medication).
- Adhere to hospital infection control policies – strict hand washing, use of clean towel with each patient and correct disposal of paper towels.
- Arrange a suitable time for the treatment. For example, choose a time when neither of you will be interrupted.
- Make sure that the environment and the position you are working in is comfortable at all times.

During and after treatment

- Check with the patient intermittently that they are comfortable and happy to continue (ongoing consent).
- If a patient's visitor wishes to be present (and the patient agrees) make sure that they are briefed before hand. Knowing that they will need to sit quietly can be useful as relatives often feel that they have to talk.
- Acknowledge background noise and distractions in busy clinical settings by noticing it but coming back to the work. (You can ask the patient to do likewise.)
- Make sure that you can monitor the patient's post-treatment responses. For example, avoid treating a patient just before finishing your shift.
- Record the treatment(s) within the patient's existing records and maintain your own confidential records.

(Adapted from Mackereth [2002])

- Discuss the aspects that need to be considered in relation to safe integration of therapies.
- A 38-year-old male patient has psoriatic arthritis. Describe the complementary therapies that may help him.

REFERENCES

Arthritis Care (2002) *The Balanced Approach – A Guide to Medicines and Complementary Therapies*. London, Arthritis Care.

Autton N (1989) *Touch: An Exploration*. London, Longman.

Astin JA (1998) Why patients use alternative medicine. *Journal of the American Medical Association* 279:1548–1553.

Ariza-Ariza R, Mestanza-Peralta M, Cardiel MH (1998) Omega – 3 fatty acids in rheumatoid arthritis: an overview. *Seminars in Arthritis and Rheumatism* 27(6):336–370.

Bions WRA (1962) Theory of Thinking. *International Journal of Psychoanalysis* 43: Parts 4–5.

British Medical Association (1993) *Complementary Medicine New Approaches to Good Practice.* London, British Medical Association.

Buckle J (1997) *Clinical Aromatherapy in Nursing.* London, Arnold, p119.

Carroll D, Seers K (1998) Relaxation for the relief of chronic pain: a systematic review. *Journal of Advanced Nursing* 27:476–487.

Cawthorn A, Carter A (2000) Aromatherapy and its application in cancer and palliative care. *Complementary Therapies in Nursing and Midwifery* 6(2):83–86.

Cawthorn A (2002) *Using Imagework for Adjustment Anxiety in a Patient Diagnosed with Advanced Cancer.* Unpublished MSc Thesis, University of Wales.

Cawthorn A (2004) Poster Presentation: *Using Imagery and Dreamwork.* International Cancer Nursing Conference. Sydney, Australia.

Cooke B, Ernst E (2000) Aromatherapy: a systematic review. *British Journal of General Practice* 493–496.

Corner J, Harewood J (2004) Exploring the use of complementary and alternative medicine by people with cancer. *Nursing Times Research* 9(2):101–109.

Department of Health, Foundation for Integrated Medicine, NHS Alliance, and the National Association of Palliative Care (2000) *Complementary Medicine: Information Pack for Primary Care Groups.* London, DoH, FIM, NHS Alliance, NAPC.

Dougans I, Ellis S (1996) *The Complete Illustrated Guide to Reflexology.* Dorset; Element Books.

Dimmock S, Troughton PR, Bird HA (1996) Factors predisposing to the resort of complementary therapies in patients with fibromyalgia. *Clinical Rheumatology:* 15:478–482.

Dryden S, Holden S, Mackereth P (1999) 'Just the ticket'; the findings of a pilot complementary therapy service (Part 11). *Complementary Therapies in Nursing and Midwifery* 5:15–18.

Ernst E, Resch KL, Mills S *et al.* (1995) Complementary medicine-a definition. *British Journal of General Practice* 45:506.

Ernst E (1998) Usage of complementary therapies in rheumatology: a systematic review. *Clinical Rheumatology* 17:301–305.

Ernst E, White A (2000) The BBC survey of complementary therapy medicine used in the UK. *Complementary Therapies in Medicine* 8:32–36.

Ernst E (2003) The current position of complementary and alternative medicine in cancer. *European Journal of Cancer* 39(16):2273–2277.

Ernst E (2004) Musculoskeletal conditions and complementary/alternative medicine. Best practice and research. *Clinical Rheumatology* 18(4):539–556.

Field T (2000) *Touch Therapy.* London, Harcourt Press.

Foundation for Integrated Medicine (1997) *Integrated Healthcare: A Way Forward for the Next Five Years.* London: FIM.

Giedt MS (1997) Guided Imagery. A psychoneuroimmunological intervention in holistic nursing practice. *Journal of Holistic Nurses' Association* 15:112–127.

Goldstone L (1999) From orthodox to complementary: the fall and rise of massage, with specific reference to orthopaedic and rheumatology nursing. *Journal of Orthopaedic Nursing,* 154–158.

Holdcroft LA, Assefi N, Buchwald D (2000) Complementary and alternative medicine in fibromyalgia and related syndromes. *Best Practice in Research Clinical Rheumatology* 17(4):667–683.

House of Lords: Select Committee on Science and Technology (2000) *Complementary and alternative medicine*. HL Paper 123.London: House of Lords.

Kearney M (2000) *A Place of Healing: Working with Suffering in Living and Dying.* Oxford, Oxford University Press.

Kunz K, Kunz B (1993) *The Complete Guide to Foot Reflexology* (revised). Albuquerque, New Mexico, Kunz and Kunz Publications.

Long L, Ernst E (2001) Homeopathic remedies for the treatment of osteoarthritis: a systematic review. *British Homeopathic Journal* 90:37–43.

Mackereth P (2000) Tough places to be tender: contracting for happy or 'good enough' endings in therapeutic massage/bodywork. *Complementary Therapies in Nursing and Midwifery* 6(3):111–115.

Mackereth P, Stringer J, Lynch B *et al.* (2003). How CAM helps at an acute cancer hospital. *Journal of Holistic Healthcare* 1(1):33–38.

Mills S, Budd S (2000) *Professional Organisation of Complementary and Alternative Medicine in the United Kingdom*. Centre for the Complementary Health Studies. University of Exeter.

Molassiotis A, Cawthorn A, Mackereth P (2004) In: Kearney A, Richardson, A (eds): *Nursing Patients with Cancer: Principles and Practice*. London, Elsevier Science.

National Center for Complementary and Alternative Medicine (2004) www.nccam.nih.gov/health/whatiscam Accessed 7 March 2004.

National Federation of Spiritual Healers (1988) *What is Spiritual Healing?* Middlesex, National Federation of Spiritual Healers.

National Institute for Clinical Excellence (2004) *Improving Supportive and Palliative Care Guidelines.* London: NICE.

National Occupational Standards for Reflexology (2005) Bristol, Skills for Health. www.skillsforhealth.org.uk/view_framework.php?id=64 Accessed 7 March 2004.

Norman L (1992) *The Reflexology Handbook.* London, Piatkus.

Ong CK, Banks B (2003) *Complementary and Alternative Medicine: The Consumer Perspective.* London, The Prince of Wales's Foundation for Integrated Health.

Oregon Hospice Association and East-West College of Healing Arts (1998) Massage as a respite intervention for primary caregivers. *American Journal of Hospice and Palliative Care* 14:43–47.

Penson J (1998) Complementary therapies making a difference in palliative care. *Complementary Therapies in Nursing and Midwifery* 4:77–81.

Pietroni P (1995) *The family guide to alternative health.* Godalming, CLB Publishing.

Price S, Price L (1995) *Aromatherapy for Health care Professionals.* London, Churchill Livingstone.

Pioro-Boisset M, Esdale JM, Fitzcharlse M (1996) *Alternative medicine use in fibromyalgic syndrome.* Arthritis Care and Research, 9:3–17.

Poole HM, Murphy P, Glenn S (2001) Evaluating the efficacy of reflexology for chronic back pain. *The Journal of Pain* 2(2):47.

Rankin-Box D (1997) Therapies in practice: a survey assessing nurses' use of complementary therapies. *Complementary Therapies in Nursing and Midwifery* 3(4):92–99.

Rankin D, McVey M (2001) Policy development. In: Rankin-Box D (ed): *The Nurse's Handbook of Complementary Therapies* (2nd edn). London, Harcourt Publishers Limited.

Rossman ML (2000) *Guided Imagery for Self-Healing*. HJ Kramer New World Library, Canada.

RCN (2003) Complementary Therapies in Nursing, Midwifery and Health Visiting Practice. *RCN guidance on Integrating Complementary Therapies into Clinical Care*. London, Royal College of Nursing.

Ryman L (1994) Relaxation and visualisation. In: Wells RJ, Tschudin V (eds): *Supportive Therapies in Health care*. London, Balliere Tindall.

Sayer-Adams J, Wright S (2001) *Therapeutic Touch*. London, Churchill Livingstone.

Stephenson NLN, Weinrich SP (2000) The effects of foot reflexology on anxiety and pain in patients with breast and lung cancer. *Oncology Nursing Forum* 27(1):67–72.

Stone J (2002) *An Ethical Framework for Complementary and Alternative Therapies*. London, Routledge.

Tavares M (2003) *National Guidelines for the Use of Complementary Therapies in Supportive and Palliative Care*. The Prince of Wales's Foundation for Integrated Health and The National Council for Hospice and Specialist Palliative Services. London, The Prince of Wales's Foundation for Integrated Health.

Thomas KT, Fall M, Nicholl J (2001) Access to complementary medicine via general practice. *British Journal of General Practice* 51(462):25–30.

Tiran D (1996) The use of complementary therapies in midwifery practice: a focus on reflexology. *Complementary Therapies in Nursing and Midwifery* 2(2):32–37.

Touch Research Institutes (1997) www.miami.edu/touch-research Accessed 7 March 2004.

Trevelyan J (1996) A true complement. *Nursing Times* 92(5):42–43.

Verity S (1996) Communicating with sedated ventilated patients in intensive care: focusing on the use of touch. *Intensive and Critical Care Nursing* 12:354–358.

Vickers A, Wilson P, Kleijnen J (2002) Acupuncture effectiveness. *Bulletin of Quality Safety Health Care* 1:92–97.

Visser GJ, Peters L, Rasker JJ (1992) Rheumatologists and their patients who seek alternative care, an agreement to disagree. *British Journal of Rheumatology* 31:485–490.

Watkins A (1997) *Mind-Body Medicine*. New York: Churchill Livingstone.

Wright S, Courtney U, Donnelly T, Kenny T, Lavin C (2002) Client's perception of benefit of reflexology on their quality of life. *Complementary Therapies in Nursing Midwifery* 8:69–76.

FURTHER READING

British Acupuncture Council – www.acupuncture.org.uk
British Medical Acupuncture Society – www.medical-acupuncture.co.uk

Centres for Reviews and Dissemination (CRD) www.york.ac.uk/inst/crd/ehcb/htm
Mackereth P, Tiran D (eds) (2003) *Clinical Reflexology: A Guide for Health Professional*. Edinburgh, Churchill Livingstong.
Reiki Method – www.reikifed.co.uk

14 Surgical Interventions

M. COX
Nuffield Orthopaedic Centre, Oxford, UK

The aim of this chapter is to enable the nurse to support and care for the patient with a rheumatic disease whilst undergoing a surgical intervention. After reading this chapter the reader should be able to:

- discuss the reasons for surgical intervention as a planned episode in the patient's management plan;
- describe the most common orthopaedic surgical procedures undertaken in the treatment of rheumatoid arthritis;
- describe the specific care required by the patient with inflammatory joint disease pre-, peri- and post-operatively;
- discuss the potential problems faced during the rehabilitative phase following surgery;
- understand the importance of multidisciplinary team care.

Advances in orthopaedic surgery have substantially improved the overall function and quality of life for patients with rheumatoid arthritis (RA). The number of patients with RA who undergo orthopaedic surgery is unknown. One study that assessed occurrence and predictive factors for orthopaedic surgery suggests that 11% of patients with recent onset RA treated, with conventional disease-modifying drug therapy, undergo large or small joint replacement surgery within five years of disease onset (James et al., 2004). Factors that have strong predictive capabilities for major joint replacement surgery at one-year follow-up include:

- low haemoglobin
- high erythrocyte sedimentation rate (ESR)
- high health assessment questionnaire (HAQ) score
- high disease activity score (DAS)
- high radiological erosion scores (James et al., 2004).

Da Silva et al. (2003) identified the risk of having joint-related surgery as increased in individuals who are younger, rheumatoid-factor positive and have rheumatoid nodules. These factors correspond with measurements known to be predictive of poor prognosis in RA, therefore it could be considered that the need for orthopaedic surgery is a marker of disease severity (Anderson, 1996).

It is unknown how the use of orthopaedic surgery has changed over time. Da Silva *et al.* (2003) determined that there was a significant decrease in the utilisation of all types of joint surgery in patients diagnosed with rheumatoid arthritis in the decade after 1985. This may well reflect improvements in disease management, and it is suggested that it could be an indication that modern therapies for rheumatoid arthritis are having a positive impact on outcome. It remains to be seen if the need for orthopaedic surgery, including major joint replacement, changes with further improvements in drug therapy and the increased use of biologic treatments. It should be remembered that whilst medical treatment might delay the onset of joint failure, surgical treatment should be regarded as part of the process of management of the disease, rather than a failure of medical therapy.

AIMS OF SURGICAL INTERVENTION

The primary aims of surgical procedures in the patient with inflammatory joint disease are to:

- relieve pain;
- prevent or correct deformity;
- prevent destruction of cartilage or tendons;
- maintain or improve function of joints by increasing or decreasing motion;
- enable individuals to maintain their independence;
- obtain cosmetic improvement.

Although not a prime consideration, cosmesis can bring benefits in the form of improved self-image and so should not be overlooked.

Relief of pain and loss of function are the primary reasons for consideration of any type of surgical intervention. If the pain cannot be controlled adequately by conservative means and the patient's life, in particular his/her sleep, is being affected, surgery should be considered (Seyfer, 1993).

COMMON SURGICAL PROCEDURES

Most patients will undergo orthopaedic surgery as an elective procedure. However, immediate surgical review is required for:

- instability of the cervical spine with resultant myelopathy and neurological symptoms;
- rupture of the extensor tendons at the wrist;
- removal of an infected prosthetic joint (Anderson, 1996).

The most common surgical procedures available to people with inflammatory joint disease include:

- arthroscopy
- synovectomy
- soft tissue release, realignment or repair
- arthroplasty
  - excision arthroplasty
  - prosthetic arthroplasty/joint replacement
- arthrodesis and stabilisation
- experimental procedures.

ARTHROSCOPY

Arthroscopy involves the visualisation of the inside of joints with the aid of an arthroscope. Progress in arthroscopic surgery has dramatically changed over the past 10–15 years. A high degree of clinical accuracy combined with low morbidity has encouraged the use of arthroscopy to:

- assist in diagnosis
- determine prognosis
- provide treatments such as arthroscopic debridement, partial meniscectomy, ligament repair including rotator cuff repair and acromioplasty.

This procedure can be performed with the patient under local, regional or general anaesthesia, and is often carried out as a day-case procedure.

SYNOVECTOMY

Synovectomy involves the excision of the synovial membrane that lines the joint or tendon sheath. This procedure has played a role in the management of RA for many years and is primarily carried out to prevent joint destruction occurring. The current indications for synovectomy are relief of pain in patients who have minimal structural damage to the joint refractory to pharmacological agents. Arthroscopic synovectomy is more often undertaken as opposed to an open procedure.

SOFT TISSUE RELEASE, REALIGNMENT OR REPAIR

Joint subluxation, dislocation and tendon rupture can occur due to inflammation of soft tissues, in particular the tenosynovium, ligaments and capsule. Joints most affected in this way include the metacarpophalangeal joints. Soft tissue reconstruction and synovectomy can realign and stabilise some joints, but fusion or replacement arthroplasty may be required for others.

ARTHROPLASTY

Arthroplasty is an operation to restore pain-free motion to a joint and function to the muscles.

There are two main types of arthroplasty.

Excision arthroplasty

This involves an operation to change the contours or mechanics of a joint with the intent of improving function. This procedure is normally carried out only when the integrity of the joint is not required for weight bearing. The two most common sites are the metatarsophalangeal joints and the radial head.

Prosthetic arthroplasty/joint replacement

Joint replacement can relieve pain and improve function for patients with moderate to severe destruction of cartilage and subchrondral bone in many joints, including the hip, knee, shoulder, elbow and more recently the ankle.

Despite being a major surgical intervention involving pain and a hospital stay, patients with RA perceive joint replacement as the most important intervention in their disease process rating it above methotrexate and early aggressive management (Fries, 1988).

ARTHRODESIS AND STABILISATION

Arthrodesis or joint fusion resolves pain within the joint but sacrifices motion. It is particularly useful in the wrist, ankle, talonavicular joint, and the interphalangeal joint of the fingers. Fusion of the thumb is also effective in improving grip strength (Anderson 1996). Arthrodesis is also used as a salvage procedure following failed joint replacement, particularly in the knee.

EXPERIMENTAL PROCEDURES

The ability to resurface areas of injured or damaged articular cartilage has led to intensive efforts to stimulate and repair both isolated and generalised articular defects, particularly in the knee. Currently operative approaches intended to preserve or restore cartilaginous articular surfaces include:

• surgical debridement of degenerated tissue
• correction of mechanical abnormalities.

When combined with implantation of artificial matrices, carbon fibre implants, growth factors and transplanted chrondrocytes or mesenchymal stem cells, these procedures have the potential to restore a joint surface (Buckwalter and Lohmander, 1994; Muckle and Minns, 1990). Long-term follow up and multicentre trials are required to confirm the effectiveness of such surgical interventions.

SURGERY OF THE LOWER LIMB

HIP

Synovectomy of the hip is only performed for symptomatic relief, and to gain improved function early in the course of juvenile RA. It is considered a time-gaining procedure to delay the need for arthroplasty.

Total hip arthroplasty/replacement

Total hip arthroplasty (THR) is currently the procedure of choice for severe pain and limitation of movement in the hip. Hip prostheses vary considerably but can be classified as:

• cemented
• uncemented (NICE 2000).

The type of prosthesis selected for use is dependent on many factors including:

• underlying pathology
• associated medical conditions
• the age of the patient
• potential postoperative activity level
• skill of the surgeon.

Long-term follow-up studies have demonstrated that THR provides excellent function for more than 15–20 years (Kavanagh et al., 1989; Severt et al., 1991), and this includes procedures in younger patients (Mulroy et al., 1995).
    The postoperative complications of THR include:

• deep-vein thrombosis
• dislocation
• infection.

Failure of the joint due to infection has been dramatically reduced to 1% due to modern surgical techniques and the use of prophylactic antibiotics (Fitzgerald, 1992).
    Prosthetic loosening predominantly causes long-term failure of THR which may necessitate revision surgery. The life expectancy of the revised hip is less

than the primary total hip replacement, with the average failure rate being 10% at five years (Lord *et al.*, 1988).

Surface replacement arthroplasty

This procedure involves using a surface replacement prosthesis following removal of the diseased surfaces of the joint. The development of metal-on-metal bearing surfaces has increased interest in this type of surgery, because the problems of excessive wear on the acetabular component and acetabular bone stock removal is reduced. If a metal-on-metal device is to be fitted, it is important to ensure that patients understand that less is known about the medium-to-long-term safety and reliability of this procedure. The likely need for revision surgery compared to conventional THR is also unknown (NICE 2002).

In young patients, resurfacing the femoral head alone (hemiarthroplasty) may be of value as an interim procedure that allows a relatively simple revision to a standard THR when required. Hungerford *et al.* (1998) found that progression to THR could be delayed by at least five years in 91% of patients undergoing resurfacing hemiarthroplasty. This procedure may also be advantageous to treat avascular necrosis of the femoral head, which can be a complication of long-term steroid use (Tooke *et al.*, 1987).

Minimally invasive THR

Using a minimally invasive technique for hip arthroplasty may be the procedure of choice for the future. A technique that avoids the need to cut muscle and tendons by using two small incisions has been developed. This allows for a quicker recovery and patients can be discharged 24 hours postoperatively (Berger, 2004). The efficacy and safety of this procedure has yet to be fully researched.

KNEE

Arthroscopic synovectomy of the knee

Early synovectomy is occasionally indicated if the disease fails to respond to appropriate medical treatment after 6–12 months. This procedure is most effective if the disease is limited to the synovial membrane, with little involvement of cartilage or bone. A review by Doets *et al.* (1989) concluded that an acceptable palliative effect could be achieved by this procedure. However progression of the degenerative process is not prevented.

The advantages of arthroscopic synovectomy include:

- reduced risk of loss of motion of the knee;
- only moderate blood loss;

- a quicker recovery from anaesthetic;
- reduced anticipated length of hospital stay.

Early mobilisation is important following this procedure to minimise the risk of loss of motion. Late synovectomy performed on knees with advanced arthritic changes has an unacceptably high failure rate and is not recommended.

Total knee arthroplasty/replacement

Total knee replacement (TKR) is the current treatment of choice for bi or tricompartmental knee arthritis. It has evolved over the past 30 years into a safe and cost-effective treatment with comparable results to THR.

Relative contraindications to total knee arthroplasty include high activity expectations and long life expectancy. Absolute contraindications include the presence of active infection, including conditions that may produce nonhealing ulcers of the ipsilateral lower extremity.

Current designs of prostheses allow only the joint to be resurfaced. There is minimal bone resection therefore bone stock is preserved, which maintains treatment options in the event of joint failure. There is little difference between cemented or uncemented prostheses at present, although Knutson et al. (1994) demonstrated slightly less loosening in the tibial component if cemented. All knee replacements now allow some rotation as well as unlimited flexion, and this freedom from constraints has been a major factor in preventing early joint failure.

A recent National Institute of Health (2003) consensus statement reports that the success of TKR is strongly supported by more than 20 years follow-up data. Postoperative mortality is approximately 0.5%, and there appears to be immediate and substantial improvement in the patient's pain, functional status, and overall health-related quality of life in about 90% of patients, with 85% being satisfied with the results of surgery.

Rodriguiz et al. (1996) reported delayed infections in 4.1% of patients, an average of seven years after primary total knee arthroplasty. It has been suggested that the role of steroids more than the disease process itself may be responsible for wound complications, including infections.

Arthrodesis of the knee

Arthrodesis or knee fusion is the treatment of choice only in the young, active or heavy patient with end-stage unilateral disease, or in those patients for whom there is a relative or absolute contraindication to arthroplasty. This is due to the high success rate of knee arthroplasty. Arthrodesis is also performed as a salvage procedure for failed arthroplasty. Although some functional limitation exists following an arthrodesis for failed TKR, Benson et al.

(1998) demonstrated a high level of function and patient satisfaction postoperatively, even when compared with primary knee replacements.

FOOT AND ANKLE

Nearly 90% of patients with RA will develop foot and ankle problems in the course of their disease (Michelson *et al.*, 1994), and the frequency and degree of involvement of the foot and ankle is directly proportional to disease duration (Spiegal and Spiegal, 1982). Pain may arise from impingement or entrapment of tendons or nerves, or from joints that are unstable, not just destroyed. Therefore it is essential to adequately examine the foot to determine the cause of the problem effectively.

Nonoperative foot care and patient education are very important aspects in the management of foot and ankle problems. This should include:

- advice regarding suitable footwear
- podiatric foot care
- the use of orthotic devices.

Synovectomy and soft tissue procedures

To delay deterioration in the ankle as in other joints, synovectomy is occasionally performed early in the disease process (Kvein *et al.*, 1987). Early decompression of the tibialis posterior tendon and other medial structures may also be undertaken to prevent rupture and subsequent deformity (Cracchiolo, 1984).

Excision arthroplasty

Surgical reconstruction of the forefoot is performed to:

- correct hammertoes and other lesser toe deformities;
- dislocation of the lesser metatarsophalangeal joints;
- severe hallux valgus deformity.

Many patients have bilateral foot difficulties and request simultaneous surgical reconstruction. However for patients with RA, convalescence following bilateral surgical procedures can be difficult.

Prosthetic arthroplasty

Treatment of end-stage ankle arthritis remains controversial with some surgeons advocating arthrodesis and others supporting the benefits of joint replacement. Problems such as wound complications and implant subsidence have improved with newer implant designs and better surgical techniques, but not all complications have been eliminated. The advantage of joint replacement is that when successful, it maintains motion and reduces strain on adjacent joints. The primary disadvantage is that if it fails, salvage can be difficult, particularly after deep infections which if painful and nonresponsive to surgical and medical treatment, may require a below-knee amputation.

Arthrodesis

Advanced hallux valgus deformity can be effectively treated with an arthrodesis of the metatarsophalangeal joint (Mann and Thompson, 1984). The benefits of this procedure include:

- stable alignment of the toe
- pain relief
- improved stability of the medial side of the foot.

Isolated painful destruction of the ankle joint in RA can be treated by arthrodesis. This is usually carried out by using internal fixation methods as seen in Figure 14.1 (Holt *et al.*, 1991; Moran *et al.*, 1991). If performed in the hindfoot for significant flat foot deformity relatively early, an isolated subtalar fusion may suffice. With longer established deformities and subluxation of the talonavicular joint, a triple arthrodesis may be required. This involves fusion of the talonavicular, calcaneocuboid and subtalar joints.

The goal of surgery is that the foot is plantigrade or flat to the ground. Postoperatively, patients are kept nonweight-bearing for a minimum of six weeks in a short leg cast, followed by a further six weeks in an ambulatory cast.

SURGERY OF THE UPPER LIMB

THE HAND AND WRIST

Involvement of the hand is common in RA, and erosive damage to the joints of the hand can occur very early in the disease process. The decision to undertake surgical treatment should be based on the patient's complaints and severity of symptoms, as a surprising level of function can often be maintained given the external appearances of the hand. However, the psychological and functional problems caused by deformities of the hand should not be underestimated as they are an ever-present, visible and an often painful reminder of disease. Good hand function is essential for maintaining most of the activities of daily living and leisure pursuits. The hands are also used in communication, to convey comfort and love by touch and as gestures in conversation and greetings.

Common deformities of the hand include:

- ulnar drift, caused by damage at the metacarpophalangeal joints aggravated by normal activities;
- swan-neck deformities;
- boutonniere deformities;
- Z deformity of the thumb.

Interventions range from synovectomy, tendon transfer, silastic implants or fusion of the affected joint. The postoperative care of hand surgery can be extensive. It involves close cooperation of a skilled hand therapist who has knowledge of splinting, as well as physical exercise techniques. Understanding of the implications of the surgery and postoperative regime is essential to ensure optimum outcome of these complex surgical procedures.

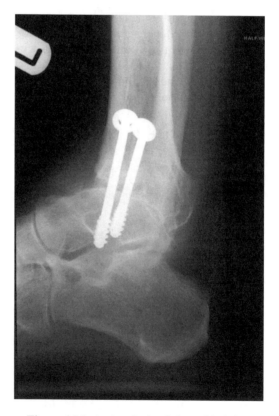

Figure 14.1 Arthrodesis of the ankle joint.

Tendon rupture/repair

Clinically the loss of finger extension at the metocarpophalangeal (MP) joint, particularly of the little finger, is the harbinger of more extensive tendon rupture if the inflammatory pathology is not addressed. Because direct repair of the tendon can only be undertaken in the acute phase, this is considered an emergency procedure (Wang and Weiland, 2001).

Prophylactic tenosynovectomy can:

- reduce pain
- increase the range of movement
- improve grip strength.

It can also help to protect the tendons from rupture, particularly when combined with resection of abnormal bony prominences at the distal radio-ulnar joint (Buckwalter et al., 1998).

Metacarpophalangeal (MCP) joint arthroplasty

Silicone implants which act as a spacer between the bones may be used for hands which are painful and have fixed deformities. Following this procedure, patients generally report a subjective functional improvement as well as greater satisfaction with the appearance of the hand. However, reported rates of fracture of implant vary between 0 and 50% (Wang and Weiland, 2001).

Synovectomy of the wrist

Synovial proliferation can destroy articular cartilage by invading surrounding soft tissue and the supporting structures. This causes instability and secondary deformity. When the articular cartilage is intact, early synovectomy can be of benefit.

Carpal tunnel decompression

Pain caused by compression of the median nerve as it passes with the flexor tendons, through the carpal tunnel at the wrist, can be relatively disabling, particularly if it is bilateral. The symptoms can vary from mild tingling on the palmer aspects of the thumb and first three fingers, to loss of motor function and intense pain which disrupts sleep. Surgical decompression is often carried out under local anaesthetic as a day-case procedure. Patients are encouraged to resume daily activities as able, and only require physiotherapy if problems are experienced regaining function. Grip strength and endurance may take three to six months to achieve, and for some may remain incomplete.

Arthrodesis of the wrist

Advanced degeneration of the interphalangeal joints, carpus and wrist, are commonly treated by arthrodesis which affords long-term pain relief and stability (Buckwalter *et al.*, 1998). To ensure that the patient can remain independent for hygiene and nutritional needs and retain the ability to use walking aids if required postoperatively, careful preoperative assessment is required.

Excision of rheumatoid nodules

These occur in 20–30% of individuals with RA. Excision of these nodules is undertaken if they become problematic to the patient but there is a tendency for them to reoccur (Wang and Weiland, 2001).

ELBOW

The elbow joint is involved in 20–50% of patients with RA. Regardless of the aetiology, a patient may complain of:

- pain
- stiffness
- weakness
- instability.

It is important to determine which symptom is paramount before planning treatment options as this improves the likelihood of patient satisfaction.

Synovectomy

In contrast with other joints, synovectomy of the elbow usually preserves or improves motion, especially forearm rotation. However, this procedure is rarely performed without excision of the radial head or where there is evidence of clinical involvement of radial humeral or radio-ulnar joint (Morrey and Adams, 1992). Mild active-assisted motion of the elbow is started approximately four days after surgery. As strength improves, pain usually decreases, and exercises progress to active motion. Pain can continue to reduce over the initial three months postoperatively, and range of motion can continue to improve for six months.

Arthroplasty of the elbow

Total elbow replacement (TER) is a common procedure. There are two types of prosthetic joint design:

- an unconstrained surface replacement (The main problem with unconstrained TER relates to instability in 20–50% of cases [O'Driscoll, 2001].);
- a linked semiconstrained prosthesis (Here the ulnar and humeral components are linked so that they do not dislocate, but the linkage allows a degree of laxity that permits the soft tissue to absorb some of the stresses that would normally be applied to the prosthesis-bone interface. This overcomes the problem of joint loosening which was seen in early hinge designs [Figure 14.2].).

The results of TER surgery are now comparable to total hip and knee arthroplasty. Pain relief is reported as being dramatic in 90% of patients (O'Driscoll, 2001), and Morrey *et al.* (1988) demonstrated functional improvement of 90% increase in strength of flexion, and 60%–70% in pronation and supination. An average postoperative functional arc of motion of 100 degrees of flexion/ extension, and 130 degrees of pronation/supination were also demonstrated.

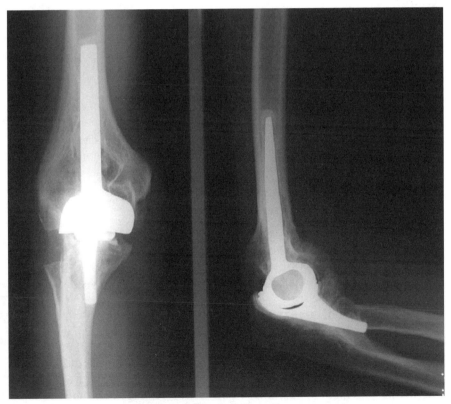

Figure 14.2 Total elbow replacement.

These ranges include the functional arcs of motion required for activities of daily living.

Infection rates following total elbow replacement have been reported to be between 2–5% (Risung, 1997). This slightly high rate is thought to be due to the relatively subcutaneous location of the elbow joint and lack of significant muscle coverage over a portion of the elbow.

SHOULDER

Although it is not affected as often as other large joints, the shoulder can suffer the destructive consequences of RA. Bilateral involvement is common, and the dominant and nondominant shoulders are equally affected. Shoulder stiffness and or muscle weakness is common preoperatively, and this can hinder or limit postoperative recovery. Careful preoperative assessment of the full extent of disease in all joints should be undertaken before shoulder surgery is undertaken.

Arthroscopy

Recent developments in the surgical management of patients with shoulder arthritis include minimally invasive procedures. The role of shoulder arthroscopy is primarily used in the surgical management of rotator cuff problems and acromioclavicular arthritis (O'Driscoll, 2001).

Hemiarthroplasty

Hemiarthroplasty involves replacement of the humeral head without resurfacing the glenonoid. This procedure is most often used in young patients or in the presence of larger rotator cuff tears.

Total shoulder arthroplasty/replacement

Total shoulder replacement (TSR) is mainly undertaken for RA of the glenohumeral joint (Figure 14.3). Pain relief and improved activities of daily living have been reported in 90% of patients (Brostrom et al., 1992). Long-term studies confirming the efficacy of TSR have indicated that revision rates can be as low as 5% (O'Driscoll, 2001).

Gentle stretch and strengthening exercises are important in the pre- and postoperative management of shoulder disease. Atrophy rapidly follows disuse and can interfere with daily function. Just 5–10 minutes of daily home exercise can help to maintain the range of movement at the shoulder as well as overhead strength. (O'Driscoll, 2001). The patient needs to understand that the postoperative rehabilitative period will be long, as it can take up to a year before the full benefit from surgery is obtained.

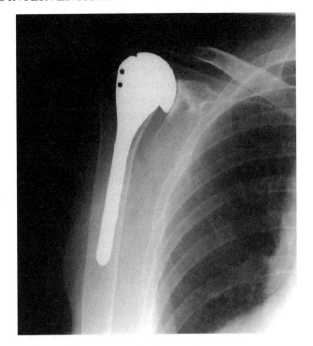

Figure 14.3 Total shoulder replacement.

SURGERY TO THE SPINE AND NECK

RA can affect the cervical spine in three ways:

- atlanto-axial subluxation
- basilar invagination
- subaxial subluxation.

Radiographic evidence of cervical spine abnormalities develop in 30–50% of patients with RA, and the incidence can be correlated with the severity of peripheral joint involvement (Reiter and Bowden, 1998). The most common indications for surgical treatment for cervical spine involvement are:

- pain which is not relieved by conservative means;
- neurological deterioration;
- radiographic evidence of impending spinal cord compression.

Patients with severe deformity or spinal canal compromise may be candidates for surgery despite an absence of pain or any neurological symptoms, as a rapid deterioration and even death are known to occur (Yaszemski and Shapler, 1990).

Considerations preoperatively must include the natural history of the disease and the potential for neurological recovery or symptomatic improvement, as well as the risks associated with surgery.

When assessing patients, symptoms such as limb heaviness, imbalance or paresthesias in the trunk and limbs associated with movement of the head and neck should be taken seriously. Physical findings such as spasticity, proprioceptive loss and early weakness may be masked. Early identification of cervical instability is important. If the myelopathy becomes severe, recovery following surgical treatment may be incomplete, and the risk of surgical mortality is increased (Casey et al., 1996).

Surgical interventions include the use of rigid devices to provide fixation of the cranium to the upper cervical spine, and sublaminar wiring at the C1 level. More recent techniques involve pedicle fixation in the cervical spine and transarticular C1–C2 screw fixation.

PLANNING SURGERY FOR THE PATIENT WITH RHEUMATOID DISEASE

Individuals who fail to gain satisfactory results from nonsurgical therapy, or who have progressive disease should be evaluated by a surgeon before they develop deformity, joint instability, contractures or advanced muscle atrophy. Delaying surgery until these problems develop can compromise the results and increase the risk of surgical complications (Buckwalter et al., 1998).

Planning surgery involves consideration of many different factors, including:

- the degree of pain and functional limitation perceived by the patient;
- the joints involved (No joint can be considered in isolation from other joints in the same limb, or other limbs.);
- the possible surgical and nonsurgical treatments, including the expected short and long-term outcomes;
- the potential risks of operative treatment, which includes the increased probability of local and systemic surgical complications associated with RA;
- the patient's individual circumstances including an understanding of their social and occupational needs;
- an understanding of the patient's goals and expectations to determine whether their goals are attainable and their expectations realistic (Any discrepancies between the patient's expectations and the likely surgical outcome should be discussed in detail before surgery. Preoperative assessment of motivation can also help predict outcome and anticipate difficulties postoperatively.).

Care is best coordinated within a combined clinic where the multidisciplinary team should ideally comprise:

- rheumatologist
- surgeon
- physiotherapist
- occupational therapist
- nurse.

Continuity of care is an important aspect in the establishment of a relationship between the patient and surgeon. This relationship enables the patient to develop trust and confidence in the surgical team, and allows the surgeon the opportunity to understand the patients individual needs.

Patients should play a role in decision-making when surgery is planned, and the joints perceived to be functionally impaired or painful should be addressed first (Wang and Weiland, 2001). Generally, large joint surgery precedes correction of hand and finger deformities. However, patients frequently rely on their upper extremities when using walking aids and so the stabilisation of a painful or unstable hand problem can facilitate rehabilitation in lower extremity surgery. Lower limb surgery should also be delayed for at least three months after shoulder or elbow replacement for the same reason (O'Driscoll, 2001).

Patients may wish to discuss proposed surgery with others who have undergone the procedure. This can be facilitated by the hospital or by contacting voluntary organisations such as Arthritis Care, or the National Rheumatoid Arthritis Society.

PREOPERATIVE EVALUATION

Although this section specifically discusses orthopaedic surgical interventions, as these form part of the management plan for many patients with RA, the nursing interventions noted can be added to care plans for any surgical procedure that the patient may be undergoing.

In the current economic climate, waiting-list times for elective surgery can vary widely, but the multidisciplinary team can do much to make this time a positive experience. The importance of a thorough preoperative history and physical examination cannot be over emphasised. The patient's general state of health should be monitored and any contraindication for surgery identified. Conditions such as reduced cardiac, renal or pulmonary function require evaluation and possible treatment before surgery is planned. It may be necessary to delay surgery to ensure optimal management of such disorders is achieved preoperatively (Buckwalter et al., 1998). All potential sources of infection should also be treated prior to surgery, such as carious teeth, pharyngitis, cystitis and skin infections including infected rheumatoid nodules (Skues and Welchew, 1993).

Smoking cessation

The cessation of smoking is a worthwhile goal for patients who are awaiting elective surgery, although it needs to be initiated at least two months before surgery for optimal effect. It can reduce the risk of cardiac ischaemia and postoperative chest infection. Heavy smoking can reduce the oxygen-carrying capacity of the blood equivalent to the loss of 2 g/dl of Hb, and so stopping smoking can produce a benefit in the postoperative period of a 1–2 unit blood transfusion (Green et al., 2003).

Weight reduction

If the patient is obese, weight reduction can produce relief of symptoms and increase the probability of a successful outcome of surgery, particularly in the lower limb. Obesity is not a contraindication for arthroplasty but there may be an increased risk of problems with:

- the anaesthetic
- intraoperative blood loss
- deep vein thrombosis
- delayed wound healing
- perioperative infection (Green et al., 2003; Wymenga et al., 1992; Lehman et al., 1994).

For some overweight patients, the pain and loss of mobility can make it more difficult to lose weight, and in these individuals the surgeon may recommend proceeding with operative treatment despite these associated risks (Buckwalter et al., 1998).

PLANNING POSTOPERATIVE CARE

Preoperative evaluation and instruction by occupational therapists should be carried out as soon as patients are placed on the waitlist. This may help individuals to cope in the interim period whilst waiting for surgery, and facilitate rehabilitation. Preoperative physiotherapy is important as it can increase strength and range of movement, and for the educational benefits that helps the patient to prepare for postoperative rehabilitation and discharge (Buckwalter et al., 1998). This is also an ideal time to determine the ability and willingness of carers to care for the patient on discharge. Assessment can then be undertaken to identify services that may be required at home in the postoperative period, and ensure these are in place to facilitate a smooth discharge from hospital.

MEDICATIONS THAT MAY AFFECT SURGERY

Aspirin

This can affect platelet adhesion and enhance intra-operative bleeding. If safe to do so, it is recommended that it be discontinued at least fourteen days prior to elective surgery (Green *et al.*, 2003).

Warfarin

Warfarin interferes with the synthesis of the vitamin K dependent clotting factors II, VII, IX and X. Unless contraindicated it should be discontinued 2–5 days preoperatively and the prothrombin time normalised prior to elective surgery (Green *et al.*, 2003). For patients who require the maintenance of anticoagulation, a continuous infusion of heparin can be established preoperatively and continued until at least day three following the reestablishment of warfarin therapy.

Steroids

Despite the known side effects of steroids, such as an increased risk of infection, delayed wound healing and thinning of the skin, it is recommended that steroid usage continue throughout the operative period (Green *et al.*, 2003). Cessation may have two adverse effects:

- If discontinued it is likely to induce a flare of an inflammatory condition, making postoperative rehabilitation difficult.
- Chronic steroid administration can cause adrenal suppression, rendering the patient less likely to deal with the stress of surgery.

Friedman *et al.* (1995) suggest that it may not be necessary to administer stress doses of corticosteriods preoperatively. However, steroid usage should always be borne in mind if the patient is unwell in the postoperative period, as they may not be able to produce the endogenous steroid surge required to enable the body to cope with trauma.

Methotrexate

It had been suggested that the continuation of methotrexate during a surgical episode of care could increase the risk of early postoperative complications (Sany *et al.*, 1993; Carpenter *et al.*, 1996). However Grennan *et al.* (2001) compared complication rates from 566 RA patients undergoing elective orthopaedic surgery. They found that there was a decreased incidence in the occurrence of infection twelve months postoperatively, in patients who had continued methotrexate throughout the surgical intervention, compared to two other groups. The first group had methotrexate discontinued two weeks pre and postoperatively, and the second group had not been taking methotrexate preoperatively. The results also demonstrated that no patients from the methotrexate group developed a flare in the year following surgery, compared to six patients in each of the comparator groups. It was concluded that methotrexate should not be stopped before elective surgery if the patient's disease is well-controlled by the drug.

Anti-TNFα

Draft guidelines drawn up by the British Society of Rheumatology (Mc Hugh, 2004), recommend that anti-TNF alpha therapy should be withheld for 2–4 weeks prior to major surgical procedures. Once wound healing is satisfactory and there is no evidence of infection, treatment may be restarted.

PREADMISSION ASSESSMENT

The National Institute for Clinical Excellence (NICE, 2003a), have issued a guidance document on the use of routine preoperative tests for all grades of elective surgery. This guidance takes the planned procedure and comorbidities into account, and recommends a preoperative testing regime that determines a patient's fitness to undergo the surgical procedure. The assessment is usually undertaken 14–21 days prior to the operation.

Orthopaedic surgical areas are considered high-risk in respect of the development of methicillin resistant staphylococcus aureus (MRSA) infection (RCN, 2004). Such an infection following a joint replacement can be catastrophic and so it is recommended that all high-risk patients are screened preoperatively. Decolonisation procedures may have to be undertaken preoperatively if an MRSA screen is positive.

CONSENT AND PATIENT EDUCATION

It is a general legal and ethical principle that valid consent must be obtained and recorded from patients before starting treatment or undergoing physical examination (DOH, 2002). This guideline supports the practice that patients should have access to sufficient information to be able to make an informed decision about whether to consent to surgery. This should include information on:

• the planned procedure
• the risks and common complication
• the type and extent of postoperative rehabilitation

- expectations for postoperative pain relief
- expectations for function
- alternative treatments.

The provision of such information has also been shown to:

- allay anxiety
- improve patient outcomes
- reduce the use of analgesia
- improve patient satisfaction (Buckwalter *et al.*, 1998).

USE OF INTEGRATED CARE PATHWAYS

Integrated care pathways are defined as: 'Locally agreed multidisciplinary practice, based on guidelines and evidence where available, for a specific patient/user group. It forms all or part of the clinical record, documents the care given and facilitates the evaluation of outcomes for continuous quality improvement.' (Du Luc, 2001).

Integrated pathways are developed and used to provide a framework for planning and delivering care by all members of the MDT within a given period. The aim of these pathways is to ensure that the patient receives appropriate care at the appropriate time, so that quality outcomes and cost are balanced.

PERIOPERATIVE CARE

For the purpose of this chapter routine peri- and postoperative care will not be discussed. However the following considerations may need to be added to care plans to ensure that the individual needs of patients are met.

INTUBATION AND MAINTENANCE OF A PATENT AIRWAY

In a study of 113 patients with RA undergoing hip or knee arthroplasty, Collins *et al.* (1991) found that 61% had evidence of cervical instability, although only 50% were symptomatic. It is suggested that routine lateral and anterior-posterior x-rays are reviewed in the preoperative assessment. Surgical intervention is rarely required but special attention is necessary during intubation to avoid neurological compromise. Nursing care may include the fitting of a soft cervical collar as a reminder of the potential for cervical damage in the peri and postoperative periods.

Temporomandibular stiffness may further complicate intubation, necessitating the use of fibre optic intubation.

POSITIONING

Whist being anaesthetised the patient must always be positioned carefully with all joints supported and not overstressed. Protection of bony surfaces, nodules and friable skin is essential (Callahan, 1996), and can be achieved by the use of gel mattresses on theatre tables. Protective bandaging may also be used for lower limbs and elbows.

EYE CARE

Sicca syndrome (dry eyes) can occur in approx 10% of patients with RA and so regular eye care may be necessary to prevent corneal damage.

PROPHYLACTIC ANTIBIOTICS

Infection rates following prosthetic joint surgery can be significantly decreased by the use of prophylactic antibiotics. Antibiotic regimes are prescribed, based on the known common infective organisms for the individual procedure. They are administered on induction and continued for 24–48 hours postoperatively (Harkness and Daniels, 2003). Although the data also supports the use of antibiotic impregnated bone cement as an additional means of reducing rates of deep wound infection, concern related to genesis of antibiotic strains of bacteria has tempered the use of this practice (NIH Draft Statement, 2003).

CIRCULATION

Any impairment to circulation may be difficult to assess due to vascular disease. The patient may require Doppler assessment to determine the presence or absence of pedal pulses following lower limb surgery.

POSTOPERATIVE CARE

Postoperatively it is important that a named professional be responsible for the coordination of care between all members of the multidisciplinary team and that patients and carers can identify their care coordinator and the key persons providing their care. Patients should be actively involved in continuously negotiating and influencing their care, and it is recommended that multidisciplinary case reviews are undertaken with the patient and that the outcomes of such meetings are fully documented (DOH, 2003).

Nurses should be fully aware of the following problems that can occur postoperatively.

HAEMORRHAGE AND SHOCK

Haemoglobin levels must be assessed preoperatively as 25% of patients with RA have a normochromic hypochromic anaemia which is resistant to treatment with iron (Callahan, 1996). If the haemoglobin is below 9 g/dl, treatment of the anaemia or blood transfusion pre or postoperatively may be required.

PAIN DUE TO SURGICAL TRAUMA

Pain assessment and management are critical skills for nurses caring for patients following surgery, particularly as postoperative pain has been identified as an important factor influencing the patient's perceptions of progress and recovery (Seers, 1987). Despite this, reports have emphasised the inadequacies of postoperative analgesia, with up to 70% of patients complaining of moderate to severe pain following surgery (Kuhns *et al.*, 1990). Research has demonstrated that nurses and patients disagree about the intensity of pain 77% of the time (Seers, 1987).

For patients with RA, it must be remembered that assessment of acute postoperative pain needs to be made alongside assessment of chronic pain in other joints. The patient's usual regime of medication, including opioids, should not be omitted for any length of time. This is particularly important preoperatively as this can affect pain control and stiffness, which restricts mobility in unoperated joints. It can even cause a flare of the disease, adversely affecting the outcome of surgery (Connelly and Panush, 1991).

Analgesia is the mainstay of postoperative pain control and should be provided according to the patient's perceived pain level and response to medication. Pain relief should be sufficient to allow mobilisation, rest and pain-free sleep, but avoid drug side effects. Patient-controlled analgesia (PCA) allows the patients to self-medicate analgesia by activating a syringe pump by pressing a button. This administers a preset amount of analgesia which enables the patient to feel in control of their analgesic requirements. The normal route of administration is intravenously, but the intramuscular or subcutaneous routes can also be used. An assessment of the patient's manual dexterity should be undertaken preoperatively, as adaptations to the administration set may need to be made to enable the patient with poor hand function to operate the pump. Careful patient education is also required in order for this type of analgesia to be successful.

Epidural analgesia is recommended in patients undergoing major lower limb surgery (Callahan, 1996). This can be continued into the immediate postoperative period if required. Close monitoring of the patient is essential as there is an increased risk of respiratory depression and urinary retention associated with this procedure. Urinary catheterisation may be required, which should be covered by prophylactic antibiotics. However it should be noted that cotrimoxazole and trimethoprim are contraindicated for patients taking methotrexate. Nurses should be fully conversant with possible complications of epidural analgesia, and be able to initiate treatment if they occur (Green et al., 2003).

The administration of nonsteroidal anti-inflammatory medication (NSAID) pre- and postarthroscopy has proven effective in reducing pain, swelling and increasing the range of movement in the early postoperative period (Phillips, 2003).

EMOTIONAL ISSUES

It is important to be aware of the emotional responses that patients may be experiencing when facing a surgical intervention. Preoperative anxiety and stress linked to uncertainty and anticipatory fear are common. Such emotional stress can have an adverse effect on the severity of symptoms of RA (Crossby, 1988). The MDT must make every effort to involve the patient in decision-making which will allow them to maintain control of their lives, and remain independent whilst in hospital. Postoperatively, it is often simple measures such as positioning bed tables and drinks within reach, and other aids to help when eating which can make a difference between dependence and independence.

It is not unusual for patients who have a chronic illness to experience an altered body image. The patient may have adjusted to the progression of the physical manifestations of the condition as the changes to appearance and function developed. However, altered body image is more often expressed in terms of the limitations imposed by the disease, such as increasing dependence on others as symptoms worsen. In this instance surgery may be viewed as a positive factor, as it aims are to relieve pain and improve function.

RESTRICTED MOBILITY OR IMPOSED BED REST

Patients who are fully independent when mobile can be almost totally dependent if confined to bed. This can contribute to a range of difficulties with activities such as:

• personal hygiene and oral care
• prevention of pressure ulcers
• manual handling.

PERSONAL HYGIENE AND ORAL CARE

It is important that the care plan documents the patient's ability to self-care and any level of assistance required to perform these activities is continually reassessed as the postoperative period progresses. This will ensure that the care provided continues to meet the needs of the individual. The occupational therapist may need to provide advice and assistive devices to help patients retain their independence.

The importance of good foot care to prevent the risk of infection from broken skin or infected toenails, should also be emphasised following joint replacement. The podiatrist may need to be consulted, particularly for patients who are unable to undertake foot care independently.

PREVENTION OF PRESSURE ULCERS

The patient with RA may be at increased risk for several reasons:

- Joint disease in the upper limbs combined with decreased strength can make it almost impossible for the patient to alter their own position in bed.
- Medication such as steroids can cause patients to have thin delicate skin which may bruise or tear easily.
- Patients undergoing surgery are more likely to have severe disease with an increase of extra-articular symptoms such as rheumatoid nodules (Da Silva et al., 2003). Their presence over pressure points such as the elbows, ischial and sacral prominences, can increase the risk of skin breakdown.

All patients undergoing surgery should be assessed by use of a recognised assessment tool, to determine their risk of developing a pressure ulcer. The plan of care should be agreed by the MDT, in partnership with the patient (NICE, 2003b). The plan should be documented, implemented and evaluated, along with evidence of ongoing reassessment throughout the pre-, peri- and postoperative period (DOH, 2003). Equipment such as pressure-relieving mattresses and cushions, electrically controlled beds etc, may need to be provided.

Poor nutritional status can also contribute to the breakdown of skin and delay wound healing. This can occur for a variety of reasons:

- Weight loss can occur as a symptom of active RA, an adverse effect of medication, or as a result of the patient experiencing difficulties in shopping, food preparation or cooking.
- Sjögren's syndrome may mean the mouth is continually dry and food cannot be swallowed or enjoyed.

Conversely weight gain can arise from steroid therapy, lack of exercise or comfort eating in response to reduced mobility and independence.

Postoperatively patients may require assistance to eat and drink, especially if recovering from upper limb surgery. Adapted crockery and cutlery may be required to enable the patients to remain independent. A dietician may be consulted to provide specific advice if the patient is malnourished or identified as at risk during their hospital stay (DOH, 2003).

MANUAL HANDLING

A manual-handling assessment should be performed preoperatively and care planned accordingly (HSE, 1992; RCN, 1996). The use of low-friction glide sheets, rolling techniques (Love, 1994) and hoists are the current recommended manual handling techniques. The use of an overhead monkey pole should be discouraged due to the potential risk of joint damage occurring in the upper limbs.

PREVENTION OF POSTOPERATIVE COMPLICATIONS

The patient is at risk for a number of complications following surgery, including:

- deep vein thrombosis
- pulmonary embolism
- chest infection
- delayed wound healing
- constipation
- restricted joint movement
- fatigue.

Deep vein thrombosis and pulmonary embolism

The development of a deep vein thrombosis (DVT) and pulmonary embolism (PE) continues to be a significant complication of major orthopaedic surgery. Studies have found that without prophylaxis, the risk of a DVT is approximately 45%–57% following THR (Geerts et al., 2001). There are two main approaches to prophylaxis.

To reduce venous stasis

Methods include leg elevation, regular dorsiflexion of the ankle when resting and early ambulation. Antiembolism stockings which work by improving venous return are also recommended. However, problems with skin fragility and poor manual dexterity means that patients with RA may find these difficult to tolerate and impossible to put on unaided.

To reduce hypercoagulability

Adequate hydration may help reduce hypercoagulability, but the main prophylactic measure is anticoagulant therapy such as low molecular weight heparin. This has a predictable plasma concentration that allows for once-a-day administration without the need for laboratory testing. It is recommended that for high-risk groups, prophylactic therapy continue for 35 days postoperatively (Hull *et al.*, 2000).

Chest infection

Patients taking immunosuppressant therapy have an increased risk of chest complications. Careful monitoring is required to detect any signs of postoperative chest infection. Those with ankylosing spondylitis may have restricted chest expansion and require intensive physiotherapy postoperatively.

Delayed wound healing

Many patients with RA have potential risk factors that contribute to delayed wound healing, including:

- poor skin condition
- poor nutritional status
- concurrent medical conditions such as respiratory and cardiovascular disease (Green *et al.*, 2003).

Wound infection is a potentially serious complication of joint replacement surgery as it can lead to an infection within the joint itself and can be a major cause of joint failure. If this occurs, the patient has to undergo a prolonged period of hospitalisation and extensive antibiotic therapy.

The type of postoperative wound dressing should also be considered carefully, as fragile skin has an increased likelihood of being torn when removing adhesive dressings. Sensitivity to the adhesive compound in some dressings can also occur.

Constipation

All bladder and bowel care should be given in an environment conducive to the patient's individual needs (DOH, 2003). Constipation is a potential problem due to the prolonged use of analgesia, particularly opioid-based medications as these reduce bowel motility and mobility. Dietary adjustments are recommended in the first instance, but aperients or suppositories could be required if symptoms persist.

Restricted joint movement

The range of movement of all joints should be assessed preoperatively as reduced mobility can cause significant problems in the postoperative period. Upper limbs must be able to support the patient when using walking aids following surgery. Pulpit/gutter rollator frames may be required initially following lower limb surgery (Figure 14.4). Patients with multiple joint involvement may be unaware of the severity of the disease in other joints as they are unable to stress those joints beyond the limits established by the one that has been operated on. This may affect the rate and success of rehabilitation.

Fatigue

Fatigue and general malaise are symptoms of RA that can affect the patient's rehabilitation. The MDT in consultation with the patient need to plan, prioritise, and pace activities and treatment, allowing time for rest.

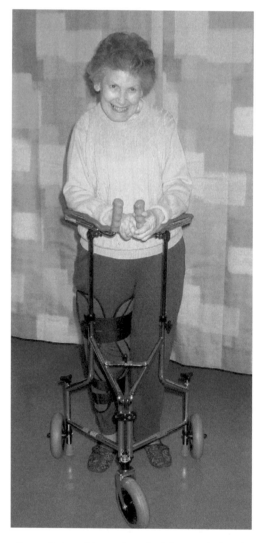

Figure 14.4 The gutter rollator. (Reproduced with permission from the patient.)

DISCHARGE PLANNING

Adjustment may have to be made to the way certain activities of daily living are carried out, depending on how the surgery affects the individual patient. Such adjustments should be anticipated preoperatively and form part of the discharge planning process.

The majority of patients who undergo major orthopaedic surgery will have more severe disease and may already be recipients of comprehensive home-care packages and social support networks in the community. A period of rehabilitation or a home visit by members of the MDT may be required to ensure the patient is discharged into a safe environment. It is also important to ascertain that the prime carer can cope with any adjustments necessary as a result of surgery.

PATIENT EDUCATION

Prior to discharge is it essential that patients are aware of who to contact if they have any questions regarding their care, or in the event of any problems arising, particularly if they happen out of hours (DOH, 2003).

Although the causal relationship between infection in joint replacements following dental treatment has been difficult to establish, it is advised that patients inform their dental surgeons if they have undergone this type of surgery as prophylactic antibiotic cover should be given following some dental procedures (American Academy of Orthopaedic Surgeons Advisory statement, 1997).

Following recent notification of problems with some forms of prosthetic components, it is recommended that patients are provided with an information card about prosthesis design and date of manufacture. This is for use in the event of any adverse knowledge about a particular prosthesis becoming available at a date following surgery.

CONCLUSION

Orthopaedic surgical interventions can have a profound impact on the quality of life for patients with RA. However the surgical management of these patients requires a carefully planned and coordinated approach, which involves all members of the MDT. It is essential for the success of surgery, to continue this collaboration during the pre-, peri-, and postoperative phases of care.

ACTION POINTS FOR PRACTICE

- Mrs Smith, a 45-year-old teacher, has RA that is causing pain and loss of function in her hands and wrists. Consider what surgical options are available to her and discuss the support that the members of the MDT could offer in the decision-making process, leading to a surgical intervention.

- Mr Jones, a 60-year-old accountant, with multiple joint involvement, is undergoing a total hip replacement. Plan his care during the postoperative period using a model of your choice.
- Mrs Brown is a 50-year-old housewife. She has had aggressive disease for many years and is wheelchair-orientated due to major destruction in her knees, which do not cause pain at rest. She has recently remarried, and her second husband devotes himself to caring for her. A year following successful bilateral knee arthroplasties, she remains dependent on the wheelchair. Consequently the improved function gained postoperatively is deteriorating. Discuss if Mrs brown was a suitable candidate for this operation.

REFERENCES

American Academy of Orthopaedic Surgeons Advisory Statement (1997). *Antibiotic prophylaxis for dental patients with joint replacements.* American Dental Association and Academy of Orthopaedic Surgeons. www.aaos.org (30 March 04).

Anderson R (1996) The orthopaedic management of rheumatoid arthritis. *Arthritis Care Research* 9:23–28.

Benson ER, Resine ST, Lewis CG (1998) Functional outcomes of arthrodesis for failed total knee arthroplasty. *Orthopaedics* 2:875–879.

Berger RA (2004) *Minimally invasive total hip arthroplasty using a two-incision technique.* American Academy of Orthopaedic Surgeons. 71st Annual Meeting Proceedings. San Francisco. 5(207):380.

Brostrom LA, Wallenstein R, Olisson E, Anderson D (1992) The Kessel prosthesis in total shoulder arthroplasty – a five year experience. *Clinical Orthopaedics* 277:155–160.

Buckwalter JA, Ballard WT, Brooks P (1998) Principles of arthritis surgery. In: Klippell JH, Dieppe P (eds) *Rheumatology* (2nd ed) London, Mosby.

Buckwalter JA, Lohmander S (1994) Operative treatment of osteoarthritis: Current practice and future development. *Journal of Bone and Joint Surgery* 76A:1405–1408.

Callahan L (1996) Perioperative care of the patient with rheumatoid arthritis. *Current Reviews PACN* 17:22:189–196.

Carpenter M, West S, Jones D (1996) Postoperative joint infections in rheumatoid arthritis patients on methotrexate therapy. *Orthopaedics* 19:207–210.

Casey AT, Crockard HA, Bland JK (1996) Surgery on the rheumatoid cervical spine for the non-ambulatory myelopathic patient – too much too late? *Lancet* 347:1004–1007.

Collins DN, Barnes CL, Fitzrandolf RL (1991) Cervical spine instability in rheumatoid patients having total hip or knee arthroplasty. *Clinical Orthopaedics* 272:127–135.

Connelly CS, Panush RS (1991) Should NSAID's be stopped before elective surgery? *Archives of International Medicine* 157:1963–1966.

Cracchiolo AD (1984) *Foot abnormalities in rheumatoid arthritis.* Academy of Orthopaedic Surgeons Instructional Course Lecture. 33:86–404.

Crossby LJ (1988) Stress factors, emotional stress, and rheumatoid disease activity. *Journal of Advanced Nursing* 10:1852–1854.

Da Silva E, Doran MF, Crowson CS, O'Fallon WM, Matteson EL (2003) Declining use of orthopaedic surgery in patients with rheumatoid arthritis? Results of a long term, population based assessment. *Arthritis & Rheumatism* 49(2):216–220.

Department of Health (2002) *Good practice in consent implementation guide: consent to examination or treatment.* London, Department of Health.

Department of Health (2003) *Essence of care. Patient focussed benchmarks for clinical governance.* London, Modernisation Agency.

Doets HC, Bierman BT, Von Soesbergen RM (1989) Synovectomy of the rheumatoid knee does not prevent deterioration. *Acta Orthopaedica Scandanavica* 60:523–525.

Du Luc K (2001) *Developing Care Pathways – The Handbook.* Oxford, Radcliffe Medical Press.

Fitzgerald FH (1992) Total hip arthroplasty sepsis. Prevention and diagnosis. *Orthopaedic Clinics of North America* 23:259–264.

Friedman RJ, Scliff CF, Bronburg JS (1995) The use of supplemental steroids in patients having orthopaedic operations. *Journal of Bone and Joint Surgery* 77A:1801–1816.

Fries JF (1988) Milestones in rheumatologic care (1965–1985). In: Fries JF (ed) *Milestones in Management: Rheumatoid Arthritis.* Puerto Rico, Syntex.

Geerts WH, Heit JA, Claggett CP, Pineo GF, Colwell CW, Anderson FA (2001) Prevention of venous thromboembolism. *Chest* 119:132S–175S.

Green D, Ervine M, White S (2003) *Fundamentals of Perioperative Management.* London, Greenwich Medical Media.

Grennan DM, Gray J, Louden J, Fear S (2001) Methotrexate and early postoperative complications in patients with rheumatoid arthritis undergoing elective orthopaedic surgery. *Annals of the Rheumatic Diseases* 60:214–217.

Harkness JW, Daniels AU (2003) Arthroplasty: Introduction and overview. In: Canale ST (ed) *Campbell's Operative Orthopaedics.* (10th ed) St Louis, Mosby.

Health and Safety Executive (1992) *Manual Handling Guidance and Regulations.* London, HMSO.

Holt ES, Hansen ST, Mayo KA, Sangeorzan BJ (1991) Ankle arthrodesis using internal screw fixation. *Clinical Orthopaedics and Related Research* 268:21–28.

Hull RD, Pineo GF, Francis C, Bergqvist D, Fellenius C, *et al.* (2000) Low molecular weight heparin prophylaxis using dalteparin extended out-of-hospital vs in-hospital warfarin/out-of-hospital placebo in hip arthroplasty patients. A double blind randomised comparison. *Archives of internal Medicine* 160:2208–2215.

Hungerford MW, Mont MA, Scott R, Fiore C, Hungerford DS, *et al.* (1998) Surface replacement hemi-arthroplasty for the treatment of osteonecrosis of the femoral head. *Journal of Bone and Joint Surgery* 80:11:1656–1664.

James D, Young E, Kulinskaya E, Knight E, Thompson W *et al.* (2004) Orthopaedic intervention in early rheumatoid arthritis. Occurrence and predictive factors in an inception cohort of 1064 patients followed for 5 years. *Rheumatology* 43(3): 369–376.

Kavanagh BF, Dewitz MA, Ilstrup DM, Stauffer RN, Coventry MB (1989) Charnley total hip arthroplasty with cement: Fifteen-year results. *Journal of Bone and Joint Surgery* 71A:1496–1503.

Knutson K, Lewold S, Robertsson O, Lidgren L (1994) The Swedish knee arthroplasty register. A nationwide study of 30,003 knees, 1976–1992. *Acta Orthopaedica Scandinavica* 65:375–386.

Kuhns S, Cook K, Collins M, Jones JM, Mucklow JC (1990) Patients perceptions of pain after surgery. *British Medical Journal* 300:1687–1690.

Kvein TK, Pahle JA, Hoyerral HM, Sandstad B (1987) Comparison of synovectomy and no synovectomy in patients with juvenile rheumatoid arthritis. A 24 month controlled study. *Scandinavian Journal of Rheumatology* 16:375–386.

Lehman DE, Capello WN, Feinburg JR (1994) Total hip arthroplasty without cement in obese patients. *Journal of Bone Joint Surgery* 76A:854–862.

Lord G, Marotife JH, Guillamon JL, Blanchard JP (1988) Cementless revision of failed aseptic cemented and cementless total hip arthroplasties. *Clinical Orthopaedics and Related Research* 235:67–74.

Love C (1994) Rolling or lifting following total hip replacement. *Professional Nurse.* 9(7):456–464.

Mann RA, Thompson FM (1984) Arthrodesis of the first metatarsophalangeal joint for hallux valgus in rheumatoid arthritis. *Bone & Joint Surgery America* 66:687–692.

McHugh (2004) *Draft Guidelines for anti-TNF alpha therapy in rheumatoid arthritis.* London, British Society of Rheumatology.

Michelson J, Easley M, Wigley FM, Hellman D (1994) Foot and ankle problems in rheumatoid arthritis. *Foot and Ankle International* 15:608.

Moran CG, Pinder IM, Smith SR (1991) Ankle arthrodesis in RA. 30 cases followed for 5 years. *Acta Orthopaedica Scandinavica* 62:538–543.

Morrey BF, Askew LJ, An KN (1988) Strength and function after elbow arthroplasty. *Clinical Orthopaedics* 234:43–50.

Morrey BF, Adams RA (1992) Semi-constrained arthroplasty for the treatment of rheumatoid arthritis of the elbow. *Journal of Bone and Joint Surgery* 74A:479–485.

Muckle DS, Minns RJ (1990) Biological response to woven carbon fibre pads in the knee: A clinical and experimental study. *Journal of Bone and Joint Surgery* 72:60–62.

Mulroy WF, Estock DM, Harris WH (1995) Total hip arthroplasty with the use of so called second generation cementing techniques: a fifteen year average follow up study. *Journal of Bone and Joint Surgery America* 77:1845.

National Institute of Clinical Excellence (2000) *Guidance on the selection of prostheses for primary total hip replacement.* (No2). London, National Institute of Clinical Excellence.

National Institute of Clinical Excellence (2002) *Guidance on the use of metal-on-metal hip resurfacing arthroplasty.* London, National Institute of Clinical Excellence.

National Institute of Clinical Excellence (2003a) *Preoperative tests. The use of routine preoperative tests for elective surgery.* London, National Institute of Clinical Excellence.

National Institute of Clinical Excellence (2003b) *Pressure ulcer prevention*. London, National Institute of Clinical Excellence.

National Institute of Health (2003) *Consensus Development Conference on Total Knee Replacement. Draft Statement,* hppt://consensus.nih.gov/cons/117/117cdc_statementn2.htm (12 December 03).

O'Driscoll S (2001) Surgery of shoulder arthritis. In: Koopman WJ (ed) *Arthritis and Allied Conditions. A Textbook of Rheumatology* (14th ed) Philadelphia, Lippincott Williams and Wilkins.

Phillips BB (2003) General principles of arthroscopy. In: Canale ST (ed) *Campbell's Operative Orthopaedics,* (10th ed) St Louis, Mosby.

Reiter MF, Bowden SD (1998) Inflammatory disorders of the cervical spine. *Spine* 23:2755–2766.

Risung F (1997) The Norway elbow replacement. Design, technique, and results after 9 years. *Journal of Bone and Joint Surgery* 79:94–402.

Rodriguiz JA, Saddler S, Edelman S, Ranawat CS (1996) Long-term results of total knee arthroplasty in class 3 and 4 rheumatoid arthritis. *Journal Arthroplasty* 11:141–145.

Royal College of Nursing (1996) *Code of practice for patient handling.* London, RCN.

Royal Collage of Nursing (2004) *Methicillin resistant staphylococcus aureus. Guidance for nursing staff.* London. RCN.

Sany J, Anaya J, Canovas F, Combe B, Jorgensen C, *et al.* (1993) Influence of methotrexate and the frequency of postoperative infections/complications in patients with rheumatoid arthritis. *Journal of Rheumatology* 20:1129–1132.

Seers K (1987) Perceptions of pain. *Nursing Times.* 83(48):37–39.

Seyfer AE (1993) Indications for upper extremity surgery in RA patients. *Seminars in Arthritis and Rheumatism* 23:125–134.

Severt R, Wood R, Cracchiolo A, Amstutz HC (1991) Long term follow up of cemented total hip arthroplasty in rheumatoid arthritis. *Clinics in Orthopaedics* 265:129–136.

Skues MA, Welchew EA (1993) Anaesthesia and RA. *Anaesthesia.* 48:989–997.

Spiegal TM, Spiegal JS (1982) Rheumatoid arthritis in the foot and ankle: Diagnosis, pathology and treatment: The relationship between foot and ankle deformity and disease duration in 50 patients. *Foot Ankle* 2:318–323.

Tooke SM, Amstutz HC, Delaunay A (1987) Hemi-resurfacing for femoral head osteonecrosis. *Journal of Arthroplasty* 2:125.

Wang AA, Weiland AJ (2001) Surgery of arthritic hand deformities. In: Koopman WJ (ed) *Arthritis and Allied Conditions. A Textbook of Rheumatology* (14th ed), Philadelphia, Lippincott, Williams and Wilkins.

Wymenga AB, Horn JR, Theeuwes A, Muytjens HL, Sloff TJ (1992) Perioperative factors associated with septic arthritis after arthroplasty. Prospective multi-centre study of 362 knee and 2651 hip operations. *Acta Orthopaedica Scandinavica* 63:665–671.

Yaszemski MJ, Shapler TR (1990) Sudden death from cord compression associated with atlanto-axial instability in rheumatoid arthritis. A case report. *Spine* 15:338–341.

15 Patient Education

J. HILL
University of Leeds, West Yorkshire, UK

Patient education can significantly improve a patient's use of self-management techniques and help to reduce the effect of disease symptoms. This makes it an essential component in the management of rheumatic disease. After reading this chapter the reader should be able to:

- understand the role of the nurse in patient education;
- underpin practice with an appropriate theoretical educational model;
- select a suitable method of delivering patient education to your patients;
- choose pertinent topics for inclusion in a patient education programme;
- discuss the merits of written literature, audio-visual and computer-assisted learning;
- assess the effectiveness of a patient education programme.

Patient education (PE) has been evolving since the late 1970s; when the term PE was synonymous with transfer of information, usually from physician to patients (Hill, 1999). Since these early beginnings, PE has developed into a potent and essential element of care for those with chronic disease. As the process has become more commonplace, research into PE has grown, and its effects have been shown to bring about:

- increases in knowledge
- changes in behaviours
- increased physical function
- increased psychosocial health.

Research into the effects of PE continues, and systematic reviews such as that undertaken by Reimsma *et al.* (2002; 2004) are pointing the way to the most effective types of intervention.

THE ROLE OF THE NURSE

The provision of information and PE is fundamental to rheumatology nursing (Hill and Hale, 2004) and clinical nurse specialists see it as one of their main

Rheumatology Nursing: A Creative Approach, 2nd edn. Edited by Jackie Hill.
Copyright 2006 by John Wiley & Sons, Ltd.

priorities (Carr, 2001). Although PE is not mentioned specifically in the commonly used conceptual theoretical nursing frameworks such as Orem's Self-Care model (Orem, 1980); Roper et al.'s Activities of Living model (Roper, et al., 1990) and Roy's Adaptational model (Roy, 1976); the underlying principles of self-care, maintaining independence and adaptation to stress outlined in these models cannot be achieved without PE. In Chapter 1, a number of beliefs that underpin the care that nurses provide are cited. They include:

- therapeutic nursing
- reciprocal care
- professional closeness.

It is important to understand the relationship of these aspects of nursing to PE.

THERAPEUTIC NURSING

Therapeutic nursing is about deliberate nursing decisions that actively promote health and healing for patients. McMahon (1991) has listed a number of activities which includes patient teaching, and this can be used as a framework for therapeutic nursing. Therapeutic nursing activities comprise:

- developing the nurse/patient relationship – partnership, intimacy, reciprocity;
- adapting the environment – interpersonal, physical;
- patient education – information, self-efficacy, behavioural changes, coping mechanisms;
- providing comfort – physical, psychological;
- complementary interventions – aromatherapy, massage;
- physical treatments – leg ulcers, pressure sores.

Nurses who deploy a therapeutic model are more likely to provide a better patient outcome than those who do not.

RECIPROCITY

Reciprocity is a key concept in nursing. It is an act of mutual exchange reflecting the belief that the nurse/patient relationship is beneficial to both parties. Reciprocity is particularly important in the process of PE because it is recognised that patients contribute a unique expertise. Only patients can assess their pain, decide how ill or well they feel and how their disease impacts on their lives. Nurses can learn from their patients and vice versa. This reciprocal teaching/learning process can assist in the solving of both current and future problems and help us to develop our practice.

PROFESSIONAL CLOSENESS

The term 'professional closeness' was first used by Peplau (1969) to differentiate between the symbiotic learning process that takes place in the nurse/patient relationship and peer learning. Professional closeness stems from the empathy that develops between the nurse and patient, and this is important in the context of PE as it helps patients to feel safe so they freely express their thoughts and feelings. This kind of relationship ensures that the patients' needs are truly met. The down side to professional closeness is that some patients and nurses can misinterpret the professional rapport for that of an interpersonal relationship in which the needs of the patient and the professional are mutual.

A DEFINITION OF PE

PE is any set of planned educational activities designed to improve patients' health behaviours, consequently their health status, and possibly their long-term outcome.

A task force of the National Arthritis Advisory Board in the USA has developed a set of standards for arthritis PE and has defined it as:

'organized learning experiences designed to facilitate voluntary adoption of behaviours or belief conducive to health. It is a set of planned educational activities that are separate from clinical patient care. The activities of a patient education program must be designed to attain goals the patient has participated in formulating. The primary focus of these activities includes acquisition of information, skills, beliefs and attitudes which impact on health status, quality of life, and possibly health care utilization.' (Burckhardt, 1994).

The process of PE can be represented schematically as shown in Figure 15.1.

However, PE is not a treatment per se and should be regarded as a treatment enhancer, magnifying the effects of standard treatments by persuading patients to adhere more closely or adopt actions that are believed to be beneficial. The ultimate success or failure in terms of health status or long-term outcome will remain dependent upon the inherent effectiveness of the treatment employed.

THEORIES AND MODELS

Theories and models do not tell us what to do or how to do things. They do however guide our practice, and the most successful PE programmes are underpinned by a combination of theories and models (Lorig, 1996).

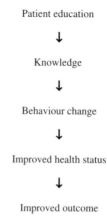

Figure 15.1 The process of patient education.

Originally, the traditional biomedical model was used. This assumes that disease can be completely explained by disordered physiology and biology. For some diseases it has worked well, but the biomedical model is not really suitable for chronic diseases and many health professionals now discount its use and follow a more pragmatic approach.

The learning and teaching theory developed to pass knowledge to children has also been tried, but it is inappropriate when teaching adults. A more interactive, didactic style is more successful when working with mixed ability adult groups (Lorig *et al.*, 1987). Patients are usually adults whose experience is one of their major resources. In general, they do not accept advice unless it is justifiable and makes sense to them. This was highlighted in a study by Donovan *et al.* (1989), where only six out of thirty-two patients took the number of drugs prescribed by their general practitioners. The other twenty-six compared their perceptions of the potential side effects and efficacy with their symptoms, and made a judgement on the required dosage. The study recommended a shift of emphasis from didactic programmes to more informal methods of PE.

The respect, intimacy and reciprocity required to bond the nurse/patient relationship, will enable the nurse to perceive the patient as a person with his or her own knowledge, belief values and experience. These must be incorporated into any system of care, including PE programmes.

Models and theories are discussed in Chapter 5, but an overview is given here of those most commonly used in PE. They are based on producing changes in behaviour and include the:

- health belief model
- learned helplessness theory

- stress and coping theory
- self-efficacy theory.

HEALTH BELIEF MODEL

The health belief model was originally put forward to explain the lack of uptake of tuberculosis screening (Becker, 1974), and it is one of the oldest and most widely used health education models. It is based on the person's perception of a combination of:

- a perceived threat
- expectations of benefit.

Before patients change their behaviour, they evaluate the perceived threat by weighing up their susceptibility to, and the severity of the danger. Lorig (1996) uses AIDS as a good example. AIDS is perceived as a severe disease. However, there are many different beliefs about susceptibility, and safe sex will only be practised by those who believe themselves to be susceptible.

Severity and susceptibility are only parts of the model. The equation is not complete without expectation. Patients must also believe that:

- a new behaviour will be beneficial;
- they are capable of carrying out the behaviour change;
- the costs of change do not outweigh the benefits.

LEARNED HELPLESSNESS THEORY

Seligman (1975) developed the learned helplessness theory following research on dogs. These animals learned that whatever their response to electric shocks, they received further shocks and subsequently they became unresponsive and helpless. This work has evolved and has been adapted to human behaviour. The individual comes to believe that their actions have no effect on eventual outcome. They do not believe they can control their disease and expect to fail in their endeavours; they become passive and unresponsive to behavioural change. This state is known as 'learned helplessness' and it is characterised by lack of:

- motivation
- cognition
- action.

A patient with severe rheumatoid arthritis who has tried many disease-modifying drugs that have caused side effects or failed to provide efficacy, may expect all drugs to fail. They tend to stop trying to overcome their problems and become nonadherent with their treatments. A typical response is, 'Why bother, what difference does it make?'

STRESS AND COPING THEORY

Any chronic, incurable disease will cause stress and coping deficits. One of the key elements of nursing is to help patients to cope with their illness (Wilson Barnett, 1984), and so stress and coping theory are relevant to rheumatological PE. There are many different coping theories, but one of the most useful focuses on the work by Lazarus and Folkman (1984). This theory has particular merit as it has practical application, works well alongside self-efficacy theory and it is recommended by respected authors (Lorig, 1996; Newbold, 1996).

Coping has been described as 'a set of cognitive and behavioural responses to events perceived as stressful' (Lazarus and Folkman, 1984). They also suggest that 'persons are constantly changing cognitions and behaviour efforts to manage specific external and/or internal demands that are appraised as taxing or exceeding the person's resources'.

This is a cognitive appraisal model that is in keeping with the concept of PE. It features:

- problem-focused coping
- emotion-focused coping.

In problem-focused coping, the acquisition of knowledge results in the belief that the stressor is controllable and its effect can be modified, avoided or minimised.

Emotion-focused coping is based on the elimination of undesirable emotions which follow on from the experience of the stressor (Auerbach, 1989).

Stress and coping strategies should be incorporated into PE programmes, but it must be borne in mind that each patient is different and what works for one may not work for another. Strategies need to be tried, their effectiveness assessed and if they are not successful, new methods explored. There is substantial literature on coping (Lazarus and Folkman, 1984) that can guide nurses on how to provide a variety of the most fitting options in their PE programmes.

SELF-EFFICACY THEORY

PE is based on the premise that patients should be active collaborators in their care and have the knowledge and skills to manage their disease. Self-efficacy is an essential component of this complex scenario, as it refers to a person's confidence in their ability to perform a specific task or achieve a certain objective (Bandura, 1977). If a person exhibits high self-efficacy in the face of a stressor, they will be more likely to carry out constructive coping behaviours and maintain a positive sense of well-being. Higher initial self-efficacy correlates with better health status two years later (Brekke *et al.*, 2001).

In a recent study, changes in self-efficacy following a stress management programme were associated with depression, pain, health status and disease activity. Enhanced self-efficacy was related to a reduction in symptoms. Self-efficacy theory is discussed in more detail in Hill, 1999, and in Chapter 5.

Many theories can be applied to PE, with their origins in the fields of adult education, communication, sociology and psychology. Each has something to offer and perhaps the most successful programmes are those which incorporate something from each.

STARTING THE PE PROCESS

The question of the best time to start the educational process has yet to be resolved, but the timing is essential if the PE programme is to meet the individual's needs. Some authors have suggested that the greatest reduction in disability can be achieved by intensive intervention at an early stage of the disease, and learning coping skills shortly after diagnosis will help patients for the rest of their lives (DeVellis and Blalock, 1993). However, there are problems with this approach. Soon after being told their diagnosis, patients commonly undergo a period of grief or bereavement reaction, leading to a period of denial. Trying to educate them under these conditions can be counterproductive and lead to further depression (Donovan *et al.*, 1989). Counselling sessions would be more helpful than PE at this stage.

When the patient starts to ask questions about their disease and treatments, it is a sign that they have begun to accept their diagnosis and the process of PE can begin. However, this information-seeking stage is only the beginning of the process. People need to be ready to move on to the next stage which is making behavioural changes (Hammond, 2003). Prochaska and Diclemente (1992) describe five stages of change:

1. precontemplation – not seriously contemplating a behaviour change;
2. contemplation – weighs the perceived benefits and cost against status quo;
3. preparation – preparation and planning stage;
4. starting to make change – actively develops skills required for behavioural change;
5. maintenance – works at sustaining long-term change.

These stages are not always sequential, patients may well revert from one stage to a former stage.

THE AIM OF PE

The aim of PE is to maintain or improve the patient's health status. Unfortunately, simply adding to their stock of knowledge does not do this. Some studies have shown that PE can change behaviour and increase health status, but the literature is not consistent (Lorig *et al.*, 1987). Even when behaviour changes occur, these actions do not automatically lead to changes in health status.

Effective self-management relies upon the patient's willingness to cooperate and their ability to comply with self-care activities; and so PE is a combined effort between the multidisciplinary team, the patient and their partner/carer (Figure 15.2). This can be difficult as disease activity can vary dramatically from day to day and so it is important that patients can tailor their therapies accordingly (Hill, 1995). They need to be able to:

- vary their drug usage according to their symptoms;
- employ coping strategies;
- regulate their daily exercise programmes;
- plan rest/activity periods.

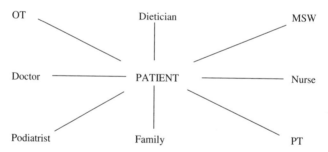

Figure 15.2 Typical multidisciplinary patient education team.

THE EFFECTS OF PE

There are many claims for the overall effectiveness of PE, but few have defined this term. A PE programme can be considered to be effective if it brings benefits that are additional to the existing treatments (Hill, 1997), and a 45-study literature review estimated that when PE is added to conventional rheumatology care, it brought about an additional 15–30% improvement (Hirano *et al.*, 1994).

A second proposal is that PE should achieve benefits comparable to those resulting from conventional therapy but with fewer side effects or at a lower cost (DeVellis and Blalock, 1993) and a number of studies have shown that PE is successful at:

- increasing knowledge
- changing behaviour
- improving physical and psychological health status.

INCREASES IN KNOWLEDGE

The acquisition of knowledge depends on a number of variables, such as:

- the skills of the teacher
- the content of the programme
- the receptiveness of the patient.

When these variables are favourable, PE can indeed increase the patient's knowledge in a number of areas. This was demonstrated in a study (Hill et al., 1994) in which patients attending a nursing clinic were taught about:

- disease aetiology
- drugs and how to take them
- exercise
- joint protection
- pain control
- coping strategies.

After six months, patients were tested for increases in knowledge, compared to study entry, using the Patient Knowledge Questionnaire (Hill et al., 1991). They had increased their scores significantly and this knowledge was further enhanced at twelve months from entry (Hill et al., 1994). This study has been replicated with similarly favourable results (Hill et al., 2003).

Another study evaluated the effectiveness of educating patients during their routine outpatient visit. It was found that overall knowledge of diagnosis and treatment was high at 86%. Knowledge of the use and likely effects of drugs ranged from 52%–92%, but many patients were unaware of the side effects of drugs and how to avoid them (Mahmud et al., 1995).

Further evidence was obtained from a literature review of 34 studies which measured changes in knowledge, in which 94% attained increases (Lorig et al., 1987).

There is of course, a difference between knowing something and acting upon it. For instance, many people know that smoking causes a wide range of health-related problems, but they continue to smoke. However, in the context of chronic diseases, knowledge is an essential precursor to behavioural change and can bridge the gap between knowing and doing.

BEHAVIOUR CHANGES

The literature review undertaken by Lorig et al. (1987), showed that PE can change behaviour patterns to a large extent. They report increases of:

- 79% in the practice of exercise;
- 33% in the practice of joint protection;
- 86% in the practice of relaxation.

Hawley (1995) used effect size to compare treatment and control groups. This is a rigorous, standardised measure of change advocated and described by Kazis et al., (1989). In the 34 studies scrutinised, self-management behaviours such as compliance with exercise and coping skills improved following PE.

IMPROVING PHYSICAL AND
PSYCHOLOGICAL HEALTH STATUS

The more serious rheumatic diseases are capable of causing pain and swelling, stiffness, joint deformity and fatigue, which inevitably lead to a deficit in mobility, energy and everyday skills. These symptoms and ensuing short-comings leave the patient feeling frustrated and inadequate which causes anxiety and depression. Weiner (1975) terms this the 'burden of arthritis'. Although medication, physical modalities and surgery can help to alleviate some of the problems, they are rarely the whole answer. PE however, has been shown to be a beneficial therapy in that it can increase both physical and psychological status. The strongest evidence is provided by the technique of meta-analysis, in which data from a number of similarly conducted studies are analysed together to provide a more robust statistical analysis.

This is the type of study undertaken by Mullen et al. (1987) who investi-gated the data from fifteen studies on the effects of PE on disability, pain and depression. Ten studies were on patients with rheumatoid arthritis, four on rheumatoid arthritis/osteoarthritis and one on osteoarthritis alone. The results showed that compared to the control groups, treatment groups had a reduction of:

- 22% in their depression
- 16% in their pain
- 8% in their disability.

The reduction in pain following the PE programmes was similar to that expe-rienced by patients following the ingestion of nonsteroidal anti-inflammatory drugs, and it is suggested that PE has an independent effect and is therefore a distinct modality.

PE can contribute to the health status of those patients with arthritis and when given in addition to other treatments provide a cumulative effect.

LONG-TERM EFFICACY

The chronic nature and lack of cure for many rheumatic diseases necessitates the assessment of long-term efficacy of treatments. However, there is a paucity of research in this area.

A 20-month follow-up study showed that patients experienced a slight decline in functional ability but retained their decrease in pain, depression and physician visits (Lorig and Holman, 1989).

Another study assessed the effect of PE four years after completion. This included patients with rheumatoid arthritis, osteoarthritis and other forms of arthritis. It was shown that the PE group:

* maintained 15% to 20% reductions in pain;
* made fewer visits to the physician;
* maintained their belief in their ability to cope.

However, their disability increased over the four years, and improvement in depression was not maintained (Lorig et al., 1993).

A controlled study which revisited patients twelve months after completion of the initial PE programme reported maintained improvement in knowledge, self-reported health behaviour and disability scores (Lindroth et al., 1989). A further follow-up to this study was undertaken at five years (Lindroth et al., 1995). The improvement in performing exercise and joint protection seen at twelve months did not persist, but those patients who had been in the PE group had more contact with their rheumatologists, physiotherapists and occupational therapists. They developed an increased sense of control and coping from twelve months to five years, resulting in a reduction in the problems they reported.

PLANNING A PE PROGRAMME

There are a number of considerations to be taken into account when planning a PE programme, for instance the physical condition of the patients who will be attending and the learning environment. Patients are usually in pain that will shorten their attention span, and they are also prone to inactivity stiffness. Those who have only recently been diagnosed are often confused about their illness and can be anxious and depressed. It is difficult to master new facts when there are physical distractions or if the environment is not conducive to learning. To overcome these problems make sure that you plan:

* easy access to the learning environment
* a comfortable temperature
* short teaching sessions

- use of appropriate seating
- exercise breaks
- some refreshment to allow patients to take their drugs.

No matter how much thought is put into the practical arrangements, it will be to no avail if the content is not seen as relevant to the individual patient. When planning the composition of a PE programme it should be borne in mind that patients are usually adults with their own beliefs and knowledge base. Adults are self-directing individuals with their own experiences; any information proffered should make sense to them and appear to be justifiable. For instance, when deciding whether or not to take drug therapy, they compare the potential efficacy and side effects with the severity of their symptoms and act accordingly.

CONTENT OF A PE PROGRAMME

PE is a complex process and the success of the programme depends heavily on the quality of the planning (Taal *et al.*, 1996). The most effective programmes will need to include the elements shown in Figure 15.3, and it is a good idea to start PE programmes with tasks that patients are sure they can achieve.

The most successful PE programmes are those which endeavour to fulfil the aspirations of both patients and health professionals, so begin by getting patients to write down their own goals in a form of contract with themselves.

There may be differences of opinion about what it is necessary to include in a PE programme, and this was highlighted in an evaluation of the Arthritis

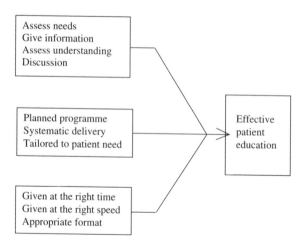

Figure 15.3 Requirements for effective patient education.

and Rheumatism Councils patient literature. Some doctors thought that giving the patients too much information could lead to undue anxiety and stress. The patients interviewed wanted more detailed information about:

- their condition
- treatments and drugs
- self-management
- dietary guidance
- exercise
- practical tips
- communication skills.

There are many PE programmes running throughout the UK and they typically contain the topics shown below:

- disease process (aetiology, symptoms, blood tests);
- drug therapy (effects, side effects, usage);
- exercise (effects, how and when to do, assessing effects);
- joint protection (what it is, use of splints, life style alterations);
- fatigue (causes, energy conservation);
- pain control (drug therapy, relaxation, distraction etc.);
- coping (practical strategies, self efficacy, contracting);
- diet (effects on health, fatigue);
- relaxation (what it is, how it works, how to do it);
- complementary therapies (acupuncture, aromatherapy, massage);
- communication (talking to doctors and health professionals);
- self-help (self-efficacy, voluntary organizations);
- goal setting (how to set achievable targets and reach them).

METHODS OF DELIVERY

PE can be delivered in a number of ways; for instance formal or informal sessions can be introduced into either the inpatient or outpatient department (Hill, 2003). The programme can be taught by health professionals or lay persons and the sessions can be given on a one-to-one basis or to a group. Each has advantages and disadvantages and each patient will have their own preference. However they are taught, it is important that the patients are provided with feedback about their performance, being careful to stress the most positive aspects first.

Opportunity education

Educating patients about their disease and treatments is one of the primary functions of the rheumatology nurse and so every encounter with the patient should be treated as an opportunity to teach (Daltroy and Liang, 1988). It is common for short encounters to take place at:

- the patient's bedside
- in outpatient clinics
- in general practitioner surgeries.

These so-called '30-second interventions' can yield positive results in the hands of a skilled practitioner. For instance a patient who is given a new drug can be asked a simple question such as, 'When are you going to take your tablets?' This will highlight any problems, such as whether they will take it with food or not. The skilled practitioner can also direct the conversation to include possible side effects and interactions with other drugs. The patient will have gained valuable knowledge and the consultation will have taken little longer than normal.

One-to-one PE

One-to-one teaching is very labour intensive which makes it the most costly. However, it is considered by some to be the most effective way of imparting information as it can be tailored to each individual's needs (Tucker and Kirwan, 1989). Because it is costly, programmes must be well-planned and the following items should be carefully thought about:

- the time needed to produce and deliver the programme;
- the content of the programme;
- the teaching methods of the programme;
- documenting what has been taught;
- assessing the effectiveness of the programme;
- the cost of the programme.

PE programmes need to be accessible to the patient. Those patients whose routine clinic consultation includes a PE session as part of their normal management find this easiest and most convenient, and research has shown it to be practical and effective (Mahmud et al., 1995).

One of the most significant aspects of one-to-one teaching is its flexibility. The educator can avoid a rigid format and can include topics that are important to the patient. The timing of introduction of the subject matter can also be varied according to the patients needs. The skilled teacher can also manipulate the session to include their own agenda alongside that of the patients. For instance, if the patient wants to talk about pain and the educator wishes to teach drug therapy, an explanation of the effect of drug therapy on pain will meet both needs.

A number of studies have demonstrated that individualised PE programmes are more effective than routinised programmes (Lorish *et al.*, 1985; Neuberger *et al.*, 1993) and wherever possible this format should be used.

Group teaching

A number of hospitals and community bases teach groups of patients through structured PE programmes. These groups can make a real difference but are not for everyone. Hammond and Badcock (2002) found that 50% of patients attending a rheumatology outpatient department would not consider attending a group programme. Despite this, many patients gain real benefit from group education.

Health professionals usually undertake teaching, but it is becoming more common for lay teachers, who have some arthritic problem to become teachers. This inspires some of the attendees, as the lay teachers act as very positive role models.

Group teaching has several advantages. Firstly it is comparatively cheap compared to one-to-one programmes. Some also believe that it is a more effective method of teaching patients skills, such as joint protection and exercise. It has a further advantage to some patients who value meeting others with the same illness and who gain benefit from sharing their experiences and meeting other patients socially.

There are of course negative aspects. Attendees will have different knowledge bases and levels of skill, which makes it difficult for the educator to meet everyone's needs.

Some patients find it difficult or expensive to attend sessions and others find it daunting to express their problems verbally for fear of failure or criticism.

THE ARTHRITIS SELF-MANAGEMENT PROGRAMME (ASMP)

This is a community-based programme that began in 1978 in the USA. The underlying theoretical basis is the patient's belief that s/he can affect the consequences of their disease (self-efficacy). It is believed that perceived self-efficacy is a significant determinant of human functioning that operates partially independently of underlying skills. The ASMP was pioneered by Lorig and her colleagues and was the first arthritis PE programme to utilise lay teachers. Over the years, the programme has been adapted as experience and research results have emerged. For instance the programmes now use pairs of teachers comprising one professional and one lay teacher rather than lay teachers alone. The lay teachers are accepted by both patients and professionals and have proved as effective as professionals in their teaching (Lorig *et al.*, 1986).

Changes have been made to the content and methodology (Lorig and Gonzalez, 1992) and at present it is usually taught as six two-hour sessions over a period of months. The format remains the same in that patients with rheumatoid arthritis, osteoarthritis or other forms of arthritis are taught in mixed groups.

The programme focuses on:

- utilising information
- problem solving
- symptom management
- use of coping skills.

The topics taught in the ASMP are similar to those listed previously, but they are taught using the techniques shown below:

- contracting
- feedback
- goal setting
- guided imagery
- principles of self help
- visualisation.

The ASMP has been very well researched in the USA. A controlled study on the effectiveness of the programme (Lorig et al., 1985) showed a significant improvement in:

- patient knowledge;
- the practice of self-management behaviours;
- pain.

The programme has become extensively used in the USA has been adapted by other teams (Lindroth et al., 1989; Taal et al., 1993; Davis et al., 1994) for use in Australia, New Zealand and Europe. The ASMP has been anglicised for use in Britain and its effects are currently being researched.

LEARNING AIDS

There are a number of techniques that can be used to enhance teaching and aid the learning process. Some, such as reiteration, are straightforward but nonetheless need to be thought about and incorporated into the programme. Others, for instance written material, needs careful research and piloting on the intended recipients.

VERBAL INFORMATION

Most patient teaching is presented verbally, but patients along with the rest of us, tend to forget a great deal of what they are told. A study from a rheumatology outpatient clinic (Anderson *et al.*, 1979) showed that patients who attended the clinic for the first time recalled about 40% of the information they were given. This figure is in broad agreement with much of the published literature.

When giving information follow some simple guidelines:

- Present the most salient points first. This is because we remember best what we are told first.
- Consider the patient's priorities. They will recall most easily what they consider to be most important.
- Do not bombard them with facts. Most people only remember the first four or five items presented to them.
- Give written backup. Oral information is easily forgotten. Written information should always be provided as a supplement. The patient can then take this material home and digest it at their leisure. They can then share it with their families/partners and use it as an aid memoir in the future.

WRITTEN INFORMATION

Patients themselves feel they need written information (Donovan and Blake, 1992) and there is some evidence to support its effectiveness. Twenty patients with rheumatoid arthritis increased their knowledge after reading information, but when the literature was combined with lectures, the knowledge gain was significantly greater (Vignos *et al.*, 1976).

A number of professional organisations produce some excellent patient literature. They include:

- Arthritis Care
- Arthritis Research Campaign
- Arthritis Foundation
- pharmaceutical companies.

Many hospitals, wards and those that organise PE programmes, prefer to produce their own literature. Producing useful written material is more difficult than it appears at first sight, and unless the material can be read and understood by those for whom it is intended, will prove to be an expensive but useless exercise.

Writing material for patients

The purpose of written information is to inform and empower the patient and so it must be:

- informative
- accurate
- understandable.

Unfortunately, medically based literature is difficult to write, as the terminology is inherently alien to the general public. Some authors have tried to address this problem (Boyd, 1987) and the following guidelines can help to make the content more user friendly:

- use lay terminology – 'knee cap' rather than 'patella', 'persistent' rather than 'chronic';
- use simple sentence structure;
- use one or two syllable words wherever possible;
- limit the number of words using three or more syllables;
- write in short paragraphs;
- personalise the material with words like I, we, us;
- use positive not negative language;
- start with the aims of the material;
- use a question and answer format;
- include what the patients want to know as well as what they need to know.

Readability

Having written the material it is important to assess whether it is easy to read (Arthur, 1995) and unfortunately this is one stage that is often left out. The readability of a document refers to the reader's ability to decipher the text (Meade and Smith, 1991).

The need for assessing readability was highlighted in a recent study (Hill and Bird, 2003), on 100 patients with rheumatoid arthritis who were attending an outpatient clinic. Twelve percent had difficulty with their reading and so drug information leaflets about penicillamine, supplied from the clinic, were rewritten to be easy or fairly easy to read. This was achieved without altering the information they contained and patients exhibited significant increases in their knowledge of their drug.

Ease of readability depends on the structure of the sentence and the length of the words used, and there a number of formulae that can be used to estimate how difficult a leaflet is to read. They are based on the:

- number of syllables per word
- number of words in each sentence.

The Flesch Reading Index (Flesch, 1948), the Dale–Chall Formula (Dale and Chall, 1948) and the 'Simple Measure of Gobbledygook' (SMOG) Grading

(McLaughlin, 1969); are the most commonly used. There is a highly positive correlation amongst formulae and so the best advice is to use what you have available. Some word processor packages now include formulae, for instance Word for Windows incorporates the Flesch Index which makes it possible to assess material as it is composed. It should be noted that most of these formulae have been developed for use with the English language and because of the differences in grammatical construction they are not suitable for use with other languages.

Although they are useful, reading ease formulae are only tools, they do not assess:

- good writing
- the accuracy of information
- the layout of the material.

Design of the material

Layout of the material is another important aspect. A well-thought-out design will encourage the patient to read it. There are a number of considerations such as:

- typeface
- type size
- colour of the paper and typeface
- size of the leaflet.

The typeface should be clear, plain, and visible; a sans-serif font is attractive and easy to read. Once you have chosen the typeface, do not try to make headings or words stand out by adding a different one. Try using larger letters of the same type face or use bold or italics.

The size of the type should not be too small, 12 point or larger is ideal and eye span should be approximately 60 or 70 characters in length. Capital letters are more difficult to read, so use lower sentence case with plenty of white space between lines.

Coloured paper can be eye catching, but beware of using colours such as yellow on white as this is difficult to read.

Finally, consider how easy the document will be to handle. If it is produced to be stored in a folder then A4 is fine, but if it is a single pamphlet, A5 or A4 is better.

Each of us learns in different way, some may find it easier to read others to watch and some to listen. It is therefore important to offer patients a variety of different modalities.

AUDIOCASSETTES

Audiocassettes provide written information in verbal format and are invaluable for those patients who have difficulty reading or are blind or partially sighted. Many people use them to practice relaxation techniques or distraction therapy, but there is no reason why information about drug therapy, pain control or other modules of a PE programme cannot be dictated on to a tape.

VIDEOS

Although written and audio formats are both excellent ways of exchanging facts, skills such as exercise and methods of joint protection are easier to demonstrate on a video. They are particularly valuable for those people who have difficulty with reading, but they should be considered a part of a PE programme rather than a substitute for it. Many voluntarily funded organisations such as the Arthritis and Rheumatism Council and Arthritis Care produce excellent videos for patients. Their value is greatly enhanced if they come with an explanatory booklet, as is the case with a programme on medications that has been well received by patients (Clayson et al., 1994).

Videos can be used in almost any setting: group sessions, one to one, wards, outpatient clinics or in the home.

COMPUTER ASSISTED LEARNING

Developments in computer technology have the potential to make enormous strides in methods of delivering patient information, and computer-assisted learning has been advocated as a way of empowering the patient rather than the educator, and therefore a positive move in the direction of self-care (Luker and Caress, 1989).

Advances in personal computer technology offer the possibility of patients having access to expert systems. Expert systems allow individuals to interrogate the computer for the information that they require. Explanations are provided in text, computer graphics and sound format. Many people now have access to the internet, and again this gives access to information from all over the world at the touch (well almost) of a switch.

Research carried out in the mideighties in the USA, assessed the effect of a computer based education lesson for patients with rheumatoid arthritis (Wetstone et al., 1985). It covered ten main topics including:

- aetiology of the disease
- dietary advice
- exercise regimes
- joint protection techniques

- medications
- other treatments.

Patients were able to access the topics of their choice in any order, and review them at will. When compared to a matched control group, the computer-educated group was shown to have enjoyed the lesson and improved significantly in a number of areas. They had:

- gained more knowledge than the controls;
- improved their outlook on life;
- were more hopeful of a good prognosis;
- reported an increase in their use of behaviours such as joint protection.

Expert systems allow PE to be genuinely patient-centred and self-directed and are therefore to be encouraged.

ACTION POINTS FOR PRACTICE

- Describe two theoretical models that you consider to be appropriate for use in a PE programme.
- Write a drug information leaflet that will be easily understood by your patients.
- Write a list of topics that would be suitable for inclusion in a PE programme for patients with systemic lupus erythematosus.
- Describe ways of assessing the effectiveness of a PE programme.
- Carry out a literature search on the effects and side effects of PE, discuss the merits and problems associated with such programmes.

REFERENCES

Anderson JL, Dodman S, Copelman M *et al.* (1979) Patient information recall in a rheumatology clinic. *Rheumatology and Rehabilitation* 18:18–22.

Arthur VAM (1995) Written patient information: a review of the literature. *Journal of Advanced Nursing* 21:1081–1086.

Auerbach SM (1989) Stress management and coping research in the health care setting: an overview and methodological commentary. *Journal of Consulting and Clinical Psychology* 57(3):388–395.

Bandura A (1977) Self-efficacy: toward a unifying theory of behavioural change. *Psychological Review* 84:191–215.

Becker M (1974) The health belief model and personal health behaviour. *Health Education Monographs* 2:236.

Boyd MD (1987) A guide to writing effective education materials. *Nursing Management* 18(7):56–57.

Brekke M, Hjortdahl P, Kvien TK (2001) Self-efficacy and health status in rheumatoid arthritis. A two year longitudinal observation study. *Rheumatology* 40:387–392.

Burckhardt CS (1994) Arthritis and musculoskeletal patient education standards. *Arthritis Care and Research* 7:1–4.

Carr A (2001) *Defining the Extended Clinical Role for Allied Health Professionals in Rheumatology.* Conference Proceedings No. 12, Chesterfield, Arthritis Research Campaign.

Clayson M, Cole A, Phillips P (1994) Medication for arthritis – an educational package for patients. *Scandinavian Journal Rheumatology* (suppl 97) Ab 113.

Dale E, Chall JS (1948) A formula for predicting readability. *Educational Research Bulletin* 27:11–20.

Daltroy LH, Liang MH (1988) Patient education in the rheumatic diseases: a research agenda. *Arthritis Care and Research* 1:161–169.

Davis P, Busch A, Lowe JC et al. (1994) Evaluation of a rheumatoid arthritis patient education program: impact on knowledge and self-efficacy. *Patient Education and Counseling* 24:55–61.

DeVellis RF, Blalock SJ (1993) Psychological and educational interventions to reduce arthritis disability. *Baillière's Clinical Rheumatology* 7:397–416.

Donovan JL, Blake D (1992) Patient compliance: deviance or reasoned decision making? *Social Science Medicine* 34:507–513.

Donovan JL, Blake DR, Fleming G (1989) The patient is not a blank sheet: lay beliefs and their relevance to patient education. *British Journal of Rheumatology* 28:58–61.

Flesch R (1948) A new readability yardstick. *Journal of Applied Psychology* 32:221–233.

Hammond A (2003) Patient education in arthritis: helping people change. *Musculoskeletal Care* 1(2):84–97.

Hammond A, Badcock L (2002) Improving education about arthritis. Identifying the educational needs of people with chronic inflammatory arthritis. *Rheumatology* 41(suppl)87:216.

Hawley D (1995) Psycho-educational interventions in the treatment of arthritis. *Baillière's Clinical Rheumatology* 9:803–823.

Hill J (1995) Patient education in rheumatic disease. *Nursing Standard* 9:25–28.

Hill J (1997) A practical guide to patient education and information giving. *Baillière's Clinical Rheumatology* 11(1):109–127.

Hill J (1999) Patient education and adherence to drug therapy. In: Ryan S (ed) Drug Therapy in Rheumatology Nursing. London, Whurr Publishers, 211–258.

Hill J (2003) An overview of education for patients with rheumatic disease. *Nursing Times* 99(19):26–27.

Hill J, Bird H (2003) The development and evaluation of a drug information leaflet for patients with rheumatoid arthritis. *Rheumatology* 42:66–70.

Hill J, Bird HA, Harmer R et al. (1994) An evaluation of the effectiveness, safety and acceptability of a nurse practitioner in a rheumatology outpatient clinic. *British Journal of Rheumatology* 33:283–288.

Hill J, Bird HA, Hopkins R (1991) The development and use of a patient knowledge questionnaire in rheumatoid arthritis. *British Journal of Rheumatology* 30:45–49.

Hill J, Hale C (2004) Clinical skills: evidence-based nursing care of people with rheumatoid arthritis. *British Journal of Nursing* 13(14):852–857.

Hill J, Thorpe R, Bird HA (2003) Outcomes for patients with RA: a rheumatology nurse practitioner clinic compared to standard outpatient care. *Musculoskeletal Care* 1(1):5–20.

Hirano PC, Laurent DD, Lorig K (1994) Arthritis patient education studies, 1987–1991: a review of the literature. *Patient Education and Counseling* 24:9–54.

Kazis LE, Anderson JJ, Meenan RF (1989) Effect sizes for interpreting changes in health status. *Medical Care* 27:S178–S189.

Lazarus RS, Folkman S (1984) *Stress appraisal and coping*. New York, Springer.

Lindroth Y, Bauman A, Barnes C *et al.* (1989) A controlled evaluation of arthritis education. *British Journal of Rheumatology* 28:7–12.

Lindroth Y, Bauman A, Brookes PM *et al.* (1995) A 5 year follow-up of a controlled trial of an arthritis education programme. *British Journal of Rheumatology* 34:647–652.

Lorig K (1996) *Patient Education a Practical Approach*, (2nd edn) Thousand Oaks, Sage.

Lorig K, Feigenbaum P, Regan C *et al.* (1986) A comparison of lay-taught and professional-taught arthritis self-management courses. *The Journal of Rheumatology* 13:763–767.

Lorig K, Gonzalez V (1992) The integration of theory with practice: a 12-year case study. *Health Education Quarterly* 19:355–368.

Lorig K, Holman HR (1989) Long-term outcomes of an arthritis self-management study: effects of reinforcement efforts. *Social Science Medicine* 29:221–224.

Lorig K, Konkol L, Gonzalez V (1987) Arthritis patient education: a review of the literature. *Patient Education and Counseling* 10:207–252.

Lorig K, Lubeck D, Kraines RG *et al.* (1985) Outcomes of self-help education for patients with arthritis. *Arthritis and Rheumatism* 28:680–685.

Lorig K, Mazonson PD, Holman HR (1993) Evidence suggesting that health education for self-management in patients with chronic arthritis has sustained health benefits while reducing health care costs. *Arthritis Rheumatism* 36:439–446.

Lorish CD, Parker J, Brown S (1985) Effective patient education: a quasi-experimental study comparing an individualized strategy with a routinized strategy. *Arthritis and Rheumatism* 28:1289–1297.

Luker K, Caress A (1989) Rethinking patient education. *Journal of Advanced Nursing* 14:711–718.

McLaughlin H (1969) SMOG grading-a new readability formula. *Journal of Reading* 12:639–646.

McMahon R (1991) Therapeutic nursing: theory, issues and practice. In: McMahon, Pearson A (eds): *Nursing as Therapy*. London, Chapman Hall.

Mahmud T, Comer M, Roberts K *et al.* (1995) Clinical implications of patients' knowledge. *Clinical Rheumatology* 14:627–630.

Meade CD, Smith CF (1991) Readability formulas: caution and criteria. *Patient Education and Counseling* 17:153–158.

Mullen PA, Laville EA, Biddle AK *et al.* (1987) Efficacy of psychoeducational interventions of pain, depression, and disability in people with arthritis: a meta-analysis. *Journal of Rheumatology* 14:33–39.

Neuberger GB, Smith KV, Black SO *et al.* (1993) Promoting self-care in clients with arthritis. *Arthritis Care and Research* 6:141–148.

Newbold D (1996) Coping with rheumatoid arthritis. How can specialist nurses influence it and promote better outcomes? *Journal of Clinical Nursing* 5:373–380.

Orem D (1980) *Nursing – Concepts of Practice* (2nd ed) New York, McGraw-Hill.

Peplau H (1969) Professional closeness. *Nursing Forum* 8(4):342–360.

Prochaska JO, Diclemente CC (1992) Stages of change in modification of problem behaviours. In: Hersen M, Eisler RM, Miller PM (eds) *Progress in Behavioural Modification*. Champaign, IL, Sycamore Press.

Reimsma R, Taal E, Kirwan J *et al.* (2002) Patient education programmes for adults with rheumatoid arthritis. *Cochrane Database of Systematic Reviews* 3: CD003688.

Reimsma RP, Taal E, Kirwan JR *et al.* (2004) Systematic review of rheumatoid arthritis patient education. *Arthritis Care and Research* 51(6):1045–1059.

Roper N, Logan W, Tiernay A (1985) *The Elements of Nursing* (2nd ed) Edinburgh, Churchill Livingstone.

Roy C (1976) *Introduction to Nursing – An Adaptational Model*. Englewood Cliffs, NJ, Prentice Hall.

Seligman M (1975) *Helplessness: on depression, development and death*. San Fransisco, W H Freeman.

Taal E, Rasker JJ, Wiegman O (1996) Patient education and self-management in the rheumatic diseases: a self efficacy approach. *Arthritis Care and Research* 9(3):229–238.

Taal E, Riemsma RP, Brus HLM *et al.* (1993) Group education for patients with rheumatoid arthritis. *Patient Education and Counseling* 20:177–187.

Tucker M, Kirwan JR (1989) Does patient education in rheumatoid arthritis have therapeutic potential? *Annals of the Rheumatic Disease* 50:422–428.

Vignos PJ, Parker WT, Thompson HM (1976) Evaluation of a clinic education programme for patients with RA. *Journal of Rheumatology* 3:155–165.

Wetstone SL, Sheehan J, Votaw RG *et al.* (1985) Evaluation of a computer based education lesson for patients with rheumatoid arthritis. *The Journal of Rheumatology* 12:907–912.

Wiener CL (1975) The burden of rheumatoid arthritis: tolerating the uncertainty. *Society of Science and Medicine* 9:97–104.

Wilson Barnett J (1984) *Key functions in nursing: the fourth Winifred Raphael memorial lecture*. London, RCN.

IV Primary and Paediatric Care

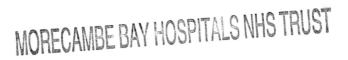

MORECAMBE BAY HOSPITALS NHS TRUST

16 Seamless Primary and Secondary Care

M. EDWARDS
Bilbrook Medical Centre, Staffordshire, UK

This chapter aims to promote an awareness of the need for adequate support mechanisms for rheumatology patients within primary care, that complement the specialist care provided by the secondary care services. After reading this chapter the reader should be able to:

- analyse the need for seamless care in the light of demographic trends, epidemiological factors and current financial resources;
- discuss the factors necessary to implement effective shared-care schemes;
- be aware of the political and financial changes introduced with the new General Medical Services (GMS) contract;
- explain the potential advantages of shared-care;
- discuss the care contribution made by the nurse to rheumatology patients in the community;
- appreciate the patient's role in self-care and management.

Orton (1994) states: 'demographic trends, changing patterns of illness and the rising cost of health care, all point to primary care as the key to the provision of effective health-care services in the future'. This statement still holds true in 2005. During the 1990's the National Health Service directed a large proportion of health-care provision to general practitioners and associated community health services. The New GMS Contract (BMA and NHS, 2003) will expand this provision, to give doctors a degree of choice in their service delivery. Close interprofessional communication and collaboration between hospital rheumatology departments and primary health-care teams is necessary for the development of a seamless rheumatology service. This combined approach can be difficult to implement, but could offer those with a rheumatic disease greater access to a cost-effective quality service.

Rheumatology Nursing: A Creative Approach, 2nd edn. Edited by Jackie Hill.
Copyright 2006 by John Wiley & Sons, Ltd.

THE SCOPE OF THE PROBLEM

In 2001, 16% of the UK population (9.4 million people) were aged over 65 years, an increase of 51% since 1961. Life expectancy at birth in 2001, was >75 years for men, and >80 years for women (Social Trends, 2003). The incidence of osteoarthritis increases with age (Hill and Ryan, 2000), and the potential consequence of this ageing population is a huge increase in workload for health and social care services.

GENERAL PRACTITIONER CONSULTATIONS

In 2001–2 almost 9 million people in the UK (19% of the population) visited their GP with arthritis-related conditions, more than 2 million of these because of osteoarthritis (OA) (ARC, 2004). Incidence rates of rheumatoid arthritis (RA) have remained steady over the past decade, but the number of people with OA has risen, as the population ages. The majority of patients do not require hospital referral and are seen in general practice. Consequently they rely on the primary health-care team (PHCT) to provide the relevant specialist advice and support. If the PHCT does not possess the necessary rheumatology and signposting knowledge, patients may be denied the benefits of appropriate treatment and education.

Research has highlighted some issues surrounding primary care management of rheumatic disease. In one study, a proportion of general practitioners overprescribed nonsteroidal anti-inflammatory drugs and underprescribed analgesics when treating patients with OA, while physiotherapy and local steroid injections were underused (Davis and Suarez-Almazor, 1995). Another study of 249 patients with RA found that only 65% of patients taking disease modifying anti-rheumatic drugs were receiving the ideal monitoring regime from their GP practice (Helliwell and O'Hara, 1995).

Patients have their own beliefs about rheumatic diseases. Vetter *et al.* (1990) reported that many patients perceived their arthritic symptoms to be normal for their age, and thus considered them to be untreatable. This view, although true for some people, would probably be less common in 2006, as patients have increased expectations about their disease management. They now present in the GP surgery with the latest internet information. Many patients want to know about their illness and methods of self-management and the community nurse may feel frustrated and inadequate if she is insufficiently knowledgeable to offer such support.

OUTPATIENT CONSULTATIONS

Having waited, sometimes for long periods to see a consultant, patients often face travelling and parking difficulties and expense when attending a hospital outpatient appointment. It has been recognised that the frustrations that this causes, coupled with the patient's anxiety and a rushed consultation, can create considerable barriers to communication (Haslock, 1987). Patient education is not always available, partly due to time constraints, but perhaps due also to inadequate ability and the unwillingness of some doctors to deliver this information. It is well-documented that nurses are better equipped than doctors with the skills required to educate and support patients.

ASPECTS OF EXISTING SERVICES

PRIMARY HEALTH-CARE TEAM (PHCT)

A survey undertaken by *Which* magazine (Consumer Association, 1992) found that the two main concerns of patients were:

- how long they had to sit in the waiting room;
- the length of time it took to get an appointment.

It is to be hoped that if this survey were to be repeated in 2006 the results would be more favourable. Recent incentives within primary care have increased accessibility for patients, and efforts are being made by primary care trusts to encourage general practices to undertake patient surveys and act on deficiencies in the service. Unfortunately, some patients do not seem to appreciate that occasionally emergencies do occur, and they may have to wait to be seen. Good communication between staff and patients should reduce patient frustrations.

Most patients prefer to see the same doctor or nurse and such personal, continuous care is linked to patient satisfaction (Freeman and Richards, 1993; Hjortdahl and Laerum, 1992). The general practitioner and other PHCT members, such as the practice nurse, district nurse and health visitor, often have a good rapport with their patients due to their close relationship. This results in:

- knowledge of the patient's physical, psychological, financial and social needs;
- the ability to visit the patient at home (district nurse and health visitor);
- the ability to make referrals to community health services such as physiotherapy, occupational therapy, social services and the voluntary sector.

Although primary prevention of many rheumatic disorders is not always possible, there are areas where health promotion can reduce morbidity from some disorders. A key area for primary prevention is to encourage weight loss for overweight and obese patients. In 2001, 27% men and 31% females were reported to be obese, with obesity peaking in both sexes in the 55–64 year age group (Social Trends, 2003). Weight loss can reduce the risk of OA of the knees (Hill and Ryan, 2000). While obesity is also a risk factor for gout, dietary calcium and Vitamin D are important for developing and maintaining strong bones and preventing osteoporosis. Simple health promotion advice supported with appropriate literature can be included in most consultations. Weight reduction prior to surgery should also be encouraged.

Increased knowledge and awareness will assist PHCT members to anticipate required support for patients and carers and encourage the promotion of self-help.

HOSPITAL RHEUMATOLOGY TEAM

Hospital rheumatology teams can offer the specialist knowledge and support required by patients with more serious conditions. Detailed clinical assessment, investigation and treatment are more easily carried out in secondary care. There is also speedier access to other health professionals such as occupational therapists and physiotherapists, and the development of rheumatology nurse specialists has enhanced patient education. The nurse specialists also coordinate activity between primary and secondary health care.

The demand for musculoskeletal services is likely to increase due to:

- an ageing population
- the development of advanced surgical techniques
- increased public expectation.

With finite resources, primary care trusts and hospital trusts have been examining ways in which services can be delivered to offer a more patient orientated experience. These are discussed below.

In 2003 the National Rheumatoid Arthritis Society (NRAS) recommended an increase in the numbers in the secondary care team. This could be a mix of consultant rheumatologist, experienced nonconsultant grade doctor and specialist nurse. One option is to develop the role of General Practitioner with a Special Interest (GPwSI). A general practitioner, who has a special interest in rheumatology, can be accredited (trained) to assist a consultant and hold clinics, thus reducing waiting lists and improving patient satisfaction. The success of the GPwSI role has been demonstrated through a pilot service at Mid Staffordshire NHS Trust between October 2002 and November 2003 (South Western Staffordshire PCT, 2004). The role resulted in:

- reduced waiting time for patients attending GPwSI clinic;
- reduced waiting time for all rheumatology patients;
- a low clinic did-not-attend rate;
- high patient and doctor satisfaction of the service;
- closer working relationships between primary and secondary care.

The data highlighted a significant number of soft tissue referrals where patients were treated with steroid injections, suggesting that not all GPs have the skills to undertake this type of injection. This may be due to lack of interest, or lack of training opportunities.

THE DEVELOPMENT OF A SEAMLESS SERVICE

Shared care has been defined as 'the joint participation of general practitioners and hospital consultants in the planned delivery of care for patients with a chronic condition, informed by an enhanced information exchange over and above routine discharge and referral letters' (Hickman *et al.*, 1994). It has been recognised that as demand for care increases, primary care doctors will need to share the care of patients with moderately severe and chronic medical problems (SMA, 2004). To do this, primary care doctors and their teams must have sufficient knowledge to advise patients competently, and be comfortable discussing treatment options with secondary care colleagues. 'Benefits for the patient comes not from providing cheap care but from greater use of primary care, where it is the appropriate level of care, as well as through shared care with our specialist colleagues' (SMA, 2004). The principles of good shared care are summarised in Table 16.1. The key to successful shared care is communication (NRAS, 2003).

Table 16.1 Principles of good outpatient shared care

- Identifying need at a local level
- Improved investment in education and training for primary care staff
- Effective joint planning initiatives
- Good communication channels between primary and secondary care

Current UK government policy has devolved health service funding to provide health care that is more responsive to local need. Consideration of the health and social data of a locality is a prerequisite to effective health-care planning and future resource allocation (Tinson, 1995). It is important that the data collected is used in conjunction with the needs expressed by individual patients, whose pain and disability can result in a vast array of problems. Aims and objectives of care can then be designed to meet the identified needs of the population. Strategies and resources can be planned and utilised more effectively and the data can contribute evidence of the need for change. A study of urban patients with rheumatic disease (Liebman *et al.*, 1986), found that the top ten expressions of need were:

- help with understanding medications
- explanations of special exercises
- provision of an arthritis doctor
- explanations of their type of arthritis

- podiatric care
- reading materials about arthritis
- help with household chores
- self-help support groups
- provision of canes and crutches
- someone to talk to about things that make them nervous.

It would be expected that these expressed needs have changed little over the years. The provision of podiatry care and help with household chores may have even deteriorated in some areas, where service provision has been reduced. These are issues which appear to receive a low priority on health and social care agendas.

INVESTMENT IN PRIMARY CARE

There is a growing recognition that the current and future demand for musculoskeletal services is likely to exceed available resources and strategies are being devised to encourage joint initiatives between primary and secondary care. Proposals aimed at providing a more efficient, effective service have included:

- provision of care close to home;
- teams of specialists in different disciplines working together;
- increased investment outside hospitals;
- a more systematic approach to incorporating research results into practice;
- promotion of collaboration rather than competition.

The new GMS contract (BMA and NHS, 2003) includes an incentive to general practitioners to set up shared-care initiatives in rheumatology. The treatment of several rheumatic diseases is reliant on drugs that require frequent blood monitoring due to potential serious side effects (BMA and NHS, 2003). The incidence of side effects can be significantly reduced if the monitoring is undertaken in an organised way, close to the patient's home. The National Enhanced Service for the provision of near-patient testing will fund a shared-care drug-monitoring service in respect of the following drugs:

- penicillamine
- auranofin
- sulphasalazine
- methotrexate
- sodium aurothiomalate.

Other key service delivery requirements are listed in Table 16.2.

Table 16.2 The National Enhanced Service funding requirements

1. Practices should be able to produce and maintain an up-to-date register of all shared-care drug-monitoring-service patients. This will include patient details and the indication and duration of treatment and last hospital appointment.
2. A system call and recall of patients is maintained.
3. All newly diagnosed/treated patients, and/or their carers, receive appropriate education and advice on management of and prevention of secondary complication of their condition.
4. Patients are offered continuing relevant information and resources.
5. Every patient will have an individual management plan, including a monitoring timetable and the recommended therapeutic range for blood results.
6. The practice will work with other appropriately trained professionals.
7. Patients will be referred promptly to other services and support agencies when necessary.
8. Practices will maintain records of service provision, including significant events, such as hospital admission.
9. All staff involved in delivering care under this scheme must have the necessary training and skills.
10. All patients should have an annual review and adult on their service provision.

(Adapted from National Enhanced Service, Provision of near-patient testing, BMA and NHS Confederation [2003])

Benefits to the patient of near-patient testing include less travelling time and expense, shorter waiting times and continuity of care by the PHCT. The NHS budget benefits from fewer attendees in the more expensive secondary care sector. However, GP practices can choose whether or not to deliver the above scheme. Where a GP declines to provide a shared care service, the Primary Care Trust will continue to commission the service, either from another surgery or from secondary care. There will inevitably be some inequity of care across a locality where GPs choose not to offer this service.

UTILISATION AND DEVELOPMENT OF MULTIDISCIPLINARY SKILLS

Doctors, nurses, managers and support staff need to recognise each other's talents, integrate their work and forge new relationships to move the new agenda for health forward. Although hospital rheumatology specialists are linked to the secondary health care team, their inclusion within the PHCT can be advantageous to the patient and colleagues.

RHEUMATOLOGISTS AND GENERAL PRACTITIONERS

General practitioners possess a wide range of medical skills that can benefit patients in the surgery or home setting. A comprehensive knowledge of the patient's physical and social situation increases the GP's ability to deal with ensuing psychological and social problems. However, GPs are generalists and not necessarily qualified to provide the specialist care required by rheumatology patients. The great majority of general practitioners acknowledge the need for postgraduate education in rheumatology and a large number would welcome education in practical skills. The provision of sufficient knowledge and skills will both enhance patient care and help to prevent unnecessary referrals to the rheumatologist, of patients with noninflammatory musculoskeletal disorders (Blaaw et al., 1995). An example of this provision is the delivery of joint injections in primary care.

Shared care offers the opportunity for mutual professional education between primary and secondary health professionals in rheumatology. This may occur through:

• regular meetings;
• primary health-care team members sitting in on hospital outpatient clinics;
• clinical assistantships where general practitioners work alongside consultant rheumatologists;
• the provision of multidisciplinary study days.

GPs have their own professional development plans for continued learning; rheumatology may be an area some may wish to develop.

RHEUMATOLOGY NURSE SPECIALIST

Rheumatology nurse specialists aim to facilitate the highest possible standards of care to rheumatology patients. They are a link between primary and secondary care, coordinating patient care after discharge and offering home visits to the housebound. This may involve undertaking joint injections at home, which can be more patient-friendly and cost-effective. Some specialist nurses also provide a telephone helpline which enables access to advice at the patient's convenience. Another advantage of the helpline is that the patient speaks to the nurse she/he knows and who knows her/his case, which may at times be more reassuring than NHS Direct. A disadvantage is the staff time commitment responding to calls.

Nurse-led clinics may be run in conjunction with consultant clinics. The patient may see the nurse six monthly and the doctor every twelve to fifteen months, but has a contact number for concerns. This ensures continuity, the patient seeing the same nurse at each visit, instead of different doctors on rotation in the speciality.

Rheumatology nurse specialists have achieved improved outcomes through their supportive educational approach to patients (Grahame and West, 1996). Such skills and knowledge are invaluable assets that could be shared with general practitioners and community nurses, providing a point of contact in dealing with particular patient problems in the community.

Currently there is no data base of specialist nurses, so numbers are unknown. However, there are never sufficient nurse specialists to participate in both hospital activities and in the development of community initiatives. In one area of the UK, this problem was addressed by the employment of a senior lecturer/consultant in community rheumatology, supported by a community rheumatology sister (Hay and Schollam, 1994 unpublished data, cited in Dargie and Proctor, 1998). Achievements in the first year included:

- receipt of over two hundred referrals from primary and secondary care sources;
- twenty-five to thirty-five home visits made per month;
- two drug monitoring clinics established in the community;
- coordination of the individual drug therapy regimes of forty patients;
- helpline established for use by patients and primary health-care teams;
- two patient education groups developed in the community;
- education meetings devised for primary health care staff;
- provision of a central information centre for community services.

These activities highlight the benefits to both patients and the primary and secondary health-care teams. It was suggested that this model could be implemented in many more areas of the country (Dargie and Proctor, 1998).

PRACTICE NURSES

As government policy increases the workload in primary care the practice nurse role has continued to develop. Many nurses work as autonomous practitioners managing chronic diseases and incorporating health promotion into their job descriptions. Their role as patient advocate has not changed, but for many nurses the confidence to deliver this role has. This is because modern training methods encourage nurses to develop their confidence.

The role of the 21st century practice nurse can be described as:

- an educator
- promoter of health
- clinical nurse
- patient advocate
- a complement to medical colleagues
- team player.

The additional role of nurse practitioner (NP) enables the nurse to make initial assessments and diagnoses. Although there are training opportunities for the NP, the majority of practices do not have this clinical expertise. However, practice nurses utilise and develop their skills in many new areas of health care. Their involvement in the management, follow up and education of rheumatology patients could therefore be a natural progression, given sufficient training and support.

DISTRICT NURSES

District nurses are trained in the essential skills to care for patients in their own environment, with the aim of achieving maximum levels of independence and comfort. Patients and their carers are encouraged and assisted to make informed choices about their healthcare needs within the context of their own lifestyles. District nurses plan and provide for episodic and continuing programmes of care for the acutely ill or chronically sick. In addition, they are involved in:

- the organisation of community resources, both professional and voluntary;
- ensuring continuity of care between the hospital and the home and the GP;
- promoting health, rehabilitation and counselling;
- ensuring quality of care is maintained.

Some district nurses may be more comfortable caring for patients with rheumatic diseases if their knowledge base was enhanced.

HEALTH VISITORS

The traditional view of health visitors' work is that it is predominantly carrying out assessments and providing preventative care on children aged five years and under. However, this role has extended to patients of all age groups, offering more public health activities, health promotion and ill health prevention, counselling and community participation in activities. The role also includes liaison with other agencies and using available resources to deal with health and welfare issues. Patients with chronic rheumatic disease may present with complex problems that affect the whole family unit, or the patient may be a child. Developing the existing skills of the health visitor could be an invaluable resource for these families.

SCHOOL NURSES

School nurses have an important role in supporting children with arthritis and their family. This role includes:

- linking the specialist nurse and the school teachers;
- supporting the child through school;
- identifying special needs;
- arranging for specialist equipment where appropriate;
- liaising with the school for extra time for exams if the child has problems with wrist joints which make writing painful and slow.

To be involved, the school nurse must be aware of potential problems, hence the importance of multidisciplinary meetings and training.

COMBINED CARE

Many patients prefer to see a nurse at regular intervals rather than a doctor only occasionally (Bird, 1985). Research has demonstrated that compared to consultant-run arthritis clinics, nurse-run clinics can result in significant improvement in patients' levels of knowledge, satisfaction and symptoms (Hill et al., 1994; Hill et al., 2003). The further development and utilisation of combined nursing skills in rheumatology across the primary/secondary care interface can be justified by the enhanced patient care it offers.

EFFECTIVE PLANNING OF COMBINED INITIATIVES

Effective combined initiatives will not evolve without meticulous planning. Barrett and Tomes (1992) believe that to achieve a smooth transition between primary and secondary care both entities must operate as one. This requires close cooperation, excellent communication and the development of common systems; a serious challenge for both primary and secondary care, but one worth surmounting.

PROTOCOLS AND GUIDELINES

Protocols and clinical guidelines provide written details of care to be administered in specific situations. Such evidence-based guidelines are thought to help decision making and standardisation of care. Where the quality of care can be maintained, patient outcomes improve (Mansfield, 1995). Shared-management protocols for rheumatic diseases may outline:

- service aims
- clinic formats
- individual roles
- clinical assessment criteria
- investigations

- education
- monitoring regimes for disease-modifying drugs
- local resources
- liaison methods
- rereferral criteria
- methods of audit.

These are incorporated into the National Enhanced Service shared-care delivery scheme described previously. Protocols and clinical guidelines can assist the primary health-care team members who may not be knowledgeable about rheumatic disease to maintain a continuity of quality care. However, in a study of attitudes and behaviours of clinicians towards clinical guidelines, it was found that 64% of clinicians did not use guidelines because they were poorly developed and 49% because they were impractical (Mansfield, 1995). If protocols and guidelines are to be utilised effectively, they should reflect local requirements and needs rather than being regimentally structured. As there is never sufficient time to reinvent the wheel, modifying existing guidelines and protocols is a realistic option. Real combined care would require representatives from all the health professional groups to be involved in this process.

THE EXPERT PATIENT

Education and patient self-management are key components to empowering patients to better manage their disease (NRAS, 2003). It has been recognised that physical, psychological, socioeconomic problems and social exclusion, often lead to a reduction in the quality of life (DoH, 2004a). The Department of Health introduced the Expert Patient Task Force in 1999, in response to the observation that patients with long-term chronic disease often understand the disease better than the doctors (DoH, 2004b). The remit was to design a new programme that would bring together the valuable work of patient and clinical organisations in developing self-management initiatives. The (DoH, 2004a) believes an expert patient will:

- feel confident and in control of his life;
- aim to manage his condition and its treatment in partnership with health-care professionals;
- communicate effectively with professionals and is willing to share responsibility and treatment;
- be realistic about the impact of his disease on himself and his family;
- use his skills and knowledge to lead a full life.

The expert patient idea has been used by several patient bodies including Arthritis Care, to design practical user-led delivery programmes. For more information see Chapter 15. It is recognised that not all patients will be comfortable in this role, but for others this form of self-management may be an inspiration.

PATIENT/PARTNERS

The patient/partner concept puts the patient as the educator, teaching and assisting doctors, medical students and nurses in musculoskeletal disease. Patients attend a pharmaceutical company-funded course where they learn about:

- anatomy
- physiology
- examining joints
- living with the disease.

They then allow the health professional to examine them and can say whether or not the method of examination, and the amount of pressure applied to the examination is correct. This can be an asset to staff learning new skills, if they are comfortable to be told their job by the patient!

The patient/partner role is very different to the expert patient, but each has its value.

SHARED-CARE SCHEMES

In their examination of shared-care schemes Hickman *et al.* (1994) devised a taxonomy of such initiatives, partly to create awareness of different schemes that may be appropriate to different settings, and to encourage their development (Table 16.3).

Community clinics

A community clinic is a clinic within a general practice attended by a hospital specialist. A variation would be the provision of a service to patients from several practices, especially useful where practices are remote from a hospital. Orton (1994) suggests that without the involvement of the primary health-care team, such a clinic could be viewed as being simply relocated, with very little improvement in the quality of care given. However, there is the opportunity for integrated teamwork, with the consultant or rheumatology nurse specialist encouraging the development of skills by the primary health-care team. Various arthritis clinic initiatives have arisen. These range from drug-monitoring clinics specifically for patients with rheumatoid arthritis, to a clinic which caters for all types of rheumatoid disease. A variation may be the community clinic based in an outpatient setting.

Table 16.3 A taxonomy of shared-care schemes for chronic disease

Classification	Description
Community clinics	Clinics run in general practice by hospital specialist and/or primary health care team
Basic model	Liaison through regular letters or standardised record sheets
Liaison model	Primary health-care teams and specialist health teams having regular patient discussions/meetings
Shared-care record card	Agreed data and results recorded on a card transferred by patients between surgery and hospital
Computer-assisted shared care	Data entered onto central hospital computer by participants, examined by consultant, with letters and recommendations for further care sent to GP
Electronic mail	A common database with multiaccess ports, available to hospital and primary health-care teams

(Adapted from Hickman, Drummond and Grimshaw *A taxonomy of shared care for chronic disease* (1994) with kind permission from Oxford University Press)

Basic model

Shared care via the basic model is described as communication by letter or standardised record sheet, to exchange information between the hospital and the general practitioner. Because of its regularity, it is viewed as an extension of normal communication. However, unless a shared-care coordinator is available to monitor the process, it may not be possible to identify when letters or sheets do not arrive at the expected time (Hickman *et al.*, 1994). This is a one-way communication channel and as such is limited in value in shared care.

Liaison model

The liaison model facilitates two-way communication through regular meetings between the hospital team and the general practitioner to discuss the care of individual patients. This may involve the development of joint management plans and guidelines and/or the initiation of jointly held clinics.

Shared-care record card

The shared-care co-op, liaison card or booklet allows the systematic recording of data, which can be carried by the patient between their general practice and hospital appointments (Figure 16.1).

Patients name:	Medication			
Address:	Drug	Dose	Date started	Date finished
Home telephone number:				
Hospital record number:				
Consultant:				
Clinical nurse specialist:				
CNS telephone no:				
General practitioner:				
Surgery address:				
Surgery telephone no:				
For important advice see back page				

IMPORTANT ADVICE

TO PATIENTS

1. Always carry this card with you and give it to your family doctor or practice nurse when you visit the surgery.

2. Tell your doctor or nurse if you have:
   a. Rash or itching
   b. Bruising or bleeding
   c. Mouth ulcers or a sore throat
   d. Stomach or abdominal pain
   e. Increased breathlessness

3. Attend regularly to have your blood and or urine tests.

Figure 16.1 Shared care liaison card.

Transfer of such valuable information could prevent tests being duplicated and provides an up-to-date picture of a patient's health status. Shared appointments may be preplanned through rereferral criteria or unplanned depending on the patient's condition. Record cards are more meaningful if there is space for the patient to include comments, particularly if experiencing pain or lack of mobility. However, they do have a potential downside. Some patients may become obsessed by the blood results and worry about raised levels, although they feel very well. They need to be taught about the meaning of the results when they are given the book and reassured that readings can vary. This patient empowerment is an integral part of shared care.

Computer-assisted shared care

Jointly agreed data is collected by the hospital laboratory and clinic and entered on to a departmental computer. The secondary care staff examine the results of each blood test and update the computerised patient record with medication changes, side effects and reasons for stopping a treatment. Letters with advice and recommendations can be sent to the general practitioner. RHEMOS is a computer package which can download data from the laboratory to the clinic. It can be programmed to highlight exceptions and trends in results and has the facility to run letters to the patient and GP if a patient has failed to attend for a blood test. Administrative support is required to run the latter part of this programme effectively.

Electronic mail

This consists of a common database where the health professionals involved in shared care can enter agreed data, so that information is accessible to all participants. The data can be entered either straight on to the computer or sent by electronic mail. Such a system could be linked to other databases in hospital or general practice to supply additional information, for example on pathology, patient administration, or general practice administration (Hickman et al., 1994). Any means of enhancing information transfer and including the patient in the care process must be welcomed. However, clinic report letters may be written several weeks after an appointment which reduces their value, especially when changes in management are suggested. Electronic messaging would be a more efficient method of data transfer or fax if this is not available. As with all methods of communication, confidentiality must be safeguarded.

ETHNICITY

As with all areas of health care, the management of musculoskeletal disease must be culturally sensitive. It has been reported that fewer people than expected access rheumatology services in Birmingham, thus showing an unmet need (Gordhan, 2003). Research carried out by Birmingham Arthritis Resource Centre (BRAC) showed a demand for a wide range of facilities, particularly educational material, in languages used locally. The ability of outreach projects to reach excluded groups has been examined (Gordhan, 2003). This highlighted the need for health-care professionals to examine the facilities they provide, if they wish to deliver a seamless, caring service.

PROFILE OF A COMMUNITY-BASED ARTHRITIS CLINIC

Dargie and Procter (1998) shared their experience in establishing and running a community-based arthritis clinic founded on a partnership between the local community health centre and local hospital. They identified a local need, developed protocols and undertook the appropriate training. Patient satisfaction was high. The arthritis clinic demonstrated that full utilisation of nurses, can reduce secondary care waiting lists, save general practitioner time and enable patients to self-manage, whilst simultaneously offering them a more individual and appropriate service.

IMPROVING SEAMLESS CARE

In the past, opportunities for training in the UK were provided through the Royal College of Nursing Rheumatology Nursing Forum and by courses in rheumatology nursing developed by the English National Board. Much of the training is now supplied through universities. This may be credits at level 3 standard, or at Master's level. Courses cover topics such as:

- joint injections;
- general rheumatology;
- specific courses for physiotherapists and podiatrists;
- splinting courses for occupational therapists.

The value of multidisciplinary training has been discussed throughout this chapter.

NONPRESCRIPTION MEDICATION

It is not uncommon for patients to present in surgery requesting glucosamine (GLS) for their joint pains, having read about its benefits in the media, or been recommended by friends. One survey found GLS was usually self-prescribed and self-managed, but participants bought a variety of products or different brands of the same product, with no dose standardisation (Blakeley and Ribeiro, 2002). Research suggests that glucosamine is effective in relieving joint pain in osteoarthritis and could be used as an alternative to anti-inflammatory drugs (Ruane and Griffiths, 2002). This would be especially beneficial for patients with asthma who are advised not to take non-steroidal anti-inflammatory drugs. This is an example of where professionals need to keep abreast of developments in nutritional supplements so that they can understand and respond to patients' queries. As research continues, the PHCT must be comfortable keeping abreast of emerging evidence.

The primary care doctor should have sufficient knowledge of the cutting edge of the speciality to be competent to advise patients and to be able to discuss management options with his colleagues.

THE FUTURE

Werrett *et al.* (2001) examined the educational needs of primary and secondary care staff for the provision of seamless care. Team-building initiatives which jointly clarify goals, define roles and responsibilities, and improve communication are likely to be invaluable in the provision of seamless care.

The need for a higher priority in primary care for training in musculoskeletal diseases has been highlighted by the NRAS (2003). The NRAS also suggests that the absence of a National Service Framework for Arthritis and musculoskeletal diseases fosters a lack of recognition of patient need within Primary Care Trusts. The GMS Contract addresses some of these issues, although there is still room for improvement. Doctors and nurses have an obligation to develop their continuing professional education; training in rheumatic disease could be incorporated into this education plan. Multidisciplinary training is preferable, where case studies can be discussed and shared learning achieved. Successful shared care requires good communication within the PHCT, between primary and secondary care, and between all other involved agencies.

In their quality guidelines, Arthritis Care (1994) supported the view that 'adequate and appropriate health care of all kinds should be readily available to all people with arthritis who need it'. The recognition of the existing problems and the adoption of the principles of good shared care by primary and secondary health-care teams can make a major contribution to meeting such a goal. Arthritis Care suggests that District Health Authorities should encourage and support joint initiatives and strategies by health providers. This will require additional investment, but only then can the concept of a seamless service be realised in practice. It has been noted that the biggest savings for the patient comes not from providing cheap care. It comes from greater use of primary care where this is the appropriate level of care as well as through shared care with specialist colleagues (SMA, 2004). The Department of Health has offered financial incentives to primary care to become more involved in rheumatology management. However, with the vast range of health agenda items contained within the GMS contract, NICE guidelines and National Service Frameworks, there is the possibility that the seamless care which will benefit our patients may not reach its potential.

ACTION POINTS FOR PRACTICE

- Briefly outline what effects the projected future demand for musculoskeletal services may have on hospital in/outpatient care and primary care.
- Make a list of outcomes that could be achieved if primary and secondary health professionals were to adopt the principles of good shared care in rheumatology.
- Mr Roberts is a sixty-eight year old man exhibiting symptoms of early osteoarthritis of the hands and knees. His present condition does not warrant a referral to the hospital rheumatology department. What support could the primary health-care team at his local surgery give?
- A community nurse would like to set up a shared-care initiative in rheumatology at their surgery. What difficulties may be encountered?
- Having read this chapter, take time to reflect upon the following questions:
  1. How could links be improved between primary and secondary rheumatology care in your area of practice?
  2. Do you envisage any difficulties in implementing shared-care schemes?
  3. What could you do to influence the support of such initiatives?

REFERENCES

Arthritis Care (1994) *Quality guidelines number three. Community health care for people with arthritis*. London, Arthritis Care.

Arthritis Research Campaign (2004) *Factfile – arthritis at a glance*. Chesterfield: ARC.

Barrett CW, Tomes J (1992) Shared care – the way forward. *Hospital Update Plus* 18(4):7–10.

Bird H (1985) Nurses: an underused resource. *British Medical Journal* 290:1589.

Blaaw A, Schuwirth I, Van Der Vleuten C, Smits F, Van Der Linden S (1995) Assessing clinical competence: recognition of case descriptions of rheumatic diseases by general practitioners. *British Journal of Rheumatology* 34:375–379.

Blakeley JS, Ribeiro V (2002) A survey of self-medication practices and perceived effectiveness of glucosamine products among older adults. *Complementary Therapies in Medicine* 10154–10160.

British Medical Association and National Health Service Confederation (2003) *New GMS Contract 2003 – Investing in General Practice*. London, BMA and NHS Confederation.

Consumer Association (1992) *GPs, your verdict. Which?* April:202–205.

Dargie L, Proctor J (1998) Seamless Care. In: Hill J (ed) *Rheumatology Nursing: A Creative Approach.* London, Churchill Livingstone.

Davis P, Suarez-Almazor M (1995) An assessment of the needs of family physicians for a rheumatology continuing medical education programme: results of a pilot project. *Journal of Rheumatology* 22(9):1762–1765.

Department of Health (2004a) *The expert patient programme – progress report.* www. doh.gov.uk/cmo/progress/expertpatientepp3.htm (28 January 2004).

Department of Health (2004b) *The expert patient programme – progress report.* www. doh.gov.uk/cmo/progress/expertpatientepp1.htm (28 January 2004).

Freeman GK, Richards SC (1993) Is personal continuity of care compatible with free choice of doctor? Patients' views on seeing the same doctor. *British Journal of General Practitioners* 43:493–497.

Gordhan C (2003) The Birmingham Arthritis Resource Centre: meeting multicultural information needs. *International Journal of Therapy and Rehabilitation* 10(9):394.

Grahame R, West J (1996) The role of the rheumatology nurse practitioner in primary care: an experiment in the further education of the practice nurse. *British Journal of Rheumatology* 35:581–588.

Haslock I (1987) The practising rheumatologist's view. In: *Bailliere's Clinical rheumatology: epidemiological, sociological and environmental aspects of rheumatology.* London, Bailliere Tindall p645–663.

Helliwell P, O'Hara M (1995) Shared care between hospital and general practice: an audit of disease-modifying drug monitoring in rheumatoid arthritis. *British Journal of Rheumatology* 34:673–676.

Hickman M, Drummond N, Grimshaw J (1994) A taxonomy of shared care for chronic disease. *Journal of Public Health Medicine* 16(4):447–454.

Hill J, Bird HA, Harmer R, Wright V, Lawton C (1994) An evaluation of the effectiveness, safety and acceptability of a nurse practitioner in a rheumatology outpatient clinic. *British Journal of Rheumatology* 33:283–288.

Hill J, Thorpe R, Bird H (2003) Outcomes for patients with RA: a rheumatology nurse practitioner clinic compared to standards outpatient care. *Musculoskeletal Care* 1(1):5–20.

Hill J, Ryan S (2000) *Rheumatology: a handbook for nurses.* London, Whurr Publishers Ltd.

Hjortdahl P, Laerum E (1992) Continuity of care in general practice: effect on patient satisfaction. *British Medical Journal* 304:1287–1290.

Liebman J, Hull A, Blauner M, Barkey J, Vignos P, Moskowitz R (1986). Identifying needs and community resources in arthritis care. *Public Health Nursing* 3(3):158–170.

Mansfield C (1995) Attitudes and behaviours towards clinical guidelines: the clinicians perspective. *Quality in Health Care* 4(4):250–255.

National Rheumatoid Arthritis Society (2003) *Rheumatoid Arthritis. The painful truth.* A consensus statement from the NRAS. London, NRAS.

Orton P (1994) Shared care. *Lancet* 344:1413–1415.

Ruane R, Griffiths P (2002) Glucosamine therapy compared to ibuprofen for joint pain. *British Journal of Community Nursing* 7(3):148–152.

Singapore Medical Association (2004) The SMA News. *General Practice and the Future.* www.sma.org.sg/sma_news/2901/news/2901N3.htm (1 February 2004).

Social Trends (2003) *National Statistics. Social Trends no 33.* London, TSO.

South Western Staffordshire Primary Care Trust (2004) Enclosure No. 28. Professional Executive Committee.

Tinson S (1995) Assessing health need: a community perspective. In: Cain P, Hyde V, Howkins E (eds) *Community Nursing: Dimensions and Dilemmas.* London, Arnold, ch7, p144.

Vetter N, Charny M, Lewis P, Farrow S (1990) Prevalence and treatment of symptoms of rheumatism and arthritis among over 65 year olds: a community profile. *British Journal of General Practice* 40:69–71.

Werrett JA, Hlem RH, Carnwell R (2001) The primary and secondary interface: the educational needs of nursing staff for the provision of seamless care. *Journal of Advanced Nursing* 34(5):629–638.

17 Paediatric Care

G. JACKSON
Leeds General Infirmary, West Yorkshire, UK

The aim of this chapter is to provide a description of the classification of juvenile idiopathic arthritis (JIA), an overview of the available treatments, and the educational and psychosocial needs of this group. After reading this chapter the reader should be able to:

- differentiate between the subclasses of juvenile idiopathic arthritis;
- describe the current treatments for JIA;
- demonstrate an understanding of the impact of JIA on a young person's education and quality of life;
- understand the importance of multiprofessional teamwork.

Paediatric rheumatology has been recognised as a subspeciality of paediatrics since 1995. It encompasses a wide range of inflammatory diseases of childhood, including:

- juvenile arthritis;
- systemic connective tissue diseases, such as lupus;
- systemic vasculitis, for example Kawasaki disease;
- arthritis related to infection, such as reactive arthritis;
- primary and acquired disorders of bone and connective tissue;
- noninflammatory conditions, such as reflex sympathetic dystrophy, chronic pain and hypermobility syndromes.

It is impossible to provide a detailed account of all the diseases involved in a single chapter, and thus this chapter will concentrate on juvenile idiopathic arthritis, its definitions and treatments and the impact it has on the child and family.

JUVENILE IDIOPATHIC ARTHRITIS (JIA)

Arthritis is defined as swelling within a joint or a limitation in the range of joint movement with joint pain or tenderness, which is not related to a primary

Rheumatology Nursing: A Creative Approach, 2nd edn. Edited by Jackie Hill.
Copyright 2006 by John Wiley & Sons, Ltd.

mechanical disorder. JIA is a heterogeneous group of autoimmune diseases characterised by persistent joint swelling, but it is genetically and clinically distinct from rheumatoid arthritis (RA). Amongst the paediatric population of the UK, its incidence is 1/10000 and its prevalence is 1/1000 (Ramanan *et al.*, 2003). The aetiology of JIA remains elusive and the diagnosis is attained by exclusion. However, it has been hypothesised that various factors, including infection, trauma and environmental elements may act as initiating agents. The diagnosis of JIA can be made when the following criteria are met:

• onset of arthritis before the age of sixteen years;
• arthritis persisting for more than six weeks;
• exclusion of all other diseases which may cause arthritis.

HISTORY AND EVOLUTION OF TERMINOLOGY

In 1897 George Fredrick Still described a number of cases of acute and chronic arthritis in children, documenting the clinical characteristics and the differing mode of onset (Schneider and Laxer, 1998). He also described a number of patients who had an acute onset with lymphadenopathy, serositis, splenomegaly and fever. On the basis of differences between childhood and adult arthritis, Still suggested that childhood arthritis may have a different aetiology or might even include more than one disease. In many areas, acute onset systemic juvenile arthritis is still referred to as Still's disease.

The classification of JA was complicated by transatlantic differences. However, in 1993 and with revision in 1997, the International League of Associations for Rheumatology (ILAR), proposed an ILAR classification to achieve as much homogeneity as possible within categories (Martin and Woo, 1999). This categorisation, termed JIA, is now recognised as the most comprehensive classification based on clinical and prognostic features and was endorsed by the World Health Organisation in 1999.

ILAR CRITERIA FOR THE CLASSIFICATION OF JUVENILE IDIOPATHIC ARTHRITIS

The principle of the ILAR classification is that each category of JIA is mutually exclusive. This is reflected in the list of exclusions for each category:

• oligoarthritis, either persistent or extended;
• polyarthritis with negative rheumatoid factor;
• polyarthritis with positive rheumatoid factor;
• psoriatic arthritis;
• systemic arthritis;
• enthesitis-related arthritis;
• undifferentiated arthritis.

The JIA classification is based on the number of joints affected in the first six months of the disease and the presence of extra-articular features. Categories 1 to 6 represent the major clinical patterns of onset of arthritis seen in children. Category 7, the undifferentiated subgroup, covers arthritis which fulfills the overall definition of JIA but does not fulfil any individual disease category or fulfils more than one. Classification is an evolving process with the ultimate goal of differentiating biologically distinct disease groups with predictable outcomes and responses to treatment.

Oligoarthritis

Oligoarthritis is defined as arthritis affecting four or fewer joints during the first six months of the disease. It is the most common form of JIA, affecting over 50% of patients and is more common in girls than in boys, usually in the preschool age group. In children it is predominantly a disease of the lower extremities, most commonly the knees and ankles. In at least half the cases only a single joint is affected, usually the knee, and it is rare to find systemic or extra-articular features. Although the joint is swollen and warm it may not be painful or red and children may seem unconcerned about the swelling or any discernable limp.

If the number of affected joints never exceeds four, it is termed persistent oligoarthritis. The articular prognosis is good and the disease is usually self-limiting with remission after a few years, although flares may reoccur many years later.

If, after the initial six months of disease, the total number of affected joints exceeds four with a progressive increase in joint involvement the term extended oligoarthritis is used. This demonstrates a pattern similar to polyarticular JIA but is more difficult to control with a poorer articular prognosis.

Antinuclear antibodies (ANA) are found in 40–80% of patients with oligoarticular JIA and are associated with the development of chronic anterior uveitis, an inflammation of the eye, often asymptomatic, which can lead to deterioration in vision and potential blindness if left untreated. Excluded from this category are:

- children with psoriasis or a family history of psoriasis or HLA-B27 associated disease;
- children with systemic arthritis and rheumatoid factor positive disease;
- boys who are HLA positive where onset of disease is after the age of eight years (Hofer and Southwood, 2002).

Polyarthritis

Polyarthritis is the second most common form of JIA, affecting 30–40% of children with arthritis. Polyarticular JIA is defined as arthritis affecting five or more joints in the first six months of the disease. It is divided into two categories rheumatoid factor (RF) negative polyarthritis and RF positive polyarthritis. The term RF positive is used when rheumatoid factor is detected on two occasions at least three months apart (Cassidy and Petty, 2001). Preschool RF negative girls form the majority of those with polyarthritis.

Although the onset may be acute, it is more often insidious, with an increasing number of joints becoming involved. It is predominately symmetrical and affects both upper and lower limbs. Prompt diagnosis and early treatment directly influences a successful outcome (Friswell and Southwood, 2004). Earlier and more aggressive treatment with a second-line agent, such as methotrexate, has been shown to be beneficial in bringing the disease under control (Ramanan et al., 2003).

Whilst most children who develop the disease are in the preschool age group, a small number develop it in late childhood or early adolescence and are RF positive. This is the juvenile form of adult rheumatoid arthritis, with often twenty or more joints involved and a much poorer articular outcome.

Psoriatic arthritis

Juvenile psoriatic arthritis (JPA) is defined as arthritis and psoriasis or as arthritis and at least two of the following:

- dactylitis;
- nail abnormalities (pitting or onycholysis);
- psoriasis confirmed by a dermatologist in at least one first degree relative.

Dactylitis may be differentiated from arthritis if swelling of one or more digits extends beyond the joint margins. It represents the combined effects of arthritis and tenosynovitis and is often described as a sausage digit.

The diagnosis of JPA is straightforward if the arthritis and the psoriasis develop and are present at the same time. However, they may not be simultaneously present and the arthritis may predate the psoriasis by many years. The onset of JPA peaks at two ages: the first, mainly in girls, during the preschool years; and the second, during mid to late childhood (Cassidy and Petty, 2001).

During the first six months, JPA usually involves the inflammation of a small number of joints, making it difficult to differentiate from oligoarticular JIA. The course of the disease is often characterised by an increasing number of affected joints and a scattered asymmetrical polyarthritis is the most common long-term finding. Swelling of a single small joint, particularly a toe, is highly suggestive of JPA because isolated small joint disease is uncommon in the other sub groups of JIA. The most commonly affected joint is the knee, accompanied by the small joints of the hands and feet. The prognosis of JPA is poorer than persistent oligoarthritis.

The presence of systemic arthritis or rheumatoid factor would exclude a patient from this category.

Systemic arthritis

Systemic arthritis is when arthritis of any number of joints occurs together with, or is preceded by, a documented quotidian fever (Figure 17.1).

This fever pattern involves one or two daily spikes of temperature, usually in late afternoon, and persists for at least two weeks. The fever rises and falls rapidly, often to subnormal temperatures in the early hours of the morning and associated symptoms may include rigors, myalgia, anorexia and fatigue. One or more of the following features must also be present to make the diagnosis:

- evanescent (quickly fading), macular, erythematous rash often at its most obvious at the height of the fever;
- generalised lymphadenopathy;
- enlargement of liver or spleen;
- serositis, involving pleurae, pericardium or abdomen, which can be life-threatening.

The associated symptoms and clinical findings often peak during the episodes of pyrexia and the child appears grossly unwell, but once the fever has subsided the child may continue with relatively normal activities and even attend school.

Systemic arthritis is the rarest form of juvenile arthritis. It can occur at any time, but it develops most commonly in early childhood, is relatively uncom-

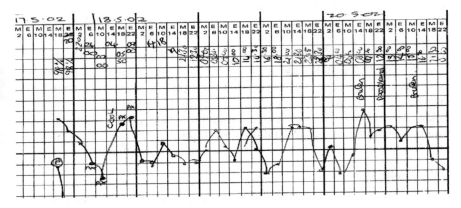

Figure 17.1 Typical temperature variations in quotidian fever.

mon in adolescence and rare in adulthood. In contrast to other subgroups of JIA, systemic onset occurs with equal frequency in boys and girls. It is often difficult to diagnose because the earliest features may be extra-articular and precede the joint involvement by many weeks or even months. The disease often mimics many other childhood conditions and the exclusion of systemic infections, malignancies and connective tissue diseases is most important in establishing the diagnosis. The number of joints involved varies and the onset is often of an oligoarticular nature with the wrists, ankles and knees most commonly affected.

One in three patients go on to develop a severe polyarthritis that is resistant to treatment and the articular outlook for these children is poor. Destructive arthritis, secondary amyloidosis and treatment complications which include infection, osteoporosis, growth retardation and the macrophage activation syndrome all contribute to the significant morbidity and mortality associated with the disease (Shneider and Laxer, 1998).

Enthesitis-related arthritis

This is defined as either arthritis and enthesitis (inflammation of tendons at insertion point to bone), or arthritis or enthesitis, plus two of the following:

- sacroiliac joint tenderness, inflammatory spinal pain or both;
- presence of HLA B27;
- family history in at least one first or second degree relative of medically confirmed HLAB27 associated disease;
- acute anterior uveitis;
- onset of arthritis in a boy after the age of eight years (Hofer and Southwood, 2002; Cassidy and Petty, 2001).

Patients with psoriasis or a family history of psoriasis in a first-degree relative would be excluded from this group.

Undifferentiated arthritis

Undifferentiated arthritis includes conditions where patients either do not meet specific criteria or meet the criteria for a number of categories. Children may develop an arthritis in association with other medical conditions such as inflammatory bowel disease, sarcoid, immunodeficiency states, Down's syndrome and other chromosomal disorders.

Chronic anterior uveitis

Some children with JIA are at a higher risk of developing chronic anterior uveitis, a clinically silent but potentially sight-threatening condition. Those at greatest risk are young girls with an early onset oligoarthritis and who are positive to antinuclear antibodies (Rosenberg, 2002). Uveitis associated with JIA can have debilitating ocular consequences. Because the majority of children do not notice any redness, discomfort or blurred vision, regular examination by an experienced ophthalmologist is necessary. If the uveitis is left untreated or poorly controlled it can result in the formation of cataracts, glaucoma or lens/iris adhesions, leading to eventual blindness. It has been suggested that up to 38% of patients with JIA associated uveitis develop severe visual impairment with 16–22% developing blindness. Currently, it is difficult to predict which children will develop uveitis and how severe it will become (Zulian et al., 2002).

The eye examination consists of a vision test followed by a slit-lamp examination. For very young children the vision test will involve pictures rather than letters and the slit lamp examination may be performed under general anaesthetic if the child is having any other procedure that involves anaesthesia, for example joint injections.

Uveitis may be unilateral or bilateral and is treated by steroid drops of various strengths which aim to control inflammation and prevent further deterioration. The frequency of application will depend on the severity of the disease and can vary from hourly to once alternate days or even once weekly. Inflammation that is unresponsive to topical applications may necessitate intraocular steroid injections under general anaesthetic. Some children, whose disease is refractory to conventional corticosteroid therapy, may be commenced experimentally on second-line agents, but there have been indications that in certain circumstances the drugs may contribute to inducing or exacerbating the uveitis (Zulian et al., 2002).

Acute anterior uveitis

Acute uveitis is associated with enthesitis-related arthritis, most commonly in boys and usually in HLA B27 positive patients. The inflammation presents acutely with pain, redness and swelling. It responds promptly to topical steroids and if treated early, there is little long-term ocular compromise.

MANAGEMENT OF CHILDHOOD ARTHRITIS

Children with rheumatic disease need a coordinated approach from an experienced multidisciplinary team (MDT) involving a nurse specialist, physiotherapist (PT), occupational therapist (OT), paediatric and adult rheumatologists, social worker, psychologist and general practitioner. There must also be firm referral pathways to the ophthalmologist, orthopaedic surgeon and paediatric endocrinologist.

The aims of immediate management are to:

- relieve pain and discomfort
- preserve function
- prevent deformities
- control inflammation.

The aims of long-term management are to:

- minimise the effects of disease and side effects of treatment;
- promote normal growth and development;
- minimise the impact of chronic illness.

Most children with chronic arthritis require treatment with a combination of drug therapy, physiotherapy and occupational therapy. The family plays a huge part in carrying out care and physical treatments at home. Family and age-appropriate patient education is paramount, commencing at diagnosis and ongoing as new therapies and drug regimes are introduced. A priority in the management of the child with JIA is to encourage normal social and psychological development and participation in school and peer group activities. This can be achieved only by a MDT approach.

MULTIDISCIPLINARY TEAMWORK

The roles of the specialist nurse, physiotherapist and occupational therapist overlap in many areas, including:

- disease education
- psychological support
- practicalities of disease management.

Regular team meetings ensure that information is shared and that the most appropriate person provides care and support for the patient and family.

Paediatric rheumatology involves a system of shared care and management, usually from a tertiary referral centre. In addition to the regional team, the MDT includes the local paediatrician, adult rheumatologists, therapists and children's community nurses. Close local and regional liaison and effective communication is a prerequisite for successful management.

CASE STUDY

The following case study provides a brief overview of team involvement following diagnosis.

Sarah Smith is ten years old and very athletic. Following a six-week history of increasing lethargy, joint pain, swelling and stiffness she is referred to the regional rheumatology centre where a diagnosis of polyarticular JIA is made. The family is shocked and Sarah is visibly upset.

An explanation of the disease and potential treatment is given by the paediatric rheumatologist and followed up separately by the nurse specialist. Driven by the family's questions, further explanations and written information about the disease and drug therapy are given. Considerable emotional support is needed at diagnosis. If this need continues, despite appropriate explanations and reassurances, Sarah and her family will be referred to the clinical psychologist who will provide more specific coping strategies relating to chronic illness. An initial assessment of Sarah's gait and foot position by the physiotherapist reveals her to be flat footed. She is referred to the podiatrist for a more detailed assessment and the provision of insoles. A combined physiotherapy/nursing visit to school is offered, to provide information about the disease and the impact it may have on her school activities, including competitive sports. A referral is also made to the local physiotherapy service, which provides initial hydrotherapy and ongoing treatment, including a home exercise programme. NSAIDs and oral steroids do not adequately control the disease and methotrexate is introduced.

Mrs Smith wants her husband involved, but he is unable to attend clinic. Consequently, a home visit is arranged to discuss the practicalities of taking methotrexate. The GP has agreed to monitor the drug and to provide repeat prescriptions. Six months later the drug is changed to the subcutaneous route to improve disease control and Sarah's mother agrees to learn to give the injection at home. Sarah is also interested in giving the drug herself. Using regional guidelines, the local children's community nurses visit Sarah at home to teach and supervise Mrs Smith giving the methotrexate.

Sarah has standard attainment tests at school and is concerned that if her wrists and fingers are sore, she may have difficulty writing for any length of time. Following a functional assessment, the occupational therapist offers specific pen grips, a writing wedge and advice regarding seating. In addition, a letter is written by the paediatric rheumatologist enabling the school to offer extra time for the exams.

Over the next twelve months Sarah's disease stabilises, the family come to terms with the diagnosis and ongoing treatment regimes and with the support of school staff she returns to sport, although at a less competitive level.

PHYSIOTHERAPY IN JIA

The physiotherapist plays an important role in the management of the paediatric rheumatology patient, providing essential skills in the assessment and treatment of musculoskeletal dysfunction. Interventions such as those detailed below, can contribute greatly to the overall management of the paediatric patient and their family.

ASSESSMENT

Initial subjective and objective assessments will be carried out to determine the following:

- presenting musculoskeletal problem and its possible mechanical origin, including aggravating and relieving factors and any 24-hour pattern of symptoms;
- level of pain/limitation to function and its relationship to joint swelling, heat, tenderness or any deformity;
- impact of any disability on home/school life and activity levels, both current and normal.

The age and maturity of the patient will usually dictate how much of this information can be obtained directly from the child and how much must be provided by parents/carers. An age-appropriate approach towards questioning and assessment techniques should enable the paediatric therapist to gain a clear picture of the disease from the child's perspective. For instance the therapist might ask, 'Are there things your friends can do that you cannot because of your arthritis?' It is important to note that what may be of significance for the child or adolescent, may not necessarily be what the therapist or carer perceives as problematic (Doherty et al., 1993; Young et al., 1995). Achieving a balance is vital in enabling the physiotherapist to formulate a treatment plan which will encourage adherence from the child and family.

TREATMENT

The nature of the problems identified in the course of the assessment will dictate which treatments are most appropriate for the child. Commonly used treatment modalities include:

- hydrotherapy
- exercise programmes
- manual therapy techniques
- heat or cold therapies
- acupuncture
- transcutaneous electrical nerve stimulation (TENS).

Hydrotherapy

Although there is little written evidence to support its use over land-based treatments hydrotherapy is an invaluable resource in the management of the paediatric rheumatology patient. The clinical reasoning behind its use include:

- Reduced or absent weight-bearing allows painful inflamed joints to be moved through a greater range of movement.
- The heat of the water can reduce pain and muscle spasm and enable the patient to exercise more effectively.
- A number of joints can be exercised simultaneously.
- The buoyancy provided by the water allows greater mobility in patients who may be struggling or reluctant to mobilise normally.
- Many children enjoy being in water and will often adhere better to treatment in this environment, perceiving the activities to be play rather than exercise.

The length of each treatment sessions is 20–25 minutes, similar to adult therapy.

If the child is very young or fearful, a parent or carer may need to accompany them in the pool until their confidence is gained.

Exercise programmes

Treatments include exercises aimed at increasing or maintaining the range of movement of joints and/or soft tissue length (Hackett et al., 1996). These may take the form of active exercises or passive stretches of varying technique. Active exercise programmes are also used to maintain or improve muscle power and recruitment, as well as to correct muscle imbalance. Exercise programmes aimed at improving or maintaining spinal posture are also used.

Studies have identified many factors that may influence adherence to treatment by the paediatric patient and parent/carer (Kyngas et al., 2000; Rapoff, 1989). In order to gain maximum adherence from the child and family, it is important that the prescribed exercise regime is both targeted and manageable. Patients and carers need a clear understanding of:

- why exercises are important;
- what the therapist is aiming to achieve;
- exactly how the exercise/stretch should be performed.

Parents may have difficulty with exercises or stretches which they perceive as causing their child discomfort. Time must be spent teaching both the child and parent the difference between safe stretching/exercising through a limited joint range and the potentially harmful effects of overzealous stretching in an acutely inflamed joint. The therapist must provide sufficient time to allow parents/carers and the child to feel fully confident in carrying out the exercise or stretch. In younger children it may be necessary, or more appropriate, to incorporate specific exercises into play or bathtime in order to achieve adherence.

In addition to specific exercises targeting problem joints as they arise, some patients may require a general programme of maintenance exercises, to be carried out on a regular basis when well. All exercise programmes must be reevaluated regularly by the physiotherapist, in order to ensure that they meet the current needs of the patient and to exclude any that may no longer be necessary.

The paediatric physiotherapist provides specific advice regarding exercise and sporting activities and also identifies which type of activity would be most beneficial for the individual. For children and young people this often involves liaison with schools either through written information or during a school visit. The aim is to encourage the child to remain as active as possible while avoiding certain high impact or contact sports, such as rugby (Malleson et al., 1996). Close liaison with schools should ensure that children are not made to participate in physical education (PE) activities that could aggravate symptoms during an acute flare. At such times it may be appropriate for PE staff to allow children to use the time to perform their home exercise programmes.

Heat and cold therapies

The application of heat or cold can reduce pain and muscle spasm and thereby increase joint range of movement and function (Low and Reed, 1990). Heat and cold can be applied in various ways, including the use of ice packs, wheat bags, cold wraps, and wax treatment. There are a variety of child-friendly versions. This encourages adherence but should always be used under adult supervision. The length of application depends on the preference of the individual. However similar to adult therapy, a minimum of ten to fifteen minutes is needed to effectively reduce pain or muscle spasm.

Acupuncture

Although there are certain cautions pertaining to the use of acupuncture in paediatric patients, for instance ensuring that anticipated adherence is sufficient to allow the safe selection and application of needle points, it can nevertheless play an important role in the reduction of pain and muscle spasm (Stux and Pomeranz, 1998). If selected carefully by assessing behaviour and level of understanding, children can be surprisingly adherent with this form of therapy. Verbal assent and written consent from the child and parent must be obtained.

Transcutaneous electrical nerve stimulation (TENS)

The lower frequency of chronic pain amongst the paediatric rheumatology population means that the use of TENS is probably less widespread than with adult patients. However, when longstanding pain is a problem, for example a child with severe arthritis of the hip awaiting surgical replacement, TENS has been shown to reduce pain levels (Fowler-Kerry, 1990).

The physiotherapist would select the most appropriate locations for application of the electrodes and these would be taught to the parent to enable independent use. Timing and selection of frequency and intensity settings are similar to adult treatments.

Foot posture and gait analysis

The physiotherapist analyses gait and foot posture in order to identify abnormalities and instigate the most appropriate treatment. Abnormal gait patterns can have a number of different causes including:

- foot position
- pain
- loss of joint/soft tissue range of movement
- muscle weakness.

A normal foot changes biomechanically from infancy to childhood and consequently age-appropriate variations of the normal must not be confused with significant abnormality. In the case of significant abnormalities, it may be necessary to refer to the paediatric orthotist or podiatrist for further specialist management.

OCCUPATIONAL THERAPY IN JIA

The aim of the occupational therapist (OT) is to achieve optimum levels of functional independence for each individual. In children, independence in activities of daily living (ADL) such as personal care, play, leisure, and education are assessed with consideration of each child's age and development. Assessment and treatment may take place in hospital, at home or at school.

DEVELOPMENT OF INDEPENDENCE

The majority of children become independent in personal care between the ages of five and seven years. If a child does not achieve this, a detailed assessment of their abilities is indicated and a graded programme is required to enable them to gain independence (Nugent, 1997). During a flare, a reduction or loss of functional independence may be experienced, but it is usually regained once the flare subsides. During this period it is important that children are encouraged to be as independent as possible within their own limitations of pain and/or joint restriction. To compensate for a temporary reduction in function, the OT may provide equipment or adaptations which enable the child to be as independent as possible.

Age-appropriate independence away from the family is encouraged, for example school trips and sleep-overs at friends' houses. The OT can alleviate fears and apprehensions about such activities by working with the child and family and ensuring that their child is supported and does not miss out.

ACTIVITIES OF DAILY LIVING

Personal care

Once the flare has subsided, every effort must be made to ensure that their preflare function is restored. When a child has gained a particular skill, for example putting on socks, it is vital that they continue with it or they may quickly forget (Nugent, 1997). If systemically unwell, help may be given initially but they should return to working independently as soon as possible. Function can be assessed using the Childhood Health Assessment Questionnaire (CHAQ). This is a reliable, subjective tool for the functional and physical assessment of children with JIA (Foster *et al.*, 2001). It identifies levels of functional ability, pain and general well-being from the perspective of both patient and parent and when completed can give valuable information about changes in condition.

If children are not given opportunities to gain and maintain independence, they will not develop age-appropriate skills. Parents can become used to performing tasks for their child and may overprotect them after a flare has subsided. They may continue to help dress a child out of habit or because it is quicker when under pressure, for example, in the morning before school. The OT can advise parents on which activities to encourage during or after a flare and how to encourage their child to return to independence and ensure that their developmental milestones are achieved.

Play and leisure

Pain, swelling and restriction of joint motion can limit a child's ability to play, interact with peers and development new skills. OTs identify these limitations and devise individual programmes to enable the child to overcome them. Programmes include:

- exercise
- stretches
- splinting
- pain management.

MANAGEMENT OF INVOLVED JOINTS

Joint stiffness

Children who experience early-morning stiffness may be slower in the morning and take longer to get ready for school. Often they will benefit from a warm bath or shower, or an alternative application of heat, such as wax treatment. During periods of flare, they may need extra assistance. Stiffness can also occur when sitting for long periods as when sitting on the floor for assemblies or at story time. In these cases, the use of chairs and regularly getting up and moving can help to reduce the stiffness. For young children, these aspects of disease management will need to be taught to parents and teachers.

Pain management

OTs advise parents and teachers on how to detect the symptoms that the child does not express. This can be due to age and inability to describe symptoms or because they will not admit to them because they do not want to be seen as different. Young children may be unable to distinguish between pain and stiffness but these can be detected by looking for signs such as grimacing or the withdrawal or avoidance of painful joints. Often children will tense the muscles around a painful joint to protect it, or compensate by over using other joints for example, over using the elbow and shoulder joints when the wrist is restricted.

Pain management techniques include wax treatment (Ayling and Marks, 2000) and cool wraps, which can be applied to the joints. The parents of younger children can be taught to administer these techniques but it is better that older children are taught to self-manage their symptoms. In addition, relaxation techniques using recorded tapes or rehearsed sequences of relaxing individual muscle groups can be taught.

Splinting

The principles of splinting for paediatric rheumatology patients are the same as for adult patients. However, the materials used are often lighter, with a shorter setting time, an important factor with young children who find it difficult to stay still long enough for some of the heavier thermoplastics to set. Adherence is greatly improved by providing a choice of colours and giving a detailed explanation to both children and parents, of the purpose of the splint. If the wrists are involved, a neoprene splint may be preferable to thermoplastic, since the material is less restrictive to joint movement and absorbs perspiration. The splint also exerts a circumferential pressure around the joint providing a feeling of increased joint stability (Figure 17.2).

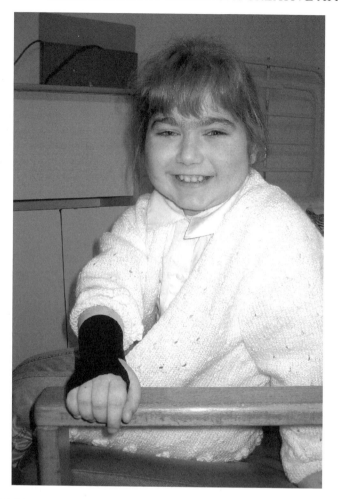

Figure 17.2 Neoprene splint (Reproduced with permission from Leeds Teaching Hospital with parent consent).

Evidence has shown that efficacy of an intra-articular steroid injection improves when the joint is rested (Sharma *et al.*, 2002). Without splints, small children would find resting a joint difficult and for this reason individual splints are provided selectively for some children in the 24-hour period following an injection (Figure 17.3).

JOINT PROTECTION AND ENERGY CONSERVATION PRINCIPLES

The joint protection and energy conservation principles for adults, described in Chapter 11, remain the same for juvenile arthritis. Young children find

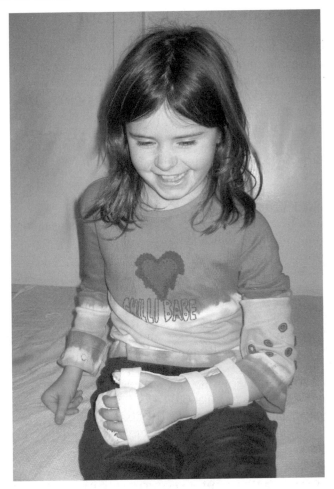

Figure 17.3 Resting splint (Reproduced with permission from Leeds Teaching Hospital with parent consent).

energy conservation techniques extremely difficult to comprehend and where a child is too young to be able to understand them, advice is given to parents. Most children do not want to be different from their peers and will often overdo things on their good days and suffer afterwards as a result. Participation in PE at school should be discussed with the physiotherapist to ensure that the activities are not detrimental to their joints. High-impact activities that involve jarring or twisting of the joints should be avoided in favour of activities such as swimming or cycling. The provision of joint protection and energy conservation principles needs to be revisited at different stages as the child becomes more mature and better able to self-manage their disease.

MEDICATION AND TREATMENT OPTIONS

The term JIA encompasses wide and varying types and severity of disease. Consequently, medication and treatments vary from simple analgesics and nonsteroidal anti-inflammatory drugs (NSAIDs) through the more complex second-line agents to the experimental stem cell transplants. The drugs, their actions and side effects have been explained in Chapter 12 and therefore this chapter will concentrate on the specific way they relate to children.

Many drugs used for children are used outside the specifications of the product license, in effect they are unlicensed. Examples are that the drug may be:

- an unlicensed medicine;
- administered by an unlicensed route (*e.g.*, subcutaneous methotrexate);
- given for an unlicensed indication;
- limited by age of patient its use for;
- unlicensed for use in children (*e.g.*, bisphosphonates).

ANALGESICS

Simple analgesia in the form of paracetamol syrup is often used in conjunction with NSAIDs to treat mild to moderate pain and inflammation. Paracetamol syrup is commonly used for a variety of childhood ailments, but parents need to be made aware that although it will relieve pyrexia and general discomfort, used in isolation it will not control the pain associated with active inflammation. Recommended dosage for ages three months to twelve years is 15 mg/kg 4–6 hourly with a maximum total dose in 24 hrs of 90 mg/kg. (RCPCH, 2003).

NONSTEROIDAL ANTI-INFLAMMATORY DRUGS (NSaids)

NSAIDs are widely used in the treatment of juvenile arthritis and when used regularly at an appropriate dose, they have both an analgesic and an anti-inflammatory effect. This has the advantage of reducing the number of medicines used in small children, where adherence and administration may be problematic. Parents are usually tolerant of the occasional use of oral analgesic and NSAIDs to treat pyrexia and pain, but are often reluctant to give medication to children on a long-term basis. In JIA, NSAIDs must be given for 3–4 weeks to have maximum clinical effect (BNF, 2004). In addition, the recommended dose for ibuprofen, the NSAID used most commonly in the paediatric population, is greater in JIA than for general paediatric use; (Table 17.1) and consequently it is important that parents and patients are given appropriate education about the drug, its administration and its effects.

Table 17.1 Formulation, dosage and administration of commonly used NSAIDs in children

Ibuprofen	30–40 mg/kg/day in 3–4 divided doses. Can be used up to 60 mg/kg/day in 6 divided doses in systemic JIA only, maximum 2.4 g per day Syrup: 100 mg/5 ml; tablets: 200 mg and 400 mg; and slow release: 800 mg
Naproxen	20–30 mg/kg/day in 2 divided doses, maximum 1 gm/day Tablets: 250 mg and 500 mg; syrup discontinued in UK
Diclofenac	1–3 mg/kg/day in 2–3 divided doses, maximum 150 mg/day Tablets: 25 mg and 50 mg; slow release: 75 mg; dispersible tablets: 50 mg (as voltarol); suppository: 100 mg
Piroxicam	Weight <15 kg: 5 mg 16–25 kg: 10 mg 26–45 kg: 15 mg >46 kg: 20 mg in single daily dose or 0.2–0.6 mg/kg/day, maximum 20 mg day

(Adapted from British Society of Paediatric and Adolescent Rheumatology [2004] and the British National Formulary [2004])

NSAIDs are generally well-tolerated in children and as in the adult population, different NSAIDs may suit different patients. Children who encounter side effects with one may be more suited to another. The most common side effect is gastrointestinal discomfort and nausea. This may resolve with the use of an H2 receptor antagonist such as ranitidine. The dosage for children aged 2–12 years is 2–4 mg/kg up to a maximum of 150 mg twice daily (RCPCH, 2003). The dosage of the proton pump inhibitor omeprazole is 700 mcg/kg once daily, increasing as necessary to 3 mg/kg/24 hrs for children aged 2–12 years. Higher doses may be given in two divided doses (RCPCH, 2003). Dosage regime and formulation also play a part in efficacy. Drugs such as naproxen, which need be given only twice a day, may be more suitable when patients are unable to take medication during school hours. Alternatively, slow release preparations given in the evening may prove advantageous to those children who are particularly stiff in the morning and have difficulty achieving school registration deadlines.

Cox II selective inhibitors have a lower incidence of gastrointestinal side effects than other NSAIDs. However, none are licensed for use with children and they are currently not mentioned in paediatric pharmacological texts. They may be used selectively in certain patients.

CORTICOSTEROID DRUGS

In JIA the use of corticosteroid therapy is mainly confined to:

- those patients with polyarticular disease with multiple joint involvement;
- treating the extra-articular features of systemic onset disease.

Oral steroids are associated with significant drug toxicity in children. When used long-term this includes growth suppression, osteoporosis and cataracts. The aim is to give the lowest dose and course duration to achieve disease control, usually 1–2 mg/kg/24 hrs (RCPCH, 2003). Administering a single daily dose in the mornings and using alternate day dosing schedules when reducing the treatment, have been shown to minimise growth suppression (Laxer and Gazarian, 2001).

The cushingoid appearance of children and young people on long-term steroid therapy can have a huge impact on their self-esteem and perception of body image (Price, 1993). Adherence may be a problem if patients feel that the steroids are making them look fat and different. Special care must be taken with drug-related patient education, emphasising the need for gradual withdrawal of steroids and not patient-driven cessation, as the disease improves.

Methylprednisolone is given where there is an acute flare of the disease and is used to achieve rapid control of disease activity often while waiting for second-line agents to take effect. It is given as a short infusion, over 30–60 minutes once daily on three consecutive days. Dosage for those aged one month to eighteen years is 30 mg/kg per once daily up to a maximum 1 g/day (RCPCH, 2003). Patients may either attend the children's ward as day cases or be fully resident. Side effects include:

- labile blood pressure
- tachycardia
- blurred vision
- flushing
- sweating
- metallic taste in the mouth
- mood changes.

DISEASE-MODIFYING ANTIRHEUMATIC DRUGS (DMARDs)

A number of DMARDs are used as second-line agents in paediatric rheumatology including sulphasalazine and cyclosporine. However methotrexate has emerged as the drug which has transformed the outlook for children with JIA and the short-to-medium term efficacy is well-established (Ramanan et al., 2003). Methotrexate therapy is not licensed in the UK for use in paediatric rheumatological diseases, but this is a common situation with many paediatric medicines (RCPCH, 2003).

Methotrexate can be administered orally, as either syrup or tablets or by injection where the recommended route is subcutaneous (RCN Guidelines, 2004). Methotrexate syrup is available commercially from a small number of manufacturers but usually has to be obtained on an individual basis by local chemists. Children normally commence therapy orally because of its convenience and ease of administration. Unlike adult care where the dose is calculated on weight, paediatric doses are based on surface area. This is derived from a combination of height and weight and is more accurate because of the variation in size of children of similar ages. The dose is increased incrementally until the standard dosage of 10 to 15 mg/m^2 per week is achieved, to maximize clinical response. However children tolerate much higher doses than adults and those with refractory disease may be prescribed doses of up to 20 to 25 mg/m^2 (Ramanan *et al.*, 2003). It has been demonstrated that subcutaneous administration of methotrexate has a 10–12% increased absorption compared to oral preparations and provides greater efficacy (Jundt *et al.*, 1993).

As with adults, the rationale for parenteral administration is based on inadequate response to oral preparations, drug toxicity and more specific to children, the problem of adherence with the oral drug. Some patients experience anticipatory nausea with symptoms occurring before the drug is taken (Murray and Lovell, 2002). Switching to the subcutaneous route may have only limited success. The use of regular folic acid may reduce side effects, although there is no clear evidence base for a dosing schedule. Some centres use 1 mg per day, six days per week, omitting a dose on the day the methotrexate is given. Others recommend 5 mg taken 48 hours after the methotrexate. It is becoming common practice for parents and children to be taught how to give subcutaneous methotrexate at home (Livermore, 2003) and the RCN guidelines advocate the use of prefilled, predosed syringes with a luer lock system.

INTRA-ARTICULAR JOINT INJECTIONS

Intra-articular corticosteroid joint injections are being used earlier in the disease process than used to be the case, particularly in children with oligoarthritis. Different preparations and dosing regimes are used for different joints. This may lead to complete resolution of the signs and symptoms of the disease (Cleary *et al.*, 2003). The majority of patients experience rapid improvement within a few days of injection and about two-thirds achieve remission for twelve months or more after a single injection. Compared to patients with polyarticular or systemic onset JIA, the duration of response appears greater in children with oligoarthritis and those who are younger and have a short disease history (Laxer and Gazarian, 2001).

Intra-articular steroids are also used in the treatment of polyarticular disease when a flare has resulted in a small number of joints becoming inflamed and the ability to inject the joints obviates the need for increasing systemic medication. Where children present with polyarticular JIA, there is no clear consensus as to whether multiple joints should be injected while simultaneously starting a DMARD such as methotrexate, or whether systemic steroid therapy alone can achieve remission.

Joint injections in small children require sedation or a short-acting general anaesthetic. Older children and teenagers may be adherent following the use of topical anaesthetic preparations and age-appropriate relaxation or distraction techniques. In some centres inhaled nitrous oxide is used. To ensure the patient is adherent and as relaxed as possible, a detailed explanation of the procedure is given to the patient and accompanying parent. Resting the joint for 24-hours following injection has been shown to be beneficial (Sharma et al., 2002).

BIOLOGIC THERAPIES IN CHILDREN

At present etanercept is the only biologic drug licensed and recommended for children aged four to seventeen years, and the National Institute of Clinical Excellence (NICE) has published guidance on its use (NICE, 2002). Eligibility for treatment in children and young people differs from that of adults and specific guidelines have been introduced (RCN, 2003).

The British Society for Paediatric and Adolescent Rheumatology Group (2003) have developed a Biologic and New Drugs Register (BNDR) for children and young people that forms part of the NICE guidance criteria and runs alongside the adult Biologics Register.

Biologic therapy is used in children who do not respond adequately to conventional management or who have unacceptable side effects to methotrexate. It is administered by subcutaneous injection twice weekly and may be used with or without methotrexate (Wilkinson et al., 2003) although anecdotal evidence suggests that maintaining a low dose of methotrexate may be advantageous.

Although it has been demonstrated that etanercept is extremely beneficial for many children, the introduction of an injectable drug therapy where the long-term safety, side effects and efficacy are unknown, causes disquiet for a number of parents. The paediatric rheumatology nurse specialist is central to the effective provision of education, support and informed consent when the drug is introduced (Wilkinson et al., 2003).

Although etanercept is the only biologic licensed at present for JIA, trials in both the UK and the USA into the use of infliximab are underway, and in the future, it is possible that anakinra and adalimumab may also become available.

AUTOLOGOUS STEM CELL TRANSPLANT (ASCT)

ASCT has been pioneered on a small number of children who have severe disease refractory to all treatments. Although it is potentially curative it is still considered experimental and the risk of death is significant. Patients with chronic inflammatory disease are at risk of opportunistic infection following transplantation because of previous long-term immunosuppression with DMARD's and steroids. Stem cells are obtained from bone marrow or mobilised from peripheral blood. Once harvested, they are purified and transplanted following intense patient immunosuppression. Autologous (patient's own) stem cells carry significant less risk of rejection than allegenic (donor) cells. It is thought that ASCT generates a resetting of the immune system rather than generating a completely new one (Wedderburn et al., 2003). Following successful transplants, children have recovered from previously devastating disease and returned to normal functional ability with an improved quality of life. In the UK there are two centres that provide ASCT for paediatric rheumatology patients: Great Ormond Street Hospital for Children NHS Trust and Newcastle upon Tyne Hospitals NHS Trust. Both are funded by the National Specialist Commisionary Advisory Group.

PSYCHOSOCIAL ISSUES FOR THE CHILD AND FAMILY

Chronic disease, pain and perceived body image abnormalities have a major impact on the social and psychological development of children with arthritis. The whole family has to adapt to the disease, having to accommodate the demands made by the condition on all aspects of their daily lives. Following diagnosis and during episodes of flare the distress and anxiety can be enormous and the family may be faced with fears of new problems, new treatment demands or the prospect of treatment failing.

Psychosocial management includes understanding the patient's and parents' needs and fears and addressing them appropriately. These may be resolved by clear and honest explanation of the disease and prognosis but more complex issues may need referral to the clinical psychologist. A trusting relationship and open honest communication are the most important requirements for effective support of families.

Children with physical disabilities and deformities and children who look different because of a rash or steroid therapy, may feel different and self-conscious. It has been suggested (Schanberg et al., 2003) that children with arthritis are at increased risk of developing psychosocial problems, including:

- depression
- decreased self-esteem

- decreased educational and social competence
- difficulty with peer relationships.

These areas need to be addressed early in the treatment pathway by the MDT so that strategies can be activated to minimise impact. Physical disability, fatigue and fluctuation in disease activity may make it difficult for the child to participate in social and family activities. Emphasis on what they can do and planning activities in which they are able to participate should help their sense of self-worth and morale. Alternative plans and backup arrangements should be made where possible.

SIBLINGS

Stress related to living with chronic illness affects every member of the family, including siblings. Siblings of patients with JIA have been found to have higher-than-expected levels of anxiety and guilt and lower self-image (Leak, 1994). Guilt that they are somehow responsible, fear of it happening to them and embarrassment that the family appears different, all impact on their perception of self. They may resent the extra time and attention given to the affected child and perceive favouritism in matters of discipline. They may be required to help more around the house or to take on responsibilities for entertaining or supervising other children in the family, including the child with arthritis. Caring for the affected child may not leave parents with sufficient time to fully satisfy the developmental needs of siblings. They may be unable to participate fully in siblings' lives, which could restrict the other children socially, in terms of being included in outings or having friends back for tea after school. Including siblings in clinic visits encourages them to understand the reasons for changes in home life, and offering them dedicated time with the nurse specialist during the clinic visit allows them to talk and explore their own needs and fears in relation to the disease. Advice may also be given about how to explain arthritis to school friends.

On the positive side, siblings can play a part in the care at home, for example, by reminding about medication and helping with exercise therapy. They often take on a more than normally protective role in school and outside the home and this builds a strong sibling relationship.

PATIENT AND FAMILY EDUCATION

Patient education has been shown to enhance adherence to drug and exercise programmes and potentiates positive outcomes of treatment (Hill, 1999). Patient and parent education and the practicalities of incorporating the needs of other family members in planning the care are essential to ensure the treatment plan is followed. In order to nurture the development of self-advocacy skills and autonomy it is vital that from an early age, children and young people are involved in decision making with respect to their illness

(McDonagh *et al.*, 2000). Children with rheumatic diseases and their parents require education and support through different stages in the disease process. Information required by families varies from the need to find out as much as possible after the initial shock of diagnosis, to specific education relating to changes in medication or physical therapy. The mode of teaching has to vary with the needs and skills of the parents and the developmental age of the child. Language barriers (where English is not the first language), cultural background and level of literacy must be taken into account. Information is readily available on the internet, but families should be made aware that not all information is reliable and should be given addresses and contact numbers of proven organisations. They also need a named member of the rheumatology team, usually the nurse specialist, to contact with queries relating to information obtained independently.

It is important to remember that for young people diagnosed during early childhood, the initial disease education will have been directed to the parents who, for a variety of reasons, may feel unable to share that knowledge with the young person. Parents often wish to protect their child from the realities and potential anxieties of chronic disease and over time, may have forgotten many of the details they were given at diagnosis. Young people should be offered the opportunity for disease education independently from their parents, so that they can explore for themselves their disease related questions and concerns.

OSTEOPOROSIS, GROWTH AND NUTRITION

Osteoporosis is a disease characterised by low bone mass and is measured in terms of bone mineral density (BMD). Bone mass is normally accumulated during childhood and adolescence when the bones are growing actively in length, width and density and reaches a peak by the third decade (Silverwood, 2003). Eating healthily during childhood and adolescence is essential to reduce the risks of osteoporosis in later life.

In JIA there are a number of risk factors associated with decreased bone mass:

- active inflammatory disease
- decreased mobility
- steroid medication
- poor calcium/vitamin D intake
- decreased sun exposure
- pubertal delay.

These create a short-term risk of growth retardation and osteopoenic/ osteoporotic bone changes and a potential long-term risk of osteoporosis and associated fractures in later life.

Poor growth is common in children with active rheumatic disease, particularly in young children. Even in low doses, steroid therapy is known to accentuate the problem. Poor nutrition, is also problematic. Some children achieve optimum height once the disease is well-controlled but others are unable to catch up. Growth hormone has been used selectively with moderate success (Rooney *et al.*, 2000) but until active inflammation is under control and oral steroid doses are minimal, it is counterproductive.

NUTRITION

Factors contributing to the nutritional problems of children with JIA include:

- Poor appetite may result from disease activity or drugs used to treat the disease.
- Mechanical feeding difficulties related to temporomandibular joint function, or micrognathia may cause practical problems (Cassidy and Petty 2001).
- Hand, wrist or jaw pain make it difficult to clean teeth and this contributes to poor dental hygiene, the potential of pain and a reluctance to eat.
- Parents may also follow fad diets in the belief that avoidance or addition of certain foodstuffs will improve their child's symptoms.

All children with rheumatic disease should have their height and weight documented regularly and be encouraged to follow a healthy balanced diet with particular emphasis on adequate amounts of calcium and vitamin D. The National Osteoporosis Society (NOS) recommends the following daily allowances for different age groups:

- 800mg calcium per day for children aged seven to twelve years;
- 1000mg calcium per day for teenagers;
- 1500mg calcium per day for pregnant or nursing teenagers.

The best and most palatable sources of calcium for young children are milk and dairy products such as cheese and yoghurt. Vitamin D, which helps the body absorb calcium, is found in margarine and cereals, but the principal source is the action of sunlight on the skin. The NOS (2002) recommends exposure to approximately fifteen minutes each day during the summer months which provides adequate amounts of vitamin D without increasing the risk of skin cancers.

The main preventative measures cited by the NOS are:

- a well-balanced calcium-rich diet
- regular weight-bearing exercise
- moderation in the use of alcohol and tobacco.

Adolescents with a rheumatological condition may not achieve these because of:

- nonadherence;
- inability or reluctance to take part in sport because of fear of pain or injury;
- peer group pressure (smoking/drinking alcohol).

Patient education through the use of teenage-friendly leaflets, appropriate websites and clear age-appropriate explanations will be necessary.

The nurse specialist is ideally placed to give general health education, information and advice about exercise, diet and appropriate foodstuffs and to refer more complex problems to the paediatric dietician. A food diary, completed at home, may give a more accurate picture of the amount and quality of the child's diet. If the calcium content is low, particularly in the presence of oral steroids, then oral supplements are recommended. Prescribed supplements containing both calcium and vitamin D are available and have a pleasant flavour that is usually acceptable to children. For the younger child, effervescent calcium can be acceptable but it does not contain additional vitamin D.

DUAL ENERGY x-RAY ABSORPTIOMETRY (DEXA) SCANNING

DEXA scanning of the axial skeleton is the accepted technique for the diagnosis of osteoporosis in adults. It is the most widely used method of measuring bone mineral density (BMD) and has led to working definitions of osteoporosis and osteopoenia. It is expressed in standard deviation units called T and Z scores. T scores compare the patient with a young adult and so are meaningless in children. BMD reported as a Z score is age and gender matched, but even here it is difficult to interpret (Fewtrell, 2003). All BMD measurements need to be interpreted in the context of the:

- child's body size
- pubertal stage;

and to a lesser extent their:

- age
- ethnic group.

Children who are small for age because of chronic illness will often have a low BMD measurement, and scores for adolescent boys and girls of the same chronological age cannot be compared because of the later onset of puberty in boys.

Children are scanned because they are thought to be at risk of low bone density due to disease activity and drug treatment, or to monitor the effects of treatment. At present, because of the difficulties interpreting results, children who have serial scans act as their own control showing individual improvement or deterioration.

USE OF BISPHOSPHNATES

Bisphosphnates are used to increase BMD in paediatric patients, and whilst the long-term risks are still unknown they have been shown to be safe in the short term (Cimaz, 2002). Although oral preparations are available, the intravenous route is often preferred because of the rigid guidelines for oral administration. Intravenous pamidronate (disodium pamidronate) is given as a 30–60 minute infusion once daily for three consecutive days, in 250mls sodium chloride 0.9%, 1mg/kg/day (up to a maximum of 60mg/day) (Leeds Hospitals NHS Trust, 2003). Patients can attend as a day case or be admitted to the children's ward. The most common side effect is a transient rise in body temperature and flu-like symptoms. This generally resolves following the infusion and the treatment is usually well-tolerated in children. Infusions are repeated every three months for one year and then the DEXA scan is repeated to monitor the bone status. Admissions are usually coordinated to coincide with school holidays or weekends to avoid regular time lost from education.

CHILDHOOD IMMUNISATION

Immunisation programmes have a significant and beneficial effect on children's health and that of the community as a whole, and currently the benefits of immunisation far outweigh any risk of exacerbation of rheumatic disease. Families should be encouraged to maintain the childhood vaccination schedule and also to take up autumn influenza immunisation. However there are a number of exceptions:

- As with all children, it is important that the child with a rheumatological condition is fit and well before being given any vaccine. An unexplained pyrexia >38C would contraindicate vaccination.
- Children taking corticosteroids at a dose of 2mg/kg/day for more than a week, or 1mg/kg/day for more than a month, or >40mg total dose for one week should avoid vaccination at this time (BSPAR, 2003). Children receiving disease-modifying (immunosuppressant) drugs and/or biologic agents should be discussed with the rheumatology team.
- No live vaccines such as bacillus calmette-guerin (BCG), measles, mumps, rubella (MMR) or oral polio should be given if a child is on immunosuppressive drugs and/or biologic agents.

- Children who have received any of the above doses for more than one week in the previous three months or received lower doses in combination with other immunosuppressant drugs, should be discussed with the rheumatology team.

Parents should be reminded that it is important that other family members should receive the MMR vaccine but should be given the inactivated form of the polio vaccine (by injection) as the oral route is excreted in faeces.

CHICKENPOX (VARICELLA)

This illness can be life-threatening in immunosuppressed children and guidance should be obtained from the rheumatology team. All children likely to need immunosuppressant drugs should have varicella zoster antibody titres measured at diagnosis. Nonimmune children should be offered immunisation with attenuated varicella vaccine (varilrix) although this may delay the start of treatment.

CONTACT WITH SHINGLES OR CHICKENPOX

Passive immunity with either oral acyclovir or zoster immune globulin (ZIG) should be given to all patients with significant exposure and those that develop chickenpox will require high dose intravenous acyclovir.

GENERAL EDUCATION AND JIA

The needs of most children are met by their local mainstream school and placement in a special school is now seen as inappropriate. The Special Educational Needs and Disability Act (2001) states that children have the right to an education in mainstream schools and colleges (Special Education Handbook, 2002). Under this act it is not permitted to treat disabled students less favourably, and educational establishments are obliged to make a reasonable amount of adjustments to improve accessibility to disabled students. The school is responsible for assessing whether a child has special educational needs (SEN). SENs are where a child finds it much harder to learn than children of a similar age, due to either a learning disability or a physical disability. All mainstream schools have a designated teacher who is the SEN coordinator (SENCO) and is responsible for the day-to-day operation of the school's SEN policy. They coordinate provision for children with SENs, maintain the SEN register and liase with parents, staff and external agencies (The Source, 2001). If a child has needs requiring special provision, they are assessed under the Education Act 1996 and this may lead to a statement of special educational needs, which is a formal document describing all the child's needs and the extra help necessary to meet them. Any pupil with a statement will be given an individual education plan (IEP), which outlines long- and short-term objectives which are assessed in the annual review meeting. This may involve the provision of a learning support assistant who works with the child for part of the day in such activities dictated by the statement. After the child's 14th birthday the annual review includes a transition plan for their move into higher education or employment.

Going to school is one of the biggest events in a child's life but for those with arthritis there may be additional difficulties and anxieties. Appropriate preparation needs to begin early. Discussion between the parents and the school to identify specific areas which may need addressing include:

- Is transport required to and from school?
- Does the child need extra time to get changed after PE or change shoes following playtime?
- Can they get up and move around if they become stiff?
- What is the school's policy on giving medication?
- Are teachers able to administer medication on a regular or *prn* basis?
- How much walking will be involved and how many flights of stairs will the child be expected to use?
- What happens if the child becomes tired and needs to rest?

There are many other points about which the teaching staff need to be aware, and the involvement of the MDT will reduce the negative impact of arthritis on the child's time at school. It is important that the staff have an understanding of JIA, its impact on education and the side effects of any drug therapy. Disease and drug education in the form of written information can be forwarded to the class teacher with the parents' permission. If necessary and with the child's agreement, this can be followed up with a school visit with an explanation to the child's peer group. Age-appropriate explanations and booklets can be used to explain the difficulties the child may have with activities, the need for splints and additional rest periods. Children often have difficulty explaining their symptoms and how they affect their school life. They may not tell teachers about painful joints or reduced function because they do not want to be perceived as different to their peers or feel they will not be believed. The aim is to equip the child with the confidence to reveal changes in physical ability but not to use it as an excuse.

The OT can undertake a formal assessment of the suitability of chairs and tables and provide guidance on alternative seating. The involvement of upper limb joints can result in difficulty with written work, neatness and completing homework on time (Southwood, 1993). An assessment of grip strength and hand range of movement will enable programmes to be devised that strengthen the muscles and improve range of movement in these joints. Wide-barrelled pens or grips can be used to ease the strain on painful, swollen fingers that have reduced grip strength and angled writing wedges are useful for decreasing the strain on extensors of the wrist (Figure 17.4).

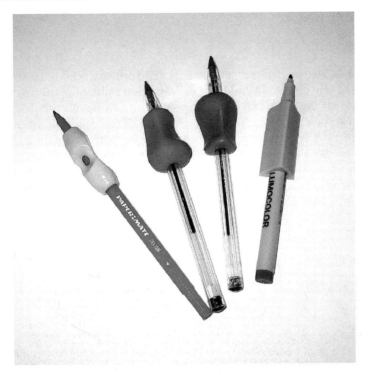

Figure 17.4 Adaptors for pens and pencils.

Children may require greater support from the MDT as they go through the transition from their inherently smaller primary school to a larger, secondary school. If a child has a Statement of SEN this will be reviewed in the summer term of Year 6, and the MDT will be asked to provide reports about the current level of function and potential complications of the child's transition.

Prior to starting secondary school, a preliminary visit may be conducted by the OT to assess the child's ability to move around the school, identify any adaptations that may be needed and to provide information for the SENCO and other teachers.

Many children find themselves the target of bullying when they have received special help or care at school, if for example they are exempted from PE or allowed to leave the class to rest if they are tired. Bullying may also occur simply because there is something different about them, such as short stature or wearing splints. All schools are required to have robust bullying policies relating to school, class and individuals and patients should be encouraged to discuss any problems with their class teacher (Karstadt, 1999).

ADOLESCENCE

SURGERY

Adolescents who are severely affected by arthritis may need to be considered for surgery. Hip disease in children is a major determinant of future disability, giving rise to the potential of hip replacement. Although this needs to be delayed to allow maximum growth of the skeleton and epiphyseal fusion, early surgery is led by the patient because of uncontrolled pain and impairment of mobility (Leak, 1994). The bones are often small, deformed and osteoporotic adding to the technical complications of surgery. However postoperatively many teenagers are able to increase their social activities significantly, complete their education and gain independence by learning to drive.

TRANSITION TO ADULT SERVICES

Adolescent health, including transitional care has been identified as a major priority in the government's National Service Framework for Children (DOH, 2003). It has also been highlighted in a major intercollegiate report by the Royal College of Paediatrics and Child Health (2003), which addresses adolescent health needs. Over one-third of patients with JIA will have active disease in adult life and over 60% will experience limitation in activities of daily living (Peterson et al., 1997). For these young people, adolescence can be a particularly challenging time. All young people have a number of developmental tasks to achieve during adolescence before they are perceived as adults (McDonagh et al., 2000):

- to consolidate their identity
- to establish relationships outside the family
- to achieve independence from family
- to find a vocation.

For the adolescent with a chronic illness these can be delayed, disrupted or even remain uncompleted. Individuals achieve these developmental tasks at different chronological ages so the transfer of patients to adult health care needs to be individual and flexible. It should also occur at a time when the young person is clinically stable. It is stressful for the patient and unfair to the adult rheumatology team to have transfer during an acute medical event, purely because hospitalisation in a paediatric area is not possible. Transferring of care is not transition. Transition is a process, not an event, and ideally should begin at diagnosis or at the latest eleven years old (McDonagh et al., 2000) and continue over a number of years. It is a process of education, preparation and planning for all parties including the patient, their family, medical, nursing and therapy staff. The term transition has been defined by the Society of Adolescent Medicine (Chira and Sandborg, 2004) as 'the purposeful, planned movement of adolescents and young adults with chronic physical and medical conditions from child-centred to adult-orientated health-care systems'. This involves not only the medical needs but also the psycho-social and educational/vocational elements of care.

Young people with a chronic illness have to achieve not only the develop-mental tasks of adolescence but also the transitional elements of education, health care and physical and emotional independence (McDonagh *et al.*, 2000) shown below:

- paediatric to adult health care
- school to work / further education / college
- family to independent living.

The Arthritis Research Campaign funded a three year multicentred project to develop and evaluate a structured and multidisciplinary programme of transitional care for adolescents with JIA. Focus groups with young people and their families clearly demonstrated that adolescent transitional needs involve more than medical issues. Education, employment, relationships and sexual health were all highlighted as important areas of need and gaining personal independence was a dominant theme (Shaw *et al.*, 2004).

These issues need to be addressed to prevent patients and families feeling ill-equipped and anxious at the time of transfer. JIA cannot be cured but many patients do go into spontaneous remission. For those who go on to have active disease in adult life, paediatric management with access to a regional multidisciplinary team and planned transitional care from an early age con-siderably improves their ability to achieve their full potential with autonomy, adult relationships and a vocation.

ACTION POINTS FOR PRACTICE

- Describe the classification of juvenile idiopathic arthritis (JIA).
- A ten-year old girl is diagnosed with polyarticular JIA and prescribed methotrexate. What are the implications for the child and family?
- A teenager being treated with a biologic therapy and approaching GCSE exams has an acute flare of her disease. What measures can be put in place to support her through the exams?

ACKNOWLEDGEMENTS

I would like to thank my fellow team members, Melanie Wright, Senior Paediatric Occupational Therapist, and Dawn Wills, Senior Paediatric

Physiotherapist (The Leeds Teaching Hospitals Trust), for their invaluable help with the section on therapy.

REFERENCES

Ayling J, Marks R (2000) Efficacy of paraffin wax baths for rheumatoid arthritis hands. *Physiotherapy* 86(4):190–201.

British National Formulary (2004) BMJ Publishing and Royal Pharmaceutical Society of Great Britain. London.

British Society for Paediatric and Adolescent Rheumatology (2003) *Guidance on immunisation of the child with a potentially impaired immune response.* Draft unpublished.

Cassidy JT, Petty RE (2001) *Textbook of Paediatric Rheumatology.* Philadelphia, WB Saunders.

Chira P, Sandborg C (2004) Adolescent rheumatology transitional care: steps to bringing health policy into practice. *Rheumatology* 43:687–689.

Cimaz R (2002) Osteoporosis in childhood rheumatic disease: prevention and therapy. *Best Practice and Research Clinical Rheumatology* 6;ch3:397–409.

Cleary AG, Murphy HD, Davidson JE (2003) Intra-articular corticosteroid injections in juvenile idiopathic arthritis. *Archives of Disease in Childhood* 88:192–196.

Department of Health (2003) *Getting the Right Start: National Service Framework for Children Standard for Hospital Services.* London, HMSO.

Doherty E, Yanni G, Conroy R et al. (1993) A comparison of child and parent ratings of disability and pain. *Journal of Rheumatology* 20:9;1563–1566.

Fewtrell MS (2003) Bone densitometry in children assessed by dual x-ray absorptiometry; uses and pitfalls. *Archives of Disease in Childhood* 88:795–798.

Friswell M, Southwood TR (2000) Juvenile Idiopathic Arthritis. In: Snaith ML (ed) *ABC of Rheumatology*, 3rd edition. London, BMJ Publishing.

Foster H, Nugent J, Woo P et al. (2001) The British version of the Childhood Health assessment questionnaire (CHAQ) and the child health Questionnaire (CHQ). *Clinical and Experimental Rheumatology* 19(4):163–167.

Fowler-Kerry SE (1990) An evaluation of TENS with children. *Pain Supplement* 5:59.

Hill J (1999) Patient education and adherence to dug therapy. In: Ryan S (ed) *Drug Therapy in Rheumatology Nursing.* London, Whurr Publishers.

Hackett J, Johnson B, Parkin A et al. (1996) Physiotherapy and occupational therapy for JCA: custom and practice in 5 centres in the UK, USA and Canada. *British Journal of Rheumatology* 35:695–699.

Hofer M, Southwood TR (2002) Classification of childhood arthritis. *Best Practice and Research Clinical Rheumatology* 16:379–396.

Jundt JW, Browne BA, Fiocco GP et al. (1993) A comparison of low dose methotrexate bioavailability: oral solution, oral tablet, subcutaneous and intramuscular dosing. *Journal of Rheumatology* 20:1845–1849.

Karstadt L, Woods S (1999) The school bullying problem. *Nursing Standard* 14(11):32–35.

Kyngas H, Kroll T, Duffy M (2000) Compliance in adolescents with chronic diseases: a review. *Journal of Adolescent Health* 26:379–388.

Laxer RM, Gazarian M (2001) Pharmacology and Drug Therapy. In: Cassidy JT, Petty RE (eds) *Textbook of Paediatric Rheumatology* 4th edition. Philadelphia, WB Saunders pp 91–46.

Leak AM (1994) The management of arthritis in adolescence. *British Journal of Rheumatology* 33:882–888.

Leeds Hospitals NHS Trust (2003) Paediatric Rheumatology Network. *Protocol for pamidronate infusions in patients with primary or secondary osteoporosis under the care of the rheumatology team.* Unpublished.

Livermore P (2003) Teaching home administration of subcutaneous methotrexate. *Paediatric Nursing* 15(3):28–32.

Low J, Reed M (1990) *Electrotherapy Explained: Principles and Practice.* Oxford, Butterworth Heinemann.

Malleson PN, Bennet SM, Mackinnon M *et al.* (1996) Physical fitness and its relationship to other indices of health status in children with chronic arthritis. *Journal of Rheumatology* 23(6):1059–1065.

Martin K, Woo P (1999) Juvenile Idiopathic Arthritides. In: Isenberg DA, Miller J (eds) *Adolescent Rheumatology* ed. London, Dunitz p71–93.

McDonagh J, E Southwood TR, Ryder CAJ (2000) Bridging the gap in rheumatology. *Annals of the Rheumatic Diseases* 59:86–93.

Murray KJ, Lovell DJ (2002) Advanced therapy for juvenile arthritis. *Best Practice and Research Clinical Rheumatology* 16(3):361–378.

National Institute of Clinical Excellence (2002) *Guidance on the use of etanercept for juvenile idiopathic arthritis.* Technology Appraisal Number 35. London, NHS NICE.

National Osteoporosis Society (2002) *Bone health and fractures in children.* Bath, NOS.

National Osteoporosis Society (2002) *Position statement on the reporting of dual energy x-ray absorptiometry (DXA) bone mineral density scans.* Bath, NOS.

Nugent J (1997) *Children Have Arthritis Too: A guide to Juvenile Chronic Arthritis.* London, Arthritis Care.

Peterson LS, Mason T, Nelson AM *et al.* (1997) Psychosocial outcomes of health status of adults who have had juvenile rheumatoid arthritis: a controlled population based study. *Arthritis and Rheumatism* 40:2235–2240.

Price B (1993) Diseases and altered body image in children. *Paediatric Nursing* 5(6):18–21.

Ramanan AV, Whitworth P, Baildam EM (2003) Use of methotrexate in Juvenile Idiopathic Arthritis. *Archives of Disease in Childhood* 88:197–200.

Rapoff MA (1989) Compliance with treatment regimens for paediatric rheumatology diseases. *Arthritis Care and Research* 2(3):1405–1406.

Rooney M, Davies UM, Reeve J *et al.* (2000) Bone mineral content and bone mineral metabolism; changes after growth hormone treatment in juvenile chronic arthritis. *Journal of Rheumatology* 27:1073–1081.

Rosenberg AM (2002) Uveitis associated with Juvenile Idiopathic Arthritis: envisioning the future. *Journal of Rheumatology* 29:2253–2255.

Royal College of Nursing (2004) *Administering subcutaneous methotrexate for inflammatory arthritis.* London, RCN.

Royal College of Nursing (2003) *Assessing, Managing and Monitoring Biological Therapies for Inflammatory Arthritis.* London, RCN.

Royal College of Paediatrics and Child Health (2003) *Bridging the Gap: Health Care for Adolescents.* RCPCH Publications Ltd.

Royal College of Paediatrics and Child Health (2003) *Pocket Medicines for Children.* London, RCPCH Publications Ltd.

Schanberg LE, Anthony KK, Gil KM *et al.* (2003) Daily pain and symptoms in children with polyarticular Arthritis. *Arthritis and Rheumatism* 48(5):1390–139.

Sharma V, Wyatt S, Chamberlain A (2002) A randomised controlled study of resting splint versus bed rest alone for 48 hours following intra-articular steroid in juvenile idiopathic arthritis. *Archive of Disease in Childhood*, 86,suppl. 1:A49.

Shaw KL, Southwood TR, McDonagh JE (2004) User perspectives of transitional care for adolescents with juvenile idiopathic arthritis. *Rheumatology* 43:770–778.

Schneider B, Laxer RM (1998) Systemic onset juvenile rheumatoid arthritis. *Balliere's Clinical Rheumatology* 12(2):245.

Silverwood B (2003) Building healthy bones. *Paediatric Nursing* 15(5):27–29.

Southwood T (1993) Schoolchildren with Arthritis. *Head Teachers Review: Winter.*

Special Education Handbook: the law on children with special educational needs (2002) 8th edition, London Advisory Centre for Education.

Stux G, Pomeranz B (1998) *Basics of Acupuncture* 4th edition. Germany, Springer.

The Source (2001) *Going to School – Parents Fact Sheet.* London, Arthritis Care.

Young NL, Yoshida KK, Williams JI *et al.* (1995) The role of children in reporting their physical disability. *Archives of Physical Medicine and Rehabilitation* 76(10): 913–918.

Wedderburn LR, Abumin M, Palmer P *et al.* (2003) Autologous haematopoietic stem cell transplantation in juvenile idiopathic arthritis. *Archives of Disease in Childhood* 88:201–204.

Wilkinson N, Jackson G, Gardner-Medwin J (2003) Biologic therapies for Juvenile Arthritis. *Archives of Disease in Childhood* 88:186–191.

Zulian F, Martini G, Falcini F *et al.* (2002) Early predictors of severe course of uveitis in oligoarticular juvenile idiopathic arthritis. *Journal of Rheumatology* 29:2446–2453.

Index

Rheumatology Nursing: A Creative Approach, 2nd edn. Edited by Jackie Hill.
Copyright 2006 by John Wiley & Sons, Ltd.